86013

Allergy

Allergy

The History of a Modern Malady

Mark Jackson

REAKTION BOOKS

For Siobhán

Love, all alike, no season knowes, nor clyme,
Nor houres, dayes, moneths, which are the rags of time.
                                        John Donne, 'The Sunne Rising'

Published by
REAKTION BOOKS LTD
33 Great Sutton Street
London EC1V ODX, UK

www.reaktionbooks.co.uk

First published 2006

Copyright © Mark Jackson 2006

All rights reserved
No part of this publication may be reproduced, stored in a retrieval system,
or transmitted, in any form or by any means, electronic, mechanical,
photocopying, recording or otherwise, without the prior permission of
the publishers.

Printed and bound in Great Britain
by Cromwell Press Ltd, Trowbridge, Wiltshire

British Library Cataloguing in Publication Data
Jackson, Mark, 1959–
    Allergy: the history of a modern malady
    1. Allergy   2. Social medicine
    I. Title
    614.5'993

ISBN–10: 1 86189 271 3

CONTENTS

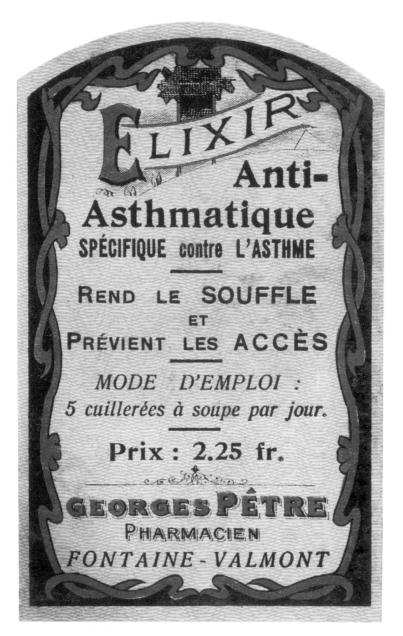

'ELIXIR Anti-Asthmatique', a French medicine label of 1920.

PREFACE

This book is fuelled by a close personal, as well as professional, interest in the dramatic emergence and astonishing tenacity of allergies in the modern world. At the turn of the millennium, an English independent commission on the organization of the school year strongly recommended adopting a six-term, rather than the traditional three-term, academic year. Within this framework, the new fifth term, stretching from early April until the end of May, was to be devoted largely to assessing and examining pupils. In addition to 'rationalising the process of assessment' and making greater space in term six for induction into the following year's programmes, this innovative educational policy was also intended to 'create more equitable assessment arrangements for 1.4 million to 1.8 million hay fever sufferers by moving assessment and examinations out of the main pollen season for grass, which is the major cause of hay fever'. Drawing strength from concurrent attempts to reform curricula and modes of assessment throughout the educational system, the commission believed that the rhythm of school life should be determined, at least in part, by the prevalence of a minor, albeit distressing, allergic disease.[1]

Such an educational strategy was not new. Throughout the 1960s, '70s and '80s contributors to the British medical and popular press regularly advocated removing examinations from the peak pollen season on the grounds that pupils with hay fever suffered both from the symptoms of their condition and from the sedative effects of medication.[2] While such arguments failed to initiate reform 30 or 40 years ago, ongoing efforts to revise the curriculum may well benefit the next generation of school pupils. In part, the greater chances of success at the start of the new millennium can be traced to dramatic shifts in the politics of education since the 1960s and '70s. More particularly, however, they can also be explained in terms of a remarkable global surge in allergic diseases, such as hay fever, asthma, food allergies and eczema, over the last century. At the start of the twentieth century, when allergy had no name, hay fever was considered to be a rare disease largely confined to the educated classes of the Western world. By the 1930s and '40s approximately 1 in 30 people in developed countries was suffering from the major manifestations of allergic reactions. In the immediate post-war decades, it was estimated not only that 10 per cent of the population in the modern industrialized world was experiencing the symptoms of allergy but also that the prevalence of allergic diseases was rising rapidly in the developing world. By the turn of the millennium, 1 in 5 British children was thought to exhibit some form of allergy, and allergic diseases had been identified as a significant threat to global health.

My own family history bears out this broad temporal trajectory. My paternal grandparents, born in 1898 and 1904, ostensibly exhibited no evidence of allergy, although my grandmother's older sister did suffer from asthma and eczema. While my father suffered from hay fever as a child (and indeed was treated for the condition by John Freeman, one of the leading British allergists) and developed both asthma and shellfish allergy as a young adult, his sister demonstrates no signs of allergic reactions except the commonly experienced reactions to horse serum. On my mother's side, not only is there a stronger tradition of allergic reactivity but allergies have also become more prominent over time. My maternal grandparents, born in 1898 and 1899, exhibited mild allergic sensitivity: in later life, my grandfather was allergic to penicillin and my grandmother had mild hay fever and reacted to certain soaps. Significantly, both children (although interestingly not their cousins) were allergic: my mother has suffered from hay fever since the age of eleven or twelve, and her brother (who died in early adulthood while exploring previously uncharted territory in Canada) had eczema during the hay fever season.

Given such a prominent family history of allergy as well as the nascent global configuration of allergies during the twentieth century, there was perhaps no prospect of escape for my own (or indeed the next) generation: my five siblings and I all enjoy some form of allergic sensitivity, whether it is hay fever, asthma, food sensitivity or skin reactions, and our children are beginning to demonstrate the characteristic rashes, wheezes and sneezes of the allergic constitution. Stimulated in part by the gradual eruption of allergic diseases within the convergent histories of the Mayhew, Haywood, Griffin, Jackson and Deehan families, this book is about the emergence of allergy in the modern world. It stretches from the first tentative formulations of the concept of allergy at the dawn of the twentieth century through to the exuberant flowering of allergy as a plague of global proportions at the turn of the millennium.

1

HISTORIES

It must first, however, be generally believed with Sydenham, that our
chronic maladies are of our own creating.

Thomas Beddoes, 1802[1]

Allergy is a modern malady, one with a relatively brief but nevertheless fertile
and tenacious history. Although clinical conditions such as asthma and
eczema had been known since antiquity and although hay fever had been
extensively described in the early nineteenth century, the notion that these
chronic afflictions might possess a common cause and a shared pathology,
conveniently captured under the rubric of allergy, emerged initially in the
early 1900s as a byproduct of rapid developments in biomedical science and
clinical practice. Allergy swiftly gained an imperious position in modern
culture. During the course of the twentieth century, the term allergy was
applied by doctors and their patients throughout the world to an expanding
range of bodily and mental symptoms; allergic reactions were thought to
determine the quintessential clinical features of hay fever, asthma, eczema,
urticaria, food sensitivities and reactions to cosmetics and other synthetic
chemicals, as well as a miscellany of diffuse physical and psychological manifestations. At the same time, allergy gained figurative currency as an expedient
and popular metaphor for a variety of personal, professional and political
antipathies and aversions; people enthusiastically, and not always ironically,
claimed to be allergic to hard work and discipline, to Mondays, to business and
sporting competitors, to other nationalities or to their mothers-in-law.

The primary purpose of this book is to trace the global history of allergy
from its roots in the comparatively limited theatre of late nineteenth- and
early twentieth-century laboratory and clinical science to its pervasive presence as an epidemiological and cultural phenomenon in the modern world. In
the process, the book charts not only evident continuities in the definition and
experience of allergic disorders but also apparent disjunctions in the manifestations and meanings of allergy across time and space. Within this ambitious
remit, the more focused aims of this introductory chapter are to establish the
theoretical, chronological and geographical parameters of the analysis and to
outline the principal evidential and structural features of the subsequent
narrative.

A modern plague

In 1906 Clemens von Pirquet (1874–1929), a young Austrian paediatrician, introduced a novel term to the scientific vocabulary. Eager to establish a constructive conceptual framework for understanding and exploring a variety of seemingly disparate clinical and experimental observations within the nascent field of immunology, von Pirquet suggested employing the term 'allergy' to denote any form of altered biological reactivity. His notion of changed reactivity encompassed not only the generation of immunity against disease but also situations in which a state of so-called hypersensitivity or supersensitivity resulted in tissue damage. Allergy was thus manifest in cases of serum sickness, hay fever, sensitivities to mosquito bites and bee stings, and various idiosyncratic food reactions as well as in individuals who had been exposed to, or successfully immunized against, common infectious diseases such as diphtheria and tuberculosis.[2]

Von Pirquet's neologism was not well received by his peers. In 1912 the eminent French physiologist Charles Richet (1850–1935) nonchalantly dismissed the new term as redundant, arguing that heightened sensitivity to foreign substances (or, more literally, for Richet, the absence of protection against such substances) was already adequately encapsulated in his own term 'anaphylaxis': 'Pirquet and Schick have termed the reaction of an organism to a foreign substance *allergy*: but it does not appear necessary to me to introduce this word in addition to the word anaphylaxis.'[3] Many years later, both the Hungarian paediatrician Béla Schick (1877–1967), who had worked closely with von Pirquet to elucidate the mechanism of serum sickness, and the Austrian-born physician Hans Selye (1907–1982) recollected the hostility with which contemporaries had responded to von Pirquet's 'superfluous publication introducing a new and useless term'.[4]

The reluctance of von Pirquet's critics to embrace the new terminology was understandable. Around the dawn of the twentieth century immunological mechanisms were almost exclusively conceived teleologically in terms of protection against disease rather than as a potential cause of pathology. As von Pirquet himself recognized, his insistence on a close biological association between immunity and supersensitivity was in many ways counter-intuitive, since 'the two terms contradict each other'.[5] There were further grounds for resisting von Pirquet's formulation of immunological disorders. Although serum sickness was rapidly becoming a major complication of administering anti-sera raised in horses in order to vaccinate against diseases such as diphtheria in humans, the various conditions identified by von Pirquet as allergic in origin were generally regarded as rare, non-fatal diseases of little immediate clinical interest. Compared with other more pressing medical and social problems facing the modern world, such as rising infant and maternal mortality rates and persistently high morbidity and mortality from acute infectious diseases, the clinical and laboratory manifestations of allergy constituted a scientific conundrum of only limited epidemiological, economic, social and political significance.

However, contemporary dismissals of von Pirquet's formulation of immunological reactivity proved premature. During the course of the twentieth century, allergy effectively installed itself not only in the lexicon of legitimate medical conditions but also in popular and political culture. By the dawn of the new millennium, allergic diseases were more common, more commonly fatal and apparently induced by an ever widening range of allergens. In the United Kingdom, as in many other developed countries, more than 1 in 3 people were at some point in their lives diagnosed either with an allergic disorder such as asthma, hay fever and eczema or with a food or drug allergy. More disturbingly, allergy was becoming increasingly prevalent in children and rising levels of allergic diseases were becoming evident in the developing world. As a result of such global trends, over the closing decades of the twentieth century allergic disorders became a prominent public health concern for international bodies such as the World Health Organization and a major drain on national and global economic resources. In the 1980s the financial cost of allergic diseases in the United States (in terms of medication, hospitalization and physician time) was estimated at $1.5 billion per annum. By the mid-1990s the burden had escalated to approximately $10 billion.[6] According to a report published by the Royal College of Physicians of London in 2003, allergy was costing the British National Health Service in the region of £900 million per annum, excluding attendance at Accident and Emergency Departments, outpatient consultations and hospital treatment. The management of allergic diseases in the community accounted for 10 per cent (£0.6 billion) of the primary care prescription budget in the United Kingdom, a figure which was 'comparable to GP prescribing costs for gastrointestinal disorders (10 per cent of overall budget) and almost half that for cardiovascular conditions (23 per cent of overall budget)'.[7]

As allergies emerged as an important focus for clinicians, epidemiologists and health care managers in the modern world, they also spawned a lucrative marketplace for the industrial sector. Although some pharmaceutical companies had been subsidizing the development of new treatments for hay fever and asthma since the late nineteenth century, after the Second World War the production of drugs for treating allergic diseases both consumed and generated massive financial resources. Concurrently, the efflorescence of allergies in the modern world also attracted investment from the cosmetic and cleaning industries, encouraged the elaboration of more careful standards of production and labelling in the food and retail industries, prompted the emergence of national and international charities aimed at promoting new research and at disseminating information and advice to patients and their families, and provoked significant media coverage of what was referred to as a 'modern plague' of allergic diseases sweeping the globe.[8]

There was a further facet to mounting preoccupations with allergy. Just as many people in the late nineteenth century claimed to be 'a little bit consumptive',[9] in the late twentieth century people routinely (perhaps even proudly) regarded themselves as 'a little bit allergic'. This transition from consumption to allergy reflected not only the shifting prevalence and incidence of the two conditions but also the manner in which allergy, like tuberculosis before it, had acquired a figurative currency which both shaped and transcended its clinical boundaries. At the turn of the millennium, allergy did not merely describe a set of clinical and experimental conditions defined strictly in terms of specific immunological reactivity; the term allergy could also denote any general state of physical or psychological antipathy or irritability, and allergic sensitivity was regarded by some commentators as a potent symbol of education and civility. At a broader political level, rising trends in allergic diseases were considered to be caused by progressive ecological imbalances and were consequently enlisted in campaigns against environmental degradation. By the early twenty-first century, therefore, the scale of allergy had shifted dramatically. In epidemiological, socio-economic, geo-political and cultural terms, allergy had effectively replaced tuberculosis (and indeed various other diseases such as gout, hysteria and neurasthenia) as an archetypal disease of modern civilization.

The eruption of allergy in the modern world constitutes a striking story, one that encompasses major transformations in theories of disease and clinical practice, the emergence and coordination of global public health interests, the growth of multi-national pharmaceutical, cosmetic and cleaning industries, remarkable modifications in domestic, atmospheric and occupational conditions, the expansion of modern ecological and environmental sensitivities, and the technical and cultural complexities of biomedical science. The history of allergy therefore sheds light on crucial transitions in modern medicine and contemporary culture. At the same time, it also raises challenging historiographical questions about how to understand the remarkable epidemiological transition from acute infectious to chronic degenerative diseases that has characterized the modern period, about how to trace the history of a disease across time doing justice both to the enduring existential reality of symptoms and to the shifting cultural meanings of disease labels, and about how to explore the relationship between patterns and meanings of disease and the processes of civilization.

Diseases of civilization

In the early nineteenth century, the physician and chemist Thomas Beddoes (1760–1808) published a series of expansive essays outlining the features of those diseases prevalent in the affluent classes. Beddoes, who had opened the Pneumatic Medical Institution in Bristol in 1799 in order to offer cures for a variety of chronic diseases (including asthma) through the inhalation of a judicious mixture of diverse gases or 'factitious airs', was particularly interested in the aetiology, treatment and prevention of consumption and scrofula, both forms of tuberculosis.[10] Although he recognized that certain sections of the labouring population were especially vulnerable, either because of their limited diet or because of poor working conditions, he also emphasized the extent to which the affluent consuming classes were prone to the disease. For Beddoes, this proclivity of the middling and upper classes to 'the giant-malady of our island' was not the product of inheritance but of a combination of sedentary lifestyles, fashionable skimpy clothing and an unhealthy material environment: 'it will appear manifest that the devastations of consumption proceed from domestic mismanagement, and not from the inalterable dispositions of nature'.[11] Beddoes was insistent that in order to 'reduce the tribute of lives we render to consumption', society needed in the first instance to acknowledge that the prevalence of tuberculosis was a self-inflicted manifestation of a tenacious and deep-seated social pathology: 'It must first, however, be generally believed with Sydenham, that our chronic maladies are of our own creating.'[12]

Beddoes's account of the aetiology and pathogenesis of consumption and his prescription for improving the health of the population can be interpreted in several ways. In the first instance, it is evident that Beddoes regarded tuberculosis as a disease of modern civilization, as a direct consequence of contemporary lifestyles and environments or, as Roy Porter has suggested, as the product of an emergent consumer economy and capitalist ideology that together promoted the pursuit of wealth at the expense of health.[13] From this perspective, diseases such as tuberculosis and gout and a wide range of nervous disorders were not caused by intractable constitutional characteristics but were firmly fashioned by the institutions, customs and organization of modern society. Of course, Beddoes's formulation of the relationship between civilization and disease in these terms was not new. Indeed, he was mobilizing traditional and familiar narratives of the pathology of progress that had previously been systematically expounded and exploited by a number of Enlightenment medical authors such as George Cheyne (1673–1743), William Cadogan (1711–1797) and Thomas Trotter (1760–1832).[14] Beddoes's account, however, accentuated the importance of sweeping social and cultural change, rather than mere individual over-indulgence, in creating new patterns of disease.[15]

There is a second strand to Beddoes's articulation of the social pathology of consumption. During the eighteenth and nineteenth centuries, several diseases such as gout, nervousness and tuberculosis carried symbolic meanings that both reflected and helped to shape contemporary formulations and experiences of the immediate clinical features of those conditions. As Roy Porter and George Rousseau have suggested, for example, gout rapidly acquired a distinct personality. In particular, the disease became desirable not only because it was seen to confer effective protection against more dangerous conditions but also because it was explicitly linked in popular and medical imaginations both to intellectual capacity and to the constitution and sensitivity of the well-educated civilized classes. Gout became a badge of honour, depicting both a disease and a state of culture.[16] Similarly, as Katherine Ott has pointed out, during the late nineteenth century 'the term "consumptive" clearly carried many meanings', not all of which could be explained simply in terms of reproducible and supposedly objective physical symptoms. Thus, consumption not only referred to the clinical features and pathological processes of tuberculosis but also conveyed romantic and artistic connotations: 'Consumption was a disease not just of body, but also of mind and of spirit.'[17] In this context, Beddoes's words allude to the manner in which metaphorical, as well as material, commitments fashion understandings of diseases and their labels.

By exposing the material and cultural determinants of disease, Beddoes was appropriating a familiar critique of modern society. As Charles Rosenberg has suggested in reference to the work of the American physician George Beard (1839–1883), it had been customary for many centuries to use 'disease incidence and theories of causation and pathology as vehicles for the articulation and legitimation of cultural criticism'.[18] Drawing on this tradition, Beddoes's approach to consumption, like that of Beard to neurasthenia and hay fever, comprised 'as much social comment as medical theory'.[19] Significantly, although Beddoes himself was optimistic that the adaptation of civilization, and more particularly advances in medicine, would eventually generate appropriate cures or prophylactics for modern maladies, many others held more pessimistic views of the downside of modernity, claiming that civilized society (including medicine) was itself now sick. Emphasizing the afflictions wrought by civilization and modern medicine as a gloomy counterpoint to the cheerful Enlightenment 'song of medical progress',[20] discontents in Europe and North America advocated a return to more simplistic and more natural rural lifestyles.[21]

Beddoes's reflections on the inherent perils of civilization reveal a further implication of his commentary on diseases of affluence, one which has been forcefully revisited and recast over subsequent centuries by Max Nordau, George Beard, Sigmund Freud, Norbert Elias, René Dubos and many others.[22] As civilizations change, so too do patterns of behaviour, health and sickness. New diseases inevitably arise to fill the vacuum left by the retreat of older disorders. In the words of the French-born and ecologically minded Pulitzer Prize-winning microbiologist and experimental pathologist René Dubos (1901–1982): 'Threats to health are inescapable accompaniments to life.'[23] From this perspective, both dreams of a world free from disease and strident fears of inevitable biological and social degeneration are exposed as either utopian or dystopian illusions, shaped and coloured by social, political and cultural contingencies. As the Polish-born sociologist Norbert Elias (1897–1990) argued many years ago in his monumental study of the civilizing process, civilization should be regarded neither as 'the most advanced of all humanly possible modes of behaviour' nor as 'the worst form of life and one that is doomed':

> We feel that we have got ourselves, through civilization, into certain entanglements unknown to less civilized peoples; but we also know that these less civilized peoples are for their part often plagued by difficulties and fears from which we no longer suffer, or at least not to the same degree.[24]

Echoes of Elias's poised and holistic vision of civilization as a complex and dynamic process rather than as a stagnant condition found occasional expression in the expansive philosophical deliberations of pathologists such as Dubos and Ludwik Hirszfeld (1884–1954) or the pioneering Polish physician

Ludwik Fleck (1896–1961), who all stressed how the inclination to figure disease merely in terms of an adversary invading from the outside appeared both unduly simplistic and misguided. Such concerns about the ecological complexity of pathological processes also surfaced in literary references to the pattern, politics and transmission of disease, most notably in Albert Camus's novel of 1947, *The Plague*, in which Jean Tarrou reminded Dr Bernard Rieux that 'each one of us has the plague within him; no one, no one on earth, is free from it'.[25] If bodies harboured (and in some circumstances depended upon) potentially pathogenic organisms or if bodies could turn upon themselves, then disease and death were integral to life and the enemy was truly within.

Although there are necessarily striking differences between early nine-teenth- and early twenty-first-century theories of disease and society, Beddoes's conception of the complex interplay between the processes of civilization and patterns of health and sickness provides a constructive framework for analysing the astonishing advent of allergy as a modern malady. At one level, rising trends in allergic diseases can clearly be linked to modern lifestyles, or more specifically to the proliferation of pollutants that have increasingly dominated modern domestic, occupational, urban and global environments. The global dimension to historical patterns of pollution and disease is partic-ularly pertinent. As Rosenberg has suggested, the prevalence of chronic diseases can no longer be viewed exclusively in terms of 'the city as a patho-genic environment' but within the context of much broader 'evolutionary and global ecological realities'.[26] At the same time, however, it is evident that allergy, like gout, was endowed with a particular personality that facilitated its global transmission and acceptance during the twentieth century. The ideo-logical links forged by some doctors and scientists between diseases such as hay fever, on the one hand, and racial, educational and cultural superiority, on the other hand, rendered allergy (or at least certain manifestations of allergy) an alluring and fashionable condition.

At another level, like the growth of nervous diseases in the eighteenth and nineteenth centuries, the proliferation of allergic diseases in the twentieth century has been mobilized by environmentalists and clinical ecologists in support of their critiques of modern commercial society and their pursuit of simpler, more harmonious lifestyles that pay greater attention to ecological balance and to the health and sustainability of the environment.[27] For some late twentieth-century commentators, for example, people with multiple allergies functioned as prophets, serving to warn society of the hazards posed by industrial pollution of the environment with toxic chemicals.[28] As in

Beddoes's time, perceived patterns of health and sickness have continued to provide suitable vehicles for the articulation of cultural criticism. Finally, as an archetypal disease of modern civilization, allergy can also be seen to have filled the epidemiological and cultural vacuum left by the retreat of infectious diseases and by the decline of other fashionable disorders such as hysteria or gout.[29] As an intimate companion of modern living, as an evocative marker (or memory) of ecological stress, and as substantive evidence of trouble from within, allergy therefore also lends credence to recurrent beliefs in the pathology, and perhaps psychopathology, of everyday life.

Histories of allergy

Like many chronic conditions, allergy has attracted little historical attention in spite of its prominent place in modern medical, political and popular culture. As Porter and Rousseau have suggested, the neglect of chronic diseases by historians 'appears rather myopic'.[30] Although studies of the epidemiological transition have focused clearly on the decline of infectious diseases, they have rarely offered any detailed insights into the rise of chronic degenerative conditions in the modern period. Apart from early excursions into the history of cancer and arthritis,[31] or recent studies in the field of occupational health history that have explored the environmental determinants and regulatory politics of chronic non-infectious diseases such as asbestosis, silicosis and lead poisoning,[32] historians have so far shown only limited interest in the dramatic downside of modern demographic and health transitions, or in 'the failures of success' as Ernest Gruenberg deftly put it many years ago in his provocative speculations on the proliferation of chronic disease and disability in the middle decades of the twentieth century.[33]

Allergy has figured only minimally in histories of immunology. Several recent constructive surveys of immunology by Ilana Löwy, Anne Marie Moulin, Alberto Cambrosio, Peter Keating, Arthur Silverstein, Leslie Brent, Pauline Mazumdar, Alfred Tauber, Thomas Söderqvist and others have outlined many crucial features in the evolution of the discipline.[34] In particular, they have identified the distinct paradigm shifts that characterized immunological approaches to bodily defence mechanisms during the nineteenth and twentieth centuries. As these accounts suggest, between approximately 1880 and 1910 both laboratory and clinical immunology were closely allied to experimental pathology and physiology, and served to encourage the development and dissemination of novel treatments such as vaccination and sero-therapy. During the early decades of the twentieth century, the perceived failure of

vaccine therapy together with the advent of 'immunochemistry' (a term introduced by the Nobel Prize-winning Swedish chemist Svante Arrhenius in
1904)[35] served to divorce immunology from physiology and pathology and to
divert attention away from clinical problems towards laboratory studies of the
biochemistry of antibodies and antigens. After 1950, however, a revival of interest in immuno-biological phenomena (such as transplant rejection and autoimmune diseases) effected a further transition in the field, and immunology
became a speciality that once again linked 'fundamental biological research
with medical practice'.[36]

It is evident, however, that within this broad historical framework many
histories of immunology have concentrated increasingly, and undoubtedly
productively, either on isolated but highly visible theoretical debates about
self/non-self discrimination or about the generation of antibody diversity and
specificity, or on the elaboration and dissemination of seminal hypotheses
and technologies, such as Paul Ehrlich's side-chain theory of antibody formation, Frank Macfarlane Burnet's clonal selection theory, Niels Jerne's notion of
an idiotype-anti-idiotype network, or the more recent production of monoclonal antibodies. As Warwick Anderson, Myles Jackson and Barbara Gutmann
Rosenkrantz have persuasively argued in their caustic plea for an 'unnatural
history of immunology', historians have thus worked largely within the conventional boundaries, or 'invented traditions', established by immunologists
themselves, and have failed to explore 'histories of vague and contingent
subjects such as immunity, infection, or allergy – topics not often identified as
part of the patrimonial legacy of the reinvented tradition'. From this perspective, there is clearly both the need and the space for 'alternative histories of
immunology, histories not of laboratories but of clinics and cultures'.[37]

Until recently, more focused historical studies of allergy have also been
dominated by accounts of intellectual and disciplinary progress, routinely
depicting developments in allergy as a series of milestones or stepping stones
of great discoveries, seminal publications and influential scientists that collectively transformed the study of immunopathology from a position of profound
ignorance in the late nineteenth century to one of enlightened knowledge and
therapeutic power at the start of the new millennium. Compiled largely by
clinical immunologists and allergists themselves, such accounts chart in
chronological sequence what have been regarded by modern practitioners as
crucial moments in the evolution of their speciality: the first use of the term
'hypersensitivity' in 1894; the identification of systemic and local anaphylaxis
in 1902 and 1903; the introduction of the term allergy in 1906; the discovery of

histamine by Henry Dale; demonstration of the passive transfer of allergic reactions and the characterization of 'atopy' in the early 1920s; the classification of hypersensitivity states according to the immunological mechanisms involved during the 1950s and '60s; the introduction of more effective chemotherapeutic approaches (such as antihistamines, bronchodilators, and inhaled steroids) in the inter-war and post-war years; the identification of IgE in 1967; and recent advances in immunological understandings of the chemical mediators involved in the pathogenesis of allergic diseases.[38]

Rectilinear narratives of the history of allergy, particularly the extensive bibliographical surveys by Hans Schadewaldt,[39] have certainly helped to identify the actors and concepts that shaped the imagination and clinical focus of allergists, and may also have operated as stabilizing influences at moments of professional anxiety.[40] Such histories, however, have often failed adequately to explore issues of particular interest to social historians. In the first place, they have tended to ignore highly contentious contemporary debates about the mechanisms of allergic phenomena, charting instead only those developments that appear to have contributed to the smooth and unproblematic creation of modern scientific knowledge. As a result, positivist accounts of the history of allergy have frequently underestimated competing explanations for allergic disorders, readily prioritizing immunological understandings of hay fever, asthma and other conditions and discounting profound contemporary interest in the possible hormonal, toxic, neurological, psychological or social ·concerns about the nature of the relationship between allergy and immunity or about the role of allergic phenomena in the evolution of the immune response, questions that divided clinicians and scientists throughout the ·immediate intellectual, institutional and pragmatic origins and determinants of clinical allergy as a medical speciality. Clinical immunology and allergy did not emerge directly or effortlessly from laboratory studies of hypersensitivity or anaphylaxis, as many positivist accounts have implicitly suggested. On the contrary, in Britain and the United States the development of allergy as a medical speciality was shaped more immediately by a constellation of practical clinical, as well as professional, considerations.

Finally, and perhaps more importantly, positivist histories have tended to disregard the manner in which the meaning of allergy changed across time and to ignore the flexibility or elasticity of the term itself. It is important to recognize that just as the meaning of tuberculosis (and many other disease categories) shifted during the nineteenth and twentieth centuries, so too the meaning of allergy changed across time. Allergy today encompasses a different set of pathological states, with different boundaries and different meanings, than it did in 1906 when the term was first conceived. Some modern formulations of hay fever, asthma and food allergies carry only distant echoes of von Pirquet's original notion of altered biological reactivity. The meanings of diagnostic categories and disease labels are never fixed. As Ludwik Fleck insisted in 1927, diseases should not be regarded as stable natural entities but as 'ideal fictitious pictures . . . round which both the individual and the variable morbid phenomena are grouped, without, however, ever corresponding completely to them'.[41] In her recent exemplary cultural history of tuberculosis, Katherine Ott reiterated Fleck's warning by emphasizing that illness is always 'a jumble of ideas that shifts among groups and over time'. Notwithstanding the existential reality of symptoms, sickness 'is a cultural artifact configured in people's bodies, in medical doctrines, and in the physical material of illness'.[42]

A small number of historians have recently begun to explore the history of clinical immunology, including allergy, in these more expansive contextual terms. Studies by Kathryn Waite and Michael Emanuel, for example, have effectively exposed the range of material and cultural factors that served to shape the clinical contours of hay fever as it emerged as a post-industrial disease of civilization in the late nineteenth century.[43] Similarly, studies of asthma by John Gabbay and Carla Keirns have examined the manner in which the disease label was constructed and how approaches to treatment were fashioned by broader ideologies of medicine and society.[44] More recently, constructive analyses of Charles Richet's formulation of anaphylaxis by Ilana Löwy and Kenton Kroker, Tilli Tansey's careful dissection of Henry Dale's discovery of histamine, and Ohad Parnes's lucid articulation of the early history of autoimmunity have suggestively drawn the history of allergy more closely into line with histories of laboratory science and the wider history of pathology.[45] Finally, Gregg Mitman's outstanding studies of the place of hay fever in nineteenth- and twentieth-century American culture have not only opened up the history of allergic diseases to greater scrutiny but also demonstrated the benefits of merging the history of medicine more effectively with burgeoning environmental histories.[46] In particular, Mitman's incisive analysis of hay fever from an environmental perspective precisely answers the call by Anderson and his colleagues for 'more ecological histories of immunity [which] would not collapse the subject into the narrow boundaries of a research school', but which would instead generate 'a more nuanced – and less linear, less filiative – understanding of how personal, social, cognitive, and technical resources and constraints shaped (and maintained) the disciplinary boundaries'.[47]

The aim of this book is to continue the process initiated by Mitman, Löwy, Kroker, Keirns and others by pursuing the history of allergy from its origins in late nineteenth- and early twentieth-century experimental physiology and paediatrics to its status as an endemic scourge of the modern world. Many of the primary sources on which this study is based are drawn from archives and libraries in Western industrialized countries and the explanatory focus is largely on Britain, North America and Western Europe, where allergic diseases first appeared as a major socio-economic and public health problem and where clinical allergy was initially forged into a distinct medical speciality. Nevertheless, given the dramatic rise in allergies in developing countries in the late twentieth century and growing concerns about the worldwide socio-economic impact of allergic diseases expressed by international health agencies, the story of the emergence of allergy as a modern malady is necessarily a global one.

The following chapter traces the origins and reception of Clemens von Pirquet's preliminary formulation of allergy in the early twentieth century. Although von Pirquet's work was closely informed by his knowledge of the natural history of infectious diseases and by his own observations of vaccination reactions and serum sickness in children being treated for scarlet fever and diphtheria, he also drew heavily on traditional notions of idiosyncracy, on late nineteenth-century accounts of hypersensitivity, and on the laboratory studies of experimental physiologists such as Charles Richet. Von Pirquet's notion eventually gained currency in Western medical and scientific circles and his preoccupation with the pragmatic clinical implications of laboratory research continued to dominate the study and practice of allergy for much of the twentieth century. Nevertheless, it is significant that initial reception of his work was marked by a number of disputes among European and North American scientists and clinicians about the meanings and mechanisms of allergy, and about the evolutionary significance of various destructive manifestations of altered biological reactivity.

The recognition that immunological mechanisms might explain certain disease processes did not immediately replace previous understandings of the aetiology of conditions such as hay fever, asthma and eczema, which continued to be conceived by some authors in terms of hormonal or psychological disturbances or as the result of toxins. However, it is clear that von Pirquet's vision did draw together a variety of previously disparate disorders that were now thought to possess a common pathology, a common epidemiology, and a common history. By highlighting the biological basis of diseases such as hay fever, the concept of allergy shifted attention away from environmental or climatic approaches to therapy and towards the manipulation of individual allergic responses. As chapter Three argues, this transition, together with developments in vaccine therapy and clinical studies of hay fever, provided the momentum for the elaboration of a pivotal new therapy, generally referred to as desensitization or immunotherapy. Although there were disagreements about the mechanism, efficacy and safety of the procedure and about the motives of its practitioners, and although the introduction of a range of pharmaceutical products such as the antihistamines eventually challenged its therapeutic status, desensitization provided the cornerstone for the construction of a new clinical speciality on both sides of the Atlantic during the middle decades of the twentieth century.

By the 1960s clinical allergy was well established in many Western countries as a distinct medical discipline that boasted its own national professional societies, a number of academic journals, and a widening network of collaborative international ventures, such as conferences, workshops, research programmes and training schemes. These international initiatives, many of which were coordinated by the newly created World Health Organization, were partly driven by, and in turn fuelled, a growing recognition that the scale of allergy was expanding dramatically. In the immediate post-war years it became apparent that allergic diseases were no longer confined to the educated, civilized classes in the Western developed world, as they were thought to have been in the early twentieth century. By the 1950s and '60s hay fever, asthma, food and drug allergies, and reactions to bee stings were acknowledged to be increasingly common and increasingly fatal in all social classes and in all parts of the world. At the same time, it had become customary for clinicians (and indeed the public) to suspect that allergy might explain a variety of seemingly non-specific clinical conditions, such as migraine, colitis, pruritis and multiple sclerosis. As a brochure produced by the Swiss pharmaceutical company CIBA, partly in order to advertise its own range of antihistamines, asked in 1948: 'Steckt eine Allergie dahinter?' ['Is there an allergy behind it?'].[48] Chapter Four explores the post-war transformation of allergy into a modern global plague and traces the concurrent efforts of national and international state and charitable agencies to chart rising trends in allergic diseases, to clarify the immunological mechanisms involved in allergic reactions, and to generate new pharmacological agents to stem mounting mortality and morbidity rates. In addition, it reveals the manner in which allergy increasingly attracted investment not only from a global pharmaceutical industry but also from cosmetic, cleaning and food industries and from the media.

As allergy blossomed in the modern world, so too did the range of explanations for its presence. Mirroring the trenchant opinions of Beddoes and Beard on the proliferation of tuberculosis and nervous diseases in previous centuries, students of allergy regarded it predominantly as a disease of modern civilization, generated by modern affluent lifestyles and environments. As the German social scientist, Ulrich Beck pointed out some years ago in his influential analysis of what he termed the 'risk society', in 'advanced modernity the social production of wealth is systematically accompanied by the social production of risks'. Inhabitants of the modern world, he suggested, were 'living on the volcano of civilization'.[49] As chapter Five argues, in the decades following the Second World War, rising trends in allergies were explained precisely in these terms. Although epidemiological assessments of risk were often plagued by shifting clinical definitions of conditions such as asthma and by the growing elasticity of the term allergy itself, in the second half of the twentieth century allergic diseases were increasingly linked to a range of modern 'pollutants' (such as cigarette smoke, vehicle exhaust fumes and house dust mites), to modern architectural and decorative fashions, to shifting patterns of breast-feeding and immunization, or to changes in domestic hygiene, diet and exercise.

Post-war debates about allergy were also marked by the resurgence of refractory disputes about the meaning or evolutionary purpose of allergic reactions. Drawing on the pioneering work of American campaigners such as Rachel Carson (1907–1964) and Theron G. Randolph (1906–1995), environmentalists and ecologists throughout the world began to challenge immunologists and clinical allergists who claimed that allergy was simply a manifestation of immunity gone wrong. On the contrary, they argued, allergy constituted an entirely appropriate protective response to dangers posed by widespread environmental and ecological damage. As I shall argue in chapter Six, in this way changing patterns of allergic disorders, and particularly the appearance of patients with multiple chemical sensitivities, were drawn implicitly into highly visible political critiques of a global consumer society. Although not the only metaphor for the pathology of progress, allergy began to figure strongly in popular protest literature and films and to gain symbolic currency as a rational and meaningful aversion to the diverse hazards of modern living. At the turn of the millennium, allergy evocatively revealed a growing dissonance between supposedly natural biological reactivity and the artifices of the modern material world.

The state of allergy

In an after-dinner address presented at a combined meeting of the two American allergy societies in Atlantic City in 1935, J. Harvey Black (1884–1958), President of the American Association for the Study of Allergy, facetiously likened the clinical field of allergy to a modern nation state. Arguing that a 'dispassionate, even pragmatic recital of the geography, topography and other characteristics' of allergy might be of some value to practitioners, Black proceeded to describe the boundaries, climate, environment, and the seemingly unlimited natural resources of this largely uncharted territory, and to recount the political and professional allegiances and manoeuvres of its inhabitants.[50] Black's analogy proved infectious. In a popular book on the subject of allergy, published in 1939 and aimed at assisting readers to 'find their way through the mazes of this strange and tantalizing state', Warren T. Vaughan (1893–1944), a leading American allergist, compared the sensitized body to that of a 'great city or state' struggling to defend itself against the recurrent threat of attack from recognized enemies. In both cases, Vaughan argued, defence of the realm was entrusted to specialist constituents 'stationed at strategic places on the frontiers, whose duty is to resist invasion'. In most instances, 'citizens' (that is the various cells) of the 'State of Allergy' lived in a harmonious and stable environment, 'bathed in a fluid which is remarkably constant and nonirritating in character'. Occasionally, however, when certain substances slipped 'unnoticed past the border patrols', the state mobilized its defence mechanisms in order to protect itself. If the enemy were to invade again, Vaughan suggested, overproduction of protective agents (antibodies and mediators such as histamine) would result in the appearance of 'the common allergic symptoms'.[51]

The discrete, but related, notions of a quasi-geographical 'state of allergy', propagated by Black and Vaughan during the 1930s, were apposite. In addition to possessing a remarkably recent and specific history, allergy (in all its various guises) has also exhibited a particular geography. At one level, this merely implies that allergic diseases have displayed an epidemiological distribution across space as well as time. In the early decades of the twentieth century, allergy was not only more common in the Western world than elsewhere but it was also more prevalent in specific locations. In North America during the 1930s and '40s, for example, estimates of the prevalence of hay fever varied from 3 per cent on the Eastern seaboard to 10 per cent in the Mississippi drainage area where ragweed was particularly prolific.[52] During the course of the twentieth century, the geographical distribution of allergic diseases changed.

Although local variations in incidence and prevalence persisted, allergy also reached epidemic proportions in the developing, as well as the developed, world. For example, while hay fever was apparently unrecognized in Japan in the early 1930s, by 1986 more than 30 per cent of children in some highly polluted districts were reported to be suffering from allergic rhinitis induced by pollen.[53]

The global spread of allergies and local geographical gradients in the prevalence of allergic diseases can partly be explained in terms of variations in the natural environment, such as the growth and dispersal of ragweed or certain grasses. It is important, however, to recognize that the environment, and therefore the risk of exposure to allergens, has been shaped not only by natural geological and environmental factors but also by political and economic forces. As Gregg Mitman, Michelle Murphy and Christopher Sellers have intimated in their temperate introduction to a fine collection of essays on the environment and health, exposures to health risks have been closely framed by socially, as well as geographically, determined patterns of production and consumption: 'Privilege and violence are built into these forms [of exposure]: from the worrisome miasmas that stalked settler societies, to the stench and filth attributed to the "great unwashed" of the urban metropolis or the colonies, to the variety of perils made possible by industrial production in the West and elsewhere.'[54] Thus, an environmental or ecological history of diseases such as hay fever and asthma needs to pay close attention to the economic and political, as well as the geographical, forces that have not only moulded urban, occupational, domestic and industrial environments but also in the process accentuated the risks of exposure to certain health hazards.

Finally, whether regarded as a category of disease or as a professional discipline, allergy has also possessed a distinct cultural geography. The clinical contours and symbolic boundaries of allergic diseases have been assembled and consumed in diverse sites, in scientific laboratories, hospital wards and clinics, in the surveys of national and international health agencies and the pages of medical journals and textbooks, in newspaper and magazine columns, in popular films and literature, in the bodies and minds of patients, and in the rhetoric of politicians, modern environmentalists and clinical ecologists. Scientific notions, clinical conceptions, political formulations and lay experiences of allergy have therefore been 'filtered through a mesh of cultural influences',[55] which have collectively conspired to define the place and purpose, as well as the symptomatic expression, of allergy in modern times. Conversely, allergy has in turn been employed to reinforce or challenge traditional geographical, political, professional and biological boundaries. Echoing Beddoes's sharp critique of the social pathology of consumption, a history of the emergence of allergy as a modern malady therefore necessarily entails a commentary on the social, political, cultural, economic and ecological forces that have shaped patterns of health and sickness, and determined the distribution of knowledge and the balance of power, in the modern world.

2

STRANGE REACTIONS

> For this general concept of a changed reactivity I propose the term allergy.
>
> Clemens von Pirquet, 1906[1]

The word allergy was first used by Clemens von Pirquet in a brief, speculative article published in a German medical journal in July 1906. Created from the conjunction of two Greek words, αλλος (meaning other or different) and εργεια (signifying energy or reactivity), the term was intended to provide a convenient means of defining various manifestations of altered biological reactivity. The roots of von Pirquet's novel approach were diverse. On the one hand, he clearly drew on scientific accounts of the strange and seemingly exaggerated physiological responses of animals to the injection of foreign substances that had been reported by experimental physiologists and pathologists working in the laboratories of some of the most prominent European and American scientific institutes. At the same time, however, von Pirquet's scheme for understanding and exploring biological reactivity was closely framed by his clinical experience of the natural history of infectious diseases and vaccination reactions evident in patients in the children's wards in Vienna. Indeed, the origins and evolution of the term testify to von Pirquet's deep commitment to exploiting insights obtained from observations made not only at the laboratory bench but also, and perhaps more importantly for von Pirquet, at the patient's bedside.

Although his formulation of altered biological reactivity was often contested by critics and although the initial broad meaning of allergy was relentlessly narrowed by subsequent investigators, Clemens von Pirquet's systematic juxtaposition of a range of diverse clinical and experimental phenomena within a distinct conceptual framework proved influential. The term itself eventually gained widespread acceptance both amongst scientists and clinicians and amongst patients and the public around the world. The clinical thrust of von Pirquet's studies of immunological reactivity also served to mould, and to some extent cast a persistent shadow over, the evolution of clinical allergy as a medical speciality. In particular, the clinical and scientific conundrums shrewdly exposed and judiciously explored by von Pirquet in his early publications continued to plague studies of allergy for much of the twentieth century. The aim of this chapter is to examine the origins of von Pirquet's formulation of allergy in late nineteenth- and early twentieth-century studies of idiosyncrasy and immunity, to analyse the immediate reception and modification of his provocative theories of biological reactivity, and to highlight the lasting impact of von Pirquet's work on the subsequent history of allergy.

Idiosyncrasy and immunity

Strange and sometimes fatal reactions to foreign substances have been reported since antiquity. Although there are ancient accounts of peculiar and severe reactions to wasp and bee stings,[2] the commonest types of idiosyncratic reaction were those described to various foods. For example, the Hippocratic Corpus, compiled both from the writings of Hippocrates (460–375 BC) and from the work of his contemporaries and followers, refers to evidence that while some people can eat cheese 'without the slightest hurt . . . others come off badly'. Significantly, the underlying cause of such reactions was not considered to be located in the nature of cheese but in the particular 'constituent of the body which is hostile to cheese, and is roused and stirred to action under its influence'.[3] Some centuries later, the Hippocratic notion of selective susceptibility was neatly expressed by the Latin philosopher and poet Lucretius (98–55 BC), who, in his expansive cogitation *De rerum natura*, asserted that 'what is food to one, is to others biting poison'.[4] These complementary concepts of unusual sensitivity to foreign substances were eventually embodied in the term idiosyncrasy, or what the London surgeon and ophthalmologist Jonathan Hutchinson (1828–1913) referred to in 1884 as 'individuality run mad'.[5]

During the early modern period, sporadic reports of idiosyncratic, harmful and occasionally life-threatening reactions to food, bee and wasp stings, and indeed to various drugs, proliferated. The first clinical observation of a systemic reaction to a bee sting was published at the end of the seventeenth century, and the earliest account of a fatality from this cause was reported by a French physician in 1765.[6] During the eighteenth and nineteenth centuries, certain drugs (such as iodides, bromides, arsenic and tobacco) were known to produce idiosyncratic cutaneous or systemic reactions analogous to those provoked by various foods.[7] In addition, a number of authors increasingly recognized that diverse disease processes could be understood in terms of functional variations or aberrations from the normal. In 1698 the Litchfield physician Sir John Floyer (1649–1734), who himself suffered from asthma, carefully recounted the range of substances that could provoke breathing difficulties in susceptible patients. In addition to noting the impact of emotional stress and exercise in asthmatics, Floyer also detailed the role of tobacco smoke, metallic vapours, foods, dust and changes in the weather in precipitating attacks.[8] In the nineteenth century, hay fever and asthma were both understood in terms of idiosyncratic sensitivity to external agents such as dust, hay, feathers and animals. Although some authors acknowledged that the identification of certain conditions in terms of an idiosyncratic response to a particular external stimulus failed to reveal the precise nature of the underlying predisposition or sensitivity, the discovery of a proximate cause of the reaction at least carried the 'immense practical advantage that the exact source of danger being known, it can be avoided'.[9]

In the closing decades of the nineteenth century, idiosyncratic reactions to foreign substances acquired a new meaning and urgency. Clinical interest was promoted partly by the proliferation of novel medicines and potential irritants to which supposedly stressed and susceptible Western civilized populations were increasingly being exposed. According to the American physician George Beard (1839–1883), for example, modern civilization was responsible for a form of nervous exhaustion (referred to by Beard as American nervousness or neurasthenia) that was not only rendering the population increasingly sensitive to climate change but also generating 'special idiosyncrasies in regard to food, medicines and external irritants'.[10] More strikingly, however, attention to the possible role of physiological idiosyncrasies in the pathogenesis of human disease was also encouraged by the elaboration and dissemination of new therapies for infectious diseases. The powerful emergence of germ theories of disease in Western Europe and North America during the Victorian period, and particularly a growing belief in the role of specific causal agents, precipitated extensive clinical and laboratory research not only into the mechanisms by which germs caused tissue damage and bodies defended themselves against injury, but also into ways of enhancing the body's defences against bacteria and their toxins.

Approaches to analysing and enhancing immunity against infectious diseases were dominated in that period by two broad, and often competing, theories. During the 1880s and '90s the Russian zoologist Elie Metchnikoff (1845–1916) suggested that immunity was essentially a cellular phenomenon, accomplished by the ability of certain white blood cells (the 'phagocytes') to devour and destroy invading microbes. While Metchnikoff's theory of cellular immunity was energetically adopted and adapted by scientists such as Alexandre

Besredka (1870–1940) working at the Pasteur Institute in France, it was vigorously challenged by German proponents of an alternative humoral theory of immunity. According to Robert Koch (1843–1910), Emil von Behring (1874–1917) and Paul Ehrlich (1854–1915), for example, effective defence against infection was mediated by specific constituents of the serum, increasingly referred to as antibodies. Although some researchers acknowledged that the two theories were not mutually exclusive and although disputes about the reality and nature of antibodies persisted, around the turn of the century researchers increasingly began to favour humoral, rather than cellular, theories of immunity and to concentrate on elucidating the precise role of antibodies in defence against infectious diseases.[11]

In the last decade of the nineteenth century, the recognition that serum from infected patients and immunized animals carried protective (or 'antitoxic') properties raised hopes that infectious diseases might be treated by the administration of specific antisera (serum containing antibodies) or antitoxins. The first demonstration of the clinical value of what became known as serum therapy or passive vaccination was achieved by Emil von Behring and Shibasaburo Kitasato (1856–1931). Working in Robert Koch's laboratory at the Institute of Hygiene in Berlin, von Behring and Kitasato raised diphtheria antitoxin by injecting animals with sublethal doses of purified toxin, and on Christmas Day in 1891 successfully used the antitoxin to treat a child suffering from diphtheria. This novel technique for combating the ravages of infectious diseases, for which von Behring received the first Nobel Prize for Medicine in 1901, was rapidly applied not only to larger groups of children with diphtheria but also to patients with tetanus.[12]

The impact of serum therapy was immediately clear. The commercial production of diphtheria antitoxin and its introduction to clinical practice in various European hospitals initiated a dramatic and sustained reduction in mortality rates from diphtheria.[13] Perhaps fuelled by reports of such successes, a number of clinicians attempted to apply serum therapy to a range of other conditions. In the early twentieth century, William Dunbar (1863–1922), an American physician and Director of the State Hygienic Institute at Hamburg, employed 'antitoxic serum' raised in horses and rabbits to counteract the effects of the 'pollen toxin' in hay fever patients.[14] In a similar vein, some doctors injected serum from patients with severe epilepsy in the hope of 'establishing immunity' in other patients suffering from milder forms of the same disorder.[15] In spite of its evident success in the treatment of infectious diseases, however, serum therapy was also attended by certain problems, related both to the difficulties of standardizing antisera and to concerns about safety. Soon after its introduction, doctors noted that some patients developed severe systemic reactions to repeated injections of antitoxin, particularly those treated with antisera raised in horses. These reactions included fevers, rashes, diarrhoea, falling blood pressure, joint pains and breathing difficulties. The first deaths from what became known as 'serum sickness' or 'serum disease' were registered not in 1896, as many historical accounts suggest, but probably the previous year.[16] In 1895 the British Medical Journal contained a report detailing the recorded deaths of three patients (in America, Norway and Hungary) who had received diphtheria antitoxin as a form of either treatment or prevention. Significantly, on the basis of post-mortem investigations into the death of a young woman in New York, physicians hinted at the possible role of the body's reaction to the antiserum (and perhaps not coincidentally deflected blame away from the procedure itself) by insisting that death could not be 'attributed in any way to the antitoxin which was employed'.[17]

While accounts of the clinical features of serum sickness provided a crucial element of the immediate context in which the notion of allergy was elaborated, a number of disparate reports of strange, idiosyncratic reactions to foreign proteins in the laboratories of experimental physiologists were equally important. During the nineteenth century, a number of sporadic observations had led scientists to suggest that, in addition to generating immunity, injection of foreign proteins into animals could also lead to a state of heightened sensitivity to the foreign substance. In 1839, for example, the influential French physiologist François Magendie (1783–1855) had noted the occasional sudden death of rabbits repeatedly injected with egg albumin.[18] Over subsequent decades, scientists recorded similar fatal reactions in animals injected with pathogens or foreign sera. In 1894 Emil von Behring introduced the term 'hypersensitivity' or 'supersensitivity' (überempfindlichkeit) to describe the exaggerated response of guinea pigs to repeated doses of diphtheria toxin.[19] Although the mechanisms were not clearly explained, the assumption was generally that death resulted from the direct effects of the foreign substance rather than from the host animal's biological reaction to that substance.

In the early twentieth century, the significance of these scattered reports was brought into greater focus by a number of studies exploring the causes and mechanisms of hypersensitivity reactions in both animals and humans. The most famous experiments were those conducted by two French physicians and physiologists, Charles Richet (1850–1935) and Paul Portier (1866–1962),

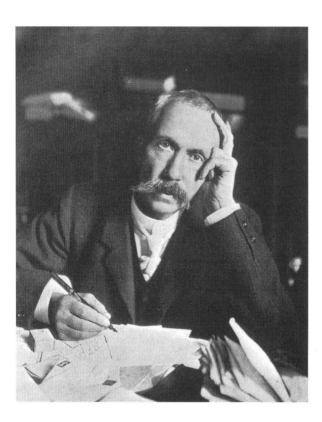

Charles Richet.

work for which Richet received the Nobel Prize in 1913. In a series of studies carried out in 1901 and 1902, in which they were attempting to immunize animals against toxin from sea anemones, Richet and Portier demonstrated that respiratory distress and death could occur when dogs were injected with a second small dose of toxin. Believing the phenomenon to be a product of reduced immunity, they introduced the term 'anaphylaxis' (literally meaning the absence of protection) in order to describe increased sensitivity to the effects of a toxin.[20]

Over the next few years, a number of investigators across Europe and North America extended Richet's and Portier's observations in crucial directions. In 1903 Maurice Arthus (1862–1945), working at the Pasteur Institute in Lille, demonstrated the possibility of inducing a form of local, as opposed to systemic, anaphylaxis in rabbits, a reaction that was generally referred to as the 'Arthus phenomenon'.[21] Three years later, two American physicians, Milton Rosenau (1869–1946) and John Anderson (1873–1958), carefully evaluated the possible role of specific anaphylactic sensitization (rather than the more general phenomenon of *status lymphaticus*) in cases of sudden death following the injection of horse serum in both guinea pigs and humans.[22] The precise pathological processes implicated in these various hypersensitivity reactions remained elusive, but early studies increasingly postulated an immunological basis for experimental anaphylaxis: the phenomenon was biologically specific; it required a latent period comparable to that required for the development of immunity; and it could be transferred passively using serum from sensitized animals. A number of researchers interpreted such findings as evidence that anaphylactic phenomena were mediated primarily not by the direct toxic properties of foreign substances (known as antigens) but by the presence of specific antibodies in the serum.[23]

When Clemens von Pirquet first introduced the term allergy in 1906, his careful formulation of the notion of altered biological reactivity drew heavily both on recent speculations about the mechanisms and meanings of hypersensitivity in animals and on growing medical interest in adverse human reactions to serum therapy. His express aim, however, was not merely to clarify the nature of a series of diverse, but putatively related, biological phenomena such as anaphylaxis, or indeed simply to enrich clinical understandings of the aetiology and pathogenesis of serum sickness, which had already benefited from his own observations of children undergoing serum therapy in the Universitäts Kinderklinik in Vienna. Rather, he was keen to expose the precise nature of the relationship between the seemingly parallel processes of immunity and hypersensitivity. Although some contemporary commentators (and indeed historians) tended to marginalize von Pirquet's contributions to medical science, favouring the eye-catching experimental work of Richet over the fanciful speculations of an Austrian paediatrician, von Pirquet's impact on the form and focus of clinical allergy was immense and enduring. In particular, his work neatly illustrates the manner in which the origins and evolution of allergy studies were

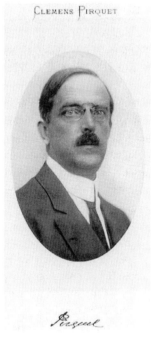

Clemens von Pirquet.

rooted in both the clinic and the laboratory, or more particularly in the complex, but integrated, histories of bacteriological, immunological, physiological, pathological and clinical investigations into idiosyncratic reactions to foreign substances.

Clemens von Pirquet and the birth of allergy

Clemens von Pirquet was born in Hirschstetten near Vienna on 12 May 1874. His father, of aristocratic Belgian descent, served in the Austrian parliament as a representative of the landowners' party and was a keen poet and playwright. His mother, a devout Catholic, was the daughter of a fashionable Viennese banker. Having been educated first at home by a private tutor and subsequently at schools in and around Vienna, Clemens von Pirquet studied theology at the University of Innsbruck and philosophy at the University of Louvain in Belgium, with the intention of entering the priesthood. Shortly after graduating, however, he abandoned theological studies and, largely against the wishes of his family who regarded medicine as an unsuitable profession for a young aristocrat, entered the University of Vienna to pursue a career as a doctor. Having spent a year in Vienna, he studied in Königsberg in Prussia (where his cousin and brother-in-law was professor of surgery) and in Graz, where he gained his MD in 1900. Perhaps influenced by Theodor Escherich, professor of paediatrics at Graz, and possibly driven by his blossoming interest in childhood infectious diseases, after six months as a medical officer in the armed forces, von Pirquet chose to specialize in paediatrics, working first in Berlin under Otto von Heubner before beginning his internship and residency in 1901 at the Universitäts Kinderklinik in Vienna, which was by then being run by Escherich.[24]

Von Pirquet's personal life was apparently plagued with difficulties. In 1904 he married Maria Christine von Husen, a young German woman whom he had met while in Berlin. Believing that Clemens had married beneath him, most of his family refused to attend the wedding and failed to accept his new wife. His choice of partner served only to crystallize evident tensions between Clemens and his siblings, tensions that had been initiated by his choice of profession and which were intensified after 1912 by unresolved legal disputes about the distribution of his mother's estate, which had been divided between her seven children rather than being handed on to the eldest son in the tradition of the Austrian nobility. According to his biographer, who worked with him in the paediatric clinics in Vienna, von Pirquet's marriage was troubled. Maria suffered from a variety of physical and mental afflictions, including increasing dependence on barbiturates, and was unable to bear children following an unsuccessful gynaecological operation. Despite his family's opposition to the marriage, however, and although friction in his domestic life was increasingly evident to his colleagues and friends, Clemens and Maria remained dedicated to, and supportive of, each other until 1929, when they committed suicide together.[25]

In spite of a turbulent private life, von Pirquet achieved considerable professional success and recognition, in terms of both his scientific research and his contributions to clinical medicine. From the outset of his career, von Pirquet's close interest in a variety of immunological problems was evident. Following the advice of Max Gruber (1835–1927), professor of hygiene at the universities of Vienna and Munich, who had suggested to him that 'a study of incubation time would furnish an important clue to the concept of immunity',[26] and conceivably influenced by contemporary preoccupations with child development, von Pirquet began to investigate the temporal characteristics of serum sickness. In particular, he started to speculate both about the character of antigen-antibody interactions and about the significance of incubation times in the natural history of childhood diseases and vaccination reactions. Together with Gruber, for example, von Pirquet published articles challenging Paul Ehrlich's account of the neutralization of toxin by antitoxin.[27]

More critically in the present context, however, von Pirquet's study of incubation times led him to question traditional views of the role of microorganisms and their toxins in human disease. In 1903 he wrote a preliminary paper on the theory of infectious diseases, in which he argued that the cardinal signs of illness (fever, skin rashes, a decrease in white cells in the blood and other constitutional symptoms and signs) were dependent not solely on the action of the invading bacteria but also on the body's ability to develop antibodies that subsequently reacted with those bacteria and their toxins. His conclusions were striking:

> 1. The length of the incubation time depends not only upon the foreign body, but also upon the organism in question.
>
> 2. The manifestations of disease appear at the moment when the antibodies formed in the organism begin to react with the causative foreign body.
>
> 3. The acquired immunity, which persists, lies in the ability of the

organism to produce the antibodies more rapidly than before, and there is a corresponding shortening of incubation time.[28]

Von Pirquet's theory was clearly outside the mainstream of pathological thinking at that time. In general, clinicians and pathologists construed disease as a product of the invasion of a host by a hostile agent and visualized the subsequent clinical course of disease in terms of a battle between external aggressors (bacteria and their toxins) and internal defence mechanisms (white blood cells and antibodies). Although it represented a departure from the dominant paradigm, however, von Pirquet's formulation of the pathogenesis of acute infectious diseases and vaccination reactions, in which the body itself played a critical role, was not entirely new. In 1881, in a series of lectures on idiosyncrasy delivered at the Royal College of Surgeons in London, Jonathan Hutchinson had hinted at the importance of recognizing individual differences in the expression of disease and had highlighted the dangers of seeking 'to make external influences explain the whole'.[29] As recent studies by Ohad Parnes and Ilana Löwy have suggested, a number of clinicians and scientists around the turn of the nineteenth into the twentieth century also understood pathology in more dynamic and holistic terms, stressing the contribution of host reactions to the manifestations of disease. According to the histologist and neuropathologist Carl Weigert (1845–1904), for example, the damage caused directly by an invading organism was often minimal compared to that caused by the processes of inflammation triggered in the host.[30] For Weigert and his followers, almost every pathological phenomenon was 'first and foremost a process of self-destruction', or what Weigert referred to as the 'Siva effect'.[31] Similar views were expressed by the Polish school of pathologists and philosophers of medicine, from Tytus Chalubinski (1820–1889) to Ludwik Fleck (1896–1961). Eager to refute static, reductionist approaches to medicine and to challenge what they regarded as naive accounts of pathogenesis, Chalubinski and his descendants developed a dynamic, ecological picture of disease that stressed both the complexity of pathological phenomena and the central role of individual physiological reactivity.[32]

Von Pirquet's formulation of the role of biological reactivity in human pathology was shaped by his extensive knowledge of the natural history of acute infectious diseases and by his meticulous studies of vaccination reactions. It was also influenced by, and in turn informed, his observations of the effects of antitoxic sera in children being treated for scarlet fever and diphtheria in the paediatric clinics in Vienna. Focusing once again on the temporal characteristics of the clinical phenomena, von Pirquet and his Hungarian co-worker, Béla Schick (1877–1967), demonstrated that serum sickness presented a familiar set of pathological features. In particular, they confirmed that the onset of symptoms after serum therapy followed a pattern analogous to that exhibited in infectious diseases: there was a reproducible interval, or incubation period, between the initial injection and the appearance of symptoms; and subsequent injections (like secondary exposure to infection) were accompanied by accelerated and exaggerated responses. Von Pirquet and Schick concluded that the clinical features of serum sickness were not the direct product of the antiserum but the outcome of a hypersensitivity reaction characterized by 'a collision of antigen and antibody'. Significantly, the results of their investigations, first tentatively announced in 1903,[33] and subsequently expounded in a book published in 1905,[34] suggested a close, albeit ostensibly paradoxical, relationship between immunity and hypersensitivity.

> The conception that the antibodies, which should protect against disease, are also responsible for the disease, sounds at first absurd. This has as its basis the fact that we are accustomed to see in disease only harm done to the organism and to see in the antibodies solely antitoxic substances. One forgets too easily that the disease represents only a stage in the development of immunity, and that the organism often attains the advantage of immunity only by means of disease.[35]

It was these observations of distinct, but related, clinical phenomena gleaned from the bedside that provided von Pirquet with both the evidence and the impetus to formulate the concept of allergy. In a brief paper published in the *Münchener Medizinische Wochenschrift* in 1906, von Pirquet proposed an elegant account of biological reactivity that not only reconciled the apparent contrast between immunity and hypersensitivity but also drew together the disparate observations of anaphylaxis reported by experimental physiologists and those made in the clinic in cases of serum sickness, observations that he pointed out 'belong to the domain of immunology but fit poorly into its framework'. Citing the work of Richet, Rosenau and Anderson, von Behring, and others, as well as his own studies with Schick (which collectively indicated the potential for 'supersensitivity in the immunized organism'), von Pirquet posed what he regarded as the central question: 'But are immunity and supersensitivity really connected with each other, or should one distinguish the processes in which pre-treatment causes immunity from those in which it leads to supersensitivity?'[36]

Although von Pirquet acknowledged that the 'two terms contradict each other', he nevertheless emphasized close parallels between immunity and hypersensitivity, particularly in terms of the shifting chronology of the response on primary and secondary exposure to antigen. Anxious to promote further research into the precise immunological features of hypersensitivity and immunity, von Pirquet attempted to simplify understandings of these diverse manifestations of biological reactivity by suggesting 'a new generalized term, which . . . expresses the change in condition which an animal experiences after contact with any organic poison, be it animate or inanimate'.[37]

> For this general concept of a changed reactivity I propose the term allergy. . . . The vaccinated, the tuberculous, the individual injected with serum becomes allergic towards the corresponding foreign substance. . . . The term immunity must be restricted to those processes in which the introduction of the foreign substance into the organism causes no clinically evident reaction, where, therefore, complete insensitivity exists.[38]

Von Pirquet recognized both the experimental and clinical implications of his approach to biological reactivity. In particular, he explicitly linked his novel formulation of immunological reactivity, or allergy, to traditional clinical notions of idiosyncrasy, thereby paving the way for new understandings of a range of both well-established and seemingly novel conditions.

> Among the allergens should be included the poisons of mosquitoes and bees in so far as their stings are followed by hypo- or hypersensitivity. For this reason we may also enrol under this term the pollen causing hay fever (Wolff-Eisner), the urticaria-producing substances of strawberries and crabs, and probably too a number of organic substances leading to idiosyncrasy.[39]

Having established a tentative framework for a new theory of disease, von Pirquet outlined the clinical parameters of allergy more expansively in a monograph published in 1911. In 1909 he had declined an offer to work at the Pasteur Institute in Paris, primarily because of the absence of a clinical appointment attached to the post, and had chosen instead to accept an invitation to become the first professor of paediatrics at The Johns Hopkins University in Baltimore. He remained in North America only for one year. In 1910 he took up a position at the University of Breslau in Germany, and the following year returned to Vienna to replace his mentor, Escherich, as professor of paediatrics at the new Kinderklinik.[40] Although he appears not to have been particularly productive while in America, he did complete two expansive articles on allergy, which were subsequently published as a book by the American Medical Association in 1911.[41]

The typical features of von Pirquet's studied approach to immunological reactivity, set out in skeleton form in 1906, are evident both throughout the text of his 1911 monograph and in the accompanying illustrations carefully charting specific patterns of biological reactivity. In the first place, he clearly retained a close interest in the seemingly paradoxical relationship between immunity and hypersensitivity. Second, his focus remained steadfastly fixed on tracing the precise temporal, qualitative and quantitative aspects of various types of altered reactivity that enabled him to compare and contrast diverse clinical and experimental observations. Finally, he also retained his strong emphasis on the broad clinical significance of allergy. Although much of the text was preoccupied with serum sickness, vaccination reactions and experimental anaphylaxis in animals as paradigmatic forms of allergy, von Pirquet considered the role of altered immunological reactivity in urticaria, food idiosyncrasies and hay fever. In addition, just as Hutchinson had done many years previously with regard to idiosyncrasy, von Pirquet speculated about the contribution of allergy to the symptomatology of various infectious diseases, such as syphilis, scarlet fever and tuberculosis.[42]

In 1911 von Pirquet also reflected more extensively on the possible mechanisms involved in the pathogenesis of these conditions, drawing both on his clinical experience and on the results of experimental studies in animals and humans. In particular, he reviewed contemporary disputes about the nature of the sensitizing substance (or allergen), summarized evidence regarding the specificity of 'serum allergy', and discussed the results of experiments demonstrating the passive transfer of anaphylaxis.[43] Although the precise character and mode of action of the serum factors responsible remained unknown, von Pirquet was convinced that most forms of allergy were mediated by specific antibodies interacting in some way with an allergen. The implications of this hypothesis, which closely echoed his own earlier deliberations on the pathogenetic significance of host reactivity, were not lost on von Pirquet.

This explanation involved also quite a new conception of an antibody. Thus far the antibodies were numbered among the protective substances, which is just the contrary of the supposition. Diphtheria antitoxin was considered as a typical antibody. The action of this antibody is to neutralize completely the antigen, i.e., the diphtheria toxin, while in my hypothesis these other antibodies form a new toxic body with the antigen. The principal new conception consisted in the suggestion that a disease might be due indirectly to an antibody, an idea to which at that time adherents of the school of Ehrlich, like Kraus, took strong exception.[44]

As von Pirquet's words suggest, his approach to immunity and hypersensitivity was not well received by many of his contemporaries, who tended to regard the results of meticulous laboratory experiments more highly than the insights to be gained from clinical observation at the bedside. In the first instance, critics scathingly dismissed von Pirquet's terminology. In promoting his own understanding of the precise mechanisms operating in anaphylaxis, for example, Charles Richet condemned the introduction of what he regarded as an unnecessary new term.[45] Richet's rejection of the term allergy was echoed elsewhere. When von Pirquet's book was reviewed in the *Lancet* in 1911, the reviewer referred to the term as 'not a happy combination', and pointed out that Richet had already coined the word anaphylaxis to describe increased sensitivity to foreign substances.[46] Some years later, in their judicious attempt to classify the phenomena of hypersensitivity, Robert A. Cooke (1880–1960) and Arthur F. Coca (1875–1959), two leading American immunologists, also expressed their dissatisfaction with the word allergy as a means of classifying clinical conditions, since adherence to von Pirquet's original definition resulted in the inclusion of 'phenomena of such different nature as to make their association valueless if not positively confusing'. In its place, Cooke and Coca advocated simply using the term hypersensitivity, which, as they explained, was already in regular use in the literature on anaphylaxis.[47]

Contemporary commentators also challenged von Pirquet's account of serum sickness and his emphasis on the role of antibodies (and, by inference, the role of bodily reactivity) in the pathogenesis of human diseases. In a short study of immune sera published in 1908, Charles F. Bolduan (b. 1873), a German-born bacteriologist working in the New York City Department of Health, discussed experiments in guinea pigs which, he argued, indicated that von Pirquet's and Schick's theory that serum disease was the direct product of an interaction between antigen and antibody was 'untenable'.[48] Cooke and Coca also disputed von Pirquet's explanation of the features of serum sickness. In particular, they cited studies that had failed to demonstrate any correlation between the symptoms of the disease and the presence or absence of either 'specific precipitins' or 'antigen' in the blood. Arguing that this lack of relationship alone was 'sufficient to overthrow von Pirquet's theory', Cooke and Coca insisted that serum disease was not directly comparable to anaphylaxis.[49]

Occasionally, von Pirquet responded to such criticism by carefully evaluating competing theories. In 1911, for example, he pointed out that Richet's belief that immunity and hypersensitivity to a particular poison were stimulated by 'two different substances' remained speculative, since 'thus far the separate existence of both these hypothetical substances has not been proved'.[50] Von Pirquet, however, was acutely aware that his work on the analogies between serum sickness, vaccination and infectious diseases 'remained unnoticed', and that 'the main point of the theory, the difference in the time of reaction, has not been understood by many scientists'.[51] Von Pirquet's assessment appears to have been accurate. While the notion of allergy, and more specifically the role of host reactivity, remained marginal to many studies in experimental physiology and clinical pathology, interest in anaphylaxis by contrast blossomed. During the first two decades of the twentieth century, an expanding stream of articles and books on anaphylaxis (rather than allergy) appeared in a number of languages.[52] In addition, contemporary commentators both in Europe and in North America noted, sometimes derisively, how anaphylaxis had become 'one of the most popular scientific terms of the day'.[53] Although scientists and clinicians acknowledged the importance of anaphylaxis 'in the field of pathology',[54] they also recognized the extent to which the term had captured the imagination of the public, becoming 'quite the fashion' as the Russian-born immunologist Alexandre Besredka put it in 1919.[55]

The systematic neglect of von Pirquet's reflections on biological reactivity was short-lived. It is noticeable that when Richet (rather than von Pirquet significantly) was awarded the Nobel Prize in 1913 for his experimental work on anaphylaxis, the linguistic tide was perhaps already beginning to turn. The previous year, the American pathologist Ludvig Hektoen (1863–1951) had published an article in the *Journal of the American Medical Association* in which he not only used the terms anaphylaxis and allergy almost interchangeably but also made explicit the links between the laboratory and the clinic that had been central to von Pirquet's formulation of the concept of altered reactivity.[56] Four years later, in an article in the *Lancet* on prophylactic vaccination against hay fever, B. P. Sormani, a lecturer in serology in Amsterdam, similarly used allergy as a shorthand for 'hypersensibility for the pollen extract'.[57] In 1923 Alexander Gunn Auld, a Scottish-trained physician who had published books on the pathology of respiratory diseases and who later wrote a monograph reporting the results of his clinical investigations into the 'subject of Allergy', outlined the possible role of anaphylaxis in reactions to peptone injections, but also used the term allergy to describe the group of clinical conditions (hay fever, asthma, migraine, epilepsy, urticaria and other skin conditions) for which he was advocating the use of peptone immunization as a treatment.[58] By the late 1920s the titles of a number of books and journal articles suggest that the word allergy was slowly superseding anaphylaxis as a more propitious, and perhaps more euphonious, means of describing a variety of experimental and clinical phenomena.[59]

The creation of a new, and increasingly convenient, clinical term was not the only legacy of Clemens von Pirquet's measured analysis of altered biological reactivity. In the first place, von Pirquet's studies led him to suggest that modified skin reactions to bacteria or their toxins might be used for diagnostic purposes. Applying his observations on altered reactivity in cases of smallpox vaccination to tuberculosis, he suggested in 1907 that the nature of the skin reaction to inoculation with tuberculin (or 'the tuberculin test') could be used to determine whether or not a patient had been in contact with the tubercle bacillus. Although the test could not necessarily distinguish between old and active infection, especially in adult patients, von Pirquet was insistent not only that the cutaneous test was preferable to the conjunctival test later introduced by Albert Calmette (1863–1933), but also that the test was important in prevention, since it could reveal which children in hospitals and schools were tuberculous and should therefore be segregated.[60] Von Pirquet was justly proud of what he termed 'the allergy test' for tuberculosis. As he pointed out in a review of the field of allergy, published in 1927, his 'finding of most practical importance, the cutaneous tuberculin reaction, is used by paediatricians all over the world with the same interpretation I devised years ago'.[61] Although there were recurrent debates about the precise role (and indeed the nature) of hypersensitivity in the evolution of immunity against tuberculosis during the middle decades of the twentieth century,[62] von Pirquet's test became a standard diagnostic tool and served as a model for the development of similar tests for other diseases, such as diphtheria, glanders and actinomycosis.[63]

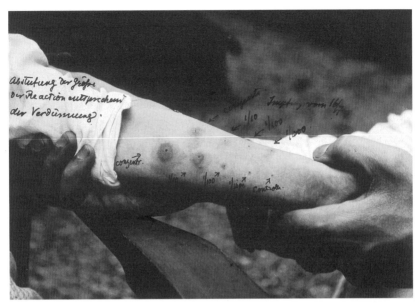

Clemens von Pirquet examining a patient's skin reaction.

Von Pirquet's notion of allergy carried other theoretical and pragmatic consequences. By postulating a clear correlation between the processes of immunity and hypersensitivity, he stimulated renewed interest in the role of what were regarded as the body's defence mechanisms in dictating the symptoms and course of human diseases. As a result, his formulation of allergy helped to sustain both conceptual and practical links between immunology and medicine, or between immunology and pathology, at a time when emergent preoccupations with the immunochemical dissection of antigens and antibodies were serving effectively to separate the laboratory from the clinic.[64] As the Nobel Prize-winning Danish immunologist Niels Jerne (1911–1994) put it many years later, as a direct result of studies on 'vaccination, allergy and serological diagnosis, immunology had a private line to medicine, which compensated for its isolation'.[65]

The ecological and biological tenor of von Pirquet's reflections on altered reactivity also shaped the intellectual context in which allergy, and later autoimmunity, emerged as distinct fields of clinical practice and scientific study. In the early decades of the twentieth century, whether framed in terms of allergy, anaphylaxis or hypersensitivity, altered immunological reactivity was implicated in the pathogenesis of hay fever, asthma, urticaria (or nettle-rash), eczema (a term derived from Greek and meaning literally to 'boil over' or 'break out'), food idiosyncrasies, supersensitivity to aspirin and other drugs, reactions to bee stings, infectious diseases such as tuberculosis, and a variety of diffuse clinical manifestations including rheumatism, eclampsia, migraine and epilepsy.[66] As studies of the role of allergy in human diseases proliferated, medical writers increasingly stressed both the extent to which these various conditions demonstrated similar pathological features and the manner in which individual patients often exhibited symptoms at more than one bodily site. From a pathological perspective, research suggested that eosinophilia (an excess of certain white blood cells) and increased capillary permeability were regular features of diseases understood in terms of anaphylaxis or allergy.[67] In the context of multiple symptoms, commentators confidently reiterated suspected links between asthma, hay fever and various dermatological and gastro-intestinal manifestations of allergy. At one level, for example, clinical studies revealed that patients with asthma were simply more likely to suffer from eczema, urticaria or hay fever.[68] At another level, medical writers not only regarded hay fever essentially as a form of asthma occurring at a different site, but also referred to 'mucous colic' as 'abdominal asthma' or 'asthma of the colon', and construed 'bilious headache' as a form of 'nervous asthma'.[69]

As Anne Marie Moulin has suggested, von Pirquet's formulation of allergy originally 'sprang from studies of the unpredicted effects of immunization'. Thus, 'the same immunology which had fostered the idea of collective immunization also harbored reflections on bodily idiosyncrasies'.[70] Subsequent consideration of the cardinal pathogenetic features of allergy encouraged clinicians and scientists to bring together a group of disparate idiosyncrasies under a single heading. Asthma, hay fever, urticaria, eczema and a range of other conditions were thought to possess a common pathology, a common aetiology and a common prognosis, and, in many cases, to be amenable to parallel forms of treatments. Although sometimes identified as the 'toxic idiopathies',[71] the 'asthma syndrome',[72] or as being representative of an 'exudative diathesis',[73] these conditions were increasingly referred to collectively as the 'allergic disorders'.[74] In this way, gradual adherence to Clemens von Pirquet's language of allergy established the foundations for the construction of a novel category of disease.

The mechanisms and meanings of allergy

In many ways, widespread application of the concepts of allergy, anaphylaxis and hypersensitivity by both clinical and laboratory researchers in Europe and North America helped to realize von Pirquet's aspiration that, by clarifying the nature of hypersensitivity and its relationship with immunity, he would enable researchers to explore the field more effectively. In the first two decades of the twentieth century, the work of von Pirquet, Richet, Arthus and others clearly motivated new studies in experimental physiology, drew together disparate fields of clinical enquiry, and provided a framework for novel approaches to treating a range of diverse conditions. However, in spite of the impetus provided by von Pirquet and his contemporaries, early studies of altered immunological reactivity were plagued by numerous problems and paradoxes.

In the first instance, although hypersensitivity to foreign substances was rapidly implicated in many pathological processes, the notion of allergy did not precipitate any clear, or immediate, revolution in theories of disease. On the contrary, well-established, alternative explanations of hay fever, asthma and a range of associated conditions persisted. A number of writers, for example, stressed the nervous origins of asthma and hay fever. In the eighth edition of his book on the principles and practice of medicine, published in 1914, the Canadian physician and Regius Professor of Medicine at Oxford, Sir William Osler (1849–1919), reiterated opinions propounded by several nineteenth-century writers (such as George Beard and Henry Hyde Salter) that there was 'in the majority of cases of bronchial asthma a strong neurotic element'.[75] Some years later, Sir Humphry Rolleston (1862–1944), Regius Professor of Physic at Cambridge and chair of the joint Ministry of Health and Medical Research Council Vaccine Committee, objected to the manner in which preoccupations with hypersensitivity often excluded consideration of the effect of 'reflex causes acting on an irritable nervous system', pointing out at the same time that the efficacy of adrenaline in treating asthma attacks was probably related to its ability to stimulate the sympathetic nervous system, thereby 'abolishing the dominance of vagotonia'.[76]

In addition to exploring the possible nervous origins of asthma and hay fever, medical writers also continued to consider a wide range of competing aetiological explanations. Thus, while they generally recognized the immediate role of pollen (or some other external agent) in precipitating attacks of hay fever and asthma in certain people, clinicians also stressed the contribution of local physical and chemical irritation of the nasal or bronchial mucous membranes,[77] the role of bacterial infections (with or without sensitization to bacterial proteins),[78] the psychological or emotional determinants of asthma in particular,[79] and increasingly the role of heredity.[80] More significantly, some commentators retained a strong interest in the possibility that so-called allergic diseases might be caused not by the patient's own immunological reactions but by the direct effect of a toxin. Indeed, as I shall argue in chapter Three, the elaboration of a novel treatment for hay fever by two British physicians in the first decade of the twentieth century was predicated on a belief that the condition was primarily 'caused by a soluble toxin found in the pollen of grasses', against which active immunity could be established.[81]

Significantly, continuing endorsements for alternative understandings of hay fever and asthma occasionally led to more direct condemnation of approaches that prioritized the role of allergy or anaphylaxis in pathogenesis. In 1913, for example, Jules Bordet (1870–1961), professor of bacteriology at the University of Brussels, pointed out that while anaphylaxis was 'suspected in a great variety of diseases', it was likely that the role of hypersensitivity in infectious diseases had been exaggerated at the expense of the 'pathogenic role of microbic poisons'.[82] In 1926 the anonymous reviewer of a book on the 'allergic diathesis' by a German author suggested not only that 'allergy will not explain all the questions' raised by various conditions occupying a 'vague hinterland of clinical medicine', but also that, for some readers, the author might have pushed 'his theories too far'.[83] While defending his use of nasal cautery for the treatment of asthma in the 1930s, Alexander Francis, a London surgeon, likewise pointed out that the role of hyperpyraemia in provoking 'a disturbance of the vasomotor system', thereby precipitating asthma, had been ignored, largely because hypersensitivity and desensitization had 'caught the popular fancy':

> The skin tests were simple and fascinating; and vaccines which were to effect immunisation when the offending protein had been found, were so popular as a cure for everything, that it was thought that the end of all asthmatic trouble was at hand.[84]

As several commentators pointed out, however, allergic theories of disease and the adoption of new methods of diagnosis frequently failed to resolve questions about aetiology. In particular, it was often difficult to correlate specific immunological reactivity with clinical symptoms, since skin reactions to foreign substances, such as the sensitization tests devised by the American allergist Isaac Chandler Walker (1883–1950), were often negative in asthma patients. As a result, physicians who used skin tests in the hope of tracing 'an attack of asthma to a sausage into which a worn-out horse has strayed' were often frustrated by their inability to identify any specific sensitivity, and were left simply with 'the old-fashioned diagnosis, bronchial or nervous asthma'.[85]

While the precise role of allergy in the pathogenesis of human diseases remained speculative, there were also disputes and doubts about the biological mechanisms and meanings of allergy. In line with emergent preoccupations with humoral, rather than cellular, forms of immunity, there was a general consensus that most, if not all, forms of hypersensitivity in both animals and humans were mediated by antibodies. Both the specificity of hypersensitivity reactions and the passive transfer of experimental anaphylaxis using serum from sensitized animals had been clearly demonstrated in early studies. In 1921 two German physicians, Carl Prausnitz (1876–1963) and Heinz Küstner (1897–1963), revealed that human idiosyncrasies to food (in this instance, fish) could similarly be transferred using serum, thereby confirming the role of antibodies in human allergies.[86] However, there were evident exceptions to the general rule. Although von Pirquet presumed that positive reactions to the tuberculin test were mediated by antibodies, Richet, among others, pointed out signal differences between anaphylaxis and heightened sensitivity to tuberculin.[87] Similarly, Rolleston later argued that 'the words anaphylaxis and anaphylactoid should be avoided in reference to drug idiosyncrasies', since the presence of antibodies to drugs had not been satisfactorily established.[88]

Even if these exceptions were disregarded, the identification of specific humoral substances (presumed to be antibodies) in cases of experimental anaphylaxis and in clinical manifestations of allergy served only to raise further questions concerning the specific mechanisms involved in hypersensitivity reactions. As one commentator in the *Lancet* pointed out in 1917, 'several theories have been from time to time propounded' to explain anaphylaxis, although most of them had 'in one respect or another been found wanting'.[89] In part, competing explanations for the biological manifestations of hypersensitivity reflected deeper uncertainties about the existence and properties of antibodies and about the precise nature of antigen-antibody reactions.[90] In addition, they were also driven by both pragmatic and philosophical concerns about the type, and possible role, of antibodies in immunopathological processes. Given the inability of researchers to demonstrate the regular presence of either precipitating or agglutinating antibodies in hypersensitivity, and given the general reluctance to accept that 'normal' antibodies might be involved in pathogenesis, commentators presumed the presence in these cases either of a previously unrecognized type of antibody, eventually referred to as 'serum reagin', 'reaginic antibody' or 'atopic reagin', or indeed of some other serum factor.[91]

However, the site and mode of action of specific antibodies (and other humoral substances, such as complement) remained elusive. In particular, there were strident disputes about whether the antibodies in question were active in the circulation or whether they were only effectual once fixed to cells. In line with increasingly dominant preoccupations with chemical approaches to immunity, a number of authors postulated a complex humoral mechanism in which initial exposure to antigen stimulated the production of a specific substance (probably reaginic antibody), variably referred to as 'toxogenin' (Richet) or 'sensibilisin' (Besredka). On subsequent exposure, this substance then reacted with the antigen to produce a toxic compound in the serum (labelled 'apotoxin' by Richet and 'anaphylatoxin' by Friedberger), which was subsequently responsible for the local and systemic manifestations of allergy or anaphylaxis.[92] For other commentators, including von Pirquet, Bordet and indeed Besredka, however, it appeared more likely that the antigen interacted with antibody either fixed to or within cells, leading to the subsequent release of active mediators from sensitized cells.[93] According to von Pirquet, for example, the delay between injection of a mixture of antibody and allergen and the appearance of symptoms suggested that 'it is probably necessary for the antibody to unite first with the cells of the organism'.[94] As the anonymous reviewer of Besredka's published critique of Friedberger's humoral theory diplomatically pointed out in 1919, these alternative approaches were 'not necessarily mutually exclusive': 'both parties are, as usual, probably more or less right, and likely the truth is that the reaction takes place inside cells, and on that account liberates poisonous substances which may act generally as well as locally'.[95]

These disputes about mechanism were partially resolved by the laboratory studies of a British scientist and clinician, Henry Dale (1875–1968). Having graduated first from Cambridge in natural sciences and then from London in medicine, in 1904 Dale accepted a post as a pharmacologist at the Wellcome Physiological Research Laboratories, of which he later became the Director. In 1910 research carried out at the Wellcome Laboratories led Dale and the chemist George Barger (1878–1939) to identify ß-iminazolyl-ethylamine, or histamine, as the active component of ergot capable of causing the contraction of cat uterine muscles *in vitro*.[96] Although histamine was not known to occur naturally in animals, further studies by Dale and his colleagues demonstrated the various physiological effects of the substance *in vivo*, including peripheral vasodilation, a drop in blood pressure, bronchial spasm and a fall in rectal temperature. The possible role of histamine in hypersensitivity reactions was immediately suspected, since, as Dale and Patrick Laidlaw (1881–1940) pointed out in 1911, a drop in rectal temperature was 'characteristic of the "anaphylactic shock"'.[97]

Two years later, and rather fortuitiously, Dale made a further significant contribution to the field, when he developed an *in vitro* model of anaphylaxis employing uterine, rather than intestinal, smooth muscle from sensitized guinea pigs. Significantly, Dale used his experimental system to test what he regarded as 'rival theories' of anaphylaxis, especially those concerning the site of the antigen-antibody reaction. In particular, his work demonstrated that extensive washing of portions of smooth muscle with Ringer's solution, thereby 'freeing them from body fluids', did not abrogate the anaphylactic contraction in response to further challenge with sensitizing antigen. Acknowledging that his work did not shed light on the precise nature of the 'anaphylactic antibody', or on its relationship with precipitin, Dale nevertheless concluded that his studies provided support for the theory that antigen interacted with cell- or tissue-fixed antibody.[98]

Although Dale received the Nobel Prize in 1936 for his work on the chemical transmission of nerve impulses, he continued to contribute regularly to debates about what he termed 'the anaphylactic process'. In particular, he demonstrated the natural presence of histamine in normal tissues and postulated a link between histamine and the H-substance identified by Thomas Lewis (1881–1945) as responsible for the characteristic 'triple response' (consisting of a red line, flare and wheal) witnessed in local tissue injury. By 1929, in a series of Croonian Lectures delivered to the Royal College of Physicians, Dale felt sufficiently confident of the accumulating evidence implicating both the role of tissue-fixed (rather than circulating) antibodies and the release of histamine in anaphylaxis to assert that:

> We may picture the anaphylactic shock, therefore, as the result of cellular injury, due to the intracellular reaction of the antigen with an aggregating antibody. Whether this is general, or localised in a particular organ, histamine will be released, and its effects will be prominent in the resulting reaction, imposing a

general resemblance to the syndrome produced by histamine itself, on the symptoms seen in each species.[99]

Significantly, Dale's reflections reiterated a familiar set of problems concerning the precise relationship between experimental anaphylaxis and clinical presentations of allergy. Although he recognized that there were differences between animal models and human clinical conditions, Dale nevertheless argued in 1929 that experimental anaphylaxis and a variety of natural or acquired human idiosyncrasies were all mediated by a similar mechanism, involving the release of histamine.[100] The connection between the two sets of conditions had been raised initially by Richet, who had hoped to establish anaphylaxis as a suitable model for exploring general pathological principles.[101] An awareness, however, that anaphylaxis manifested itself in different forms in different species, together with evidence that anaphylaxis was far more difficult to induce in humans than in animals, raised provocative and largely unresolved questions about the relationship between the laboratory and clinical manifestations of altered biological reactivity. Indeed, for many years, John Freeman (1876–1962), the doyen of clinical allergy in Britain during the first half of the twentieth century, continued to question the meaning and utility of the term anaphylaxis, suggesting in 1950 that the concept 'barely comes into human medicine at all'.[102]

In a number of publications, Henry Dale also paid close attention to two related conundrums within the field, namely the relationship between immunity and hypersensitivity and the biological and evolutionary significance or meaning of anaphylaxis.[103] Of course, it had been precisely these questions that had prompted Clemens von Pirquet's initial formulation of the concept of allergy many years previously, and in the intervening decades many commentators had regularly returned to the topic. Contemporary bacteriological conceptualizations of immunological processes primarily as a form of defence against invading organisms, combined with Paul Ehrlich's belief that in normal circumstances antibodies directed against self antigens were either not produced or were eliminated,[104] encouraged some authors to suggest that hypersensitivity constituted merely an immunological malfunction, or what Carl Prausnitz later referred to in a lecture delivered at St George's Hospital in London as 'immunity gone astray'.[105] Not only did medical writers envisage the presence of different types of antibodies in immunity and anaphylaxis but they also suggested, in Darwinian terms, that anaphylaxis constituted a failure of the natural defence mechanisms to adapt appropriately to new substances.[106]

However, scientists and clinicians increasingly challenged this conception of allergy and anaphylaxis as somehow antithetical to immunity. According to Hektoen in 1912, for example, there was 'no contradiction between immunity and allergy, which is a form of antibody reaction and, so to speak, an incident in the course of immunization'.[107] Similarly, Bordet insisted that anaphylaxis was not 'the contrary of immunity', but rather that it was 'an accident in the course of defence' that testified 'to the fact that the struggle against the foreign element is taking place'.[108] Richet and others pushed the argument further, maintaining that anaphylaxis was a necessary stage in the evolution of immunity and therefore part of a universal defence mechanism.[109] Indeed, Richet made more grandiose claims for the biological significance of anaphylaxis. During his Nobel Lecture in 1913, Richet argued that anaphylaxis operated as a means of preserving the integrity of 'the humoral personality', which (in parallel with the psychological personality) comprised the 'chemical composition of our humours' that 'makes us different from others'. From this perspective, anaphylaxis served to protect the chemical 'integrity of the race', sometimes at the expense of the individual.

> Anaphylaxis is thus necessary to the species, often to the detriment of the individual. The individual may perish, but this does not matter. The species must at all times retain its organic integrity. Anaphylaxis defends the species against the peril of adulteration.[110]

Richet's formulation of the evolutionary significance of anaphylaxis clearly contained echoes of earlier, and indeed enduring, racialist theories of idiosyncratic diseases such as hay fever.[111] In addition, it was suffused with contemporary eugenic concerns about the erection and maintenance of social, political and geographical boundaries between classes and about the preservation of racial purity in an age manifestly troubled by deep-seated anxieties about safeguarding national identities and resisting blatant threats to imperialism.[112] Although Richet's distinctive approach remained outside the mainstream of clinical and scientific writing on allergy and anaphylaxis, many of his ideas persisted, albeit in modified and attenuated forms. For example, his suggestion that the humoral personality comprised (like its psychological counterpart) a form of chemical memory, both of the evolution of the species and the history of the individual, was reformulated after the Second World War by leading immunologists and microbiologists such as Frank Macfarlane Burnet (1899–1985) and René Dubos. In addition, his emphasis on biological individuality, and his plea for 'another kind of physiology' of the individual rather than the species, preserved the notion of idiosyncrasy in the face of growing interest in collective, statistical approaches to disease.[113] Although, by the 1920s, many immunologists and clinicians regarded biological individuality as 'an obsolete topic',[114] proponents of the nascent field of allergy continued to explore the nature and treatment of idiosyncratic responses to foreign substances, thereby sowing the seeds for approaches to treatment that were aimed not at allergen avoidance (such as climate therapy for hay fever and asthma) but at modifying or effacing the destructive elements of altered biological reactivity.

The death of allergy

On 28 February 1929 Clemens von Pirquet and his wife, Maria, committed suicide. Their deaths remain an enigma. In many ways, von Pirquet appears to have pursued an immensely successful career as a paediatrician. Having returned to Europe from Baltimore, he worked for a short period in Breslau before being appointed as Professor of Paediatrics at the Kinderklinik in Vienna in which he had started his training. During the course of his career he had published extensively on a wide range of clinical and scientific topics. In particular, he maintained a strong and productive interest in anthropometrics, designed isolation beds to use in the children's wards, contributed to paediatric psychiatry, and devised a new means of calculating the nutritional status of food, which he referred to as the 'nutritional equivalent of milk', or 'nem', and which he claimed offered a more constructive measure of nutritional value than calories.[115]

Given his apparent professional success, von Pirquet's decision to terminate his life appears even more striking. It is possible that alienation from his family during the protracted law suit relating to his mother's estate, his wife's longstanding physical and psychological troubles, and the increasingly parlous state of his homeland collectively encouraged thoughts of suicide. It is also feasible that von Pirquet's sense of isolation was deepened by contemporary scepticism about the scientific and clinical value of some of his major contributions, since both allergy and the 'nem' were greeted with hostility by his peers. In addition, there is evidence in his intellectual output that von Pirquet was increasingly preoccupied with death. With a growing interest in biostatistics, he spent much time and effort during the 1920s calculating what he referred to as 'the centre of gravity' (that is, the day with the highest frequency of deaths) for different diseases. His studies, which demonstrated considerable statistical expertise and graphical imagination, were published in 1927. While acute infections were strongly seasonal, he declared, peak periods of death varied significantly according to the site and nature of the infection. By contrast, deaths from malignant tumours were unrelated to season.[116] Such obsession with charting patterns of mortality led his biographer to suggest that von Pirquet's suicide might have been linked to a fear of the ageing process itself.[117]

During the middle years of his career, von Pirquet published only a limited number of articles on allergy and its manifestations, restricting himself particularly to discussing the pathogenesis and distribution of the typical skin rash in measles, which he characteristically interpreted in terms of a reaction between antibody and antigen, and to distinguishing between normal vaccination reactions and the phenomenon of 'paravaccine'.[118] In the late 1920s, however, he returned with some vigour to the set of intellectual problems that had in many ways launched his career. In 1927 he published an overview of the emergence of scientific and clinical interest in allergy in the years following Richet's identification of anaphylaxis, focusing especially on his own contributions to the field. Noting that both his tuberculin test and Schick's test for diphtheria had become common diagnostic tools, he also suggested, with evident satisfaction, that the 'term serum sickness and the concept of allergy had become generally accepted'.[119]

During the same period, von Pirquet's resurgent interest in allergy and his growing preoccupation with the processes of ageing and dying emerged in a study of what he referred to as 'Allergie des Lebensalters', or 'allergy of the life phases'. Although a preliminary publication introducing his ideas in embryonic form appeared shortly before his death in 1929, he failed to complete an atlas setting out the age distribution for a range of diseases before he committed suicide, and his monograph addressing the impact of age on cancer mortality was published posthumously. In these studies, von Pirquet proposed that the 'characteristic age curve' for 'almost every well-defined cause of death' could be attributed to an age-dependent form of altered biological reactivity or allergy.[120]

Significantly, von Pirquet's work on the biology of ageing, like his earlier formulation of the concept of allergy and his later reflections on historical developments in the field, demonstrates the extent to which he retained throughout his life an expansive and inclusive notion of allergy as a manifestation of general altered biological reactivity. However, it is apparent that, by the time of his death, the precise meaning of the term had been substantially narrowed by his contemporaries. Increasingly, allergy was not construed in broad biological terms but was considered to be analogous to anaphylaxis and other types of hypersensitivity, that is to specific forms of immunological reactivity leading only to tissue damage. In 1927, for example, Humphry Rolleston noted that allergy had by then become 'commonly regarded as synonymous with hypersensitivity and anaphylaxis, which is not the original meaning attached to it'.[121] Two years later, in the year of von Pirquet's demise, Rolleston's words were echoed by the editors of the newly founded *Journal of Allergy*, published jointly by the two leading American societies for the study of asthma, hay fever and allied conditions. Pointing out that their approach was consistent with 'current medical usage', the editors explained that the journal had been launched 'as a medium for the presentation of papers concerning the clinical aspects of specific hypersensitiveness in human beings'.[122] This more limited meaning of the term allergy was indeed regularly adopted by scientists and clinicians. In 1933 the prominent and eccentric American pathologist Arnold Rice Rich (1893–1968), renowned for his work on immunity and hypersensitivity in relation to tuberculosis, deliberately distanced himself from von Pirquet's broad definition of allergy:

> Regardless of what Pirquet's concept of the term allergy may have been, although there is no strict uniformity in the usage of the word at present, nevertheless allergy to-day in the minds of most medical men is synonymous with acquired hypersensitiveness, as any examination of the many papers published every year on the subject will at once disclose; and it is in this sense only that I shall use the term in the present paper.[123]

Clemens von Pirquet's formative impact on the emergence of scientific and clinical studies of hypersensitivity and immunity has often been overshadowed by the Nobel Prize-winning work of his European contemporaries, such as Emil von Behring, Paul Ehrlich, Charles Richet and Jules Bordet. However, as I shall argue in subsequent chapters, although von Pirquet's original meaning of the term allergy may well have declined, reverberations from the conceptual insights and clinical focus that defined his approach to allergy continued, sometimes covertly, to shape the study of idiosyncratic reactions to foreign substances throughout the twentieth century. More particularly, the founding of the *Journal of Allergy* in 1929, the introduction of postgraduate courses in 'allergic disorders' in some European countries around the same time,[124] and the successful creation of 'allergy clinics' in hospitals on both sides of the Atlantic during the 1920s, provide dramatic testimony to the rich and immediate legacy of von Pirquet's contributions to science and medicine. At the very moment of his death, a new speciality of clinical allergy was being born in the laboratories and hospitals of Western Europe and North America.

3

ALLERGY IN THE CLINIC

> I think it might be exaggeration to say that the study of these toxic
> idiopathies will open a new field of medicine, but I feel confident that
> they throw light from a new angle across a very large field of the
> old medicine.
>
> John Freeman, 1920[1]

During the inter-war years, Clemens von Pirquet's notion of allergy proved
infectious. In spite of evident ambiguities in its meaning, the term allergy was
increasingly applied by Western scientists, clinicians and patients not only to
explain and classify a miscellany of scattered symptoms and recognizable
diseases but also to define the therapeutic focus and experimental parameters
of a new medical speciality. In particular, by emphasizing the centrality of
biological reactivity in human disease, the dynamic and holistic assumptions
embedded in von Pirquet's vision of pathological processes served to deflect
clinical attention away from merely environmental or climatic treatments for
conditions such as hay fever and asthma towards attempts to manipulate
immunological responses to specific and identifiable allergens. In the early
decades of the twentieth century, allergists (as they came to be known) on
both sides of the Atlantic concentrated predominantly on developing and
perfecting a novel treatment for allergic diseases, generally referred to as inoculation therapy, desensitization or allergen immunotherapy, which was aimed
at rendering sensitive patients more tolerant of allergenic foreign substances.

While Clemens von Pirquet's insights undoubtedly provided a sound
semantic and conceptual basis for specialization, the elaboration of new treatments and the construction of a new speciality were also clearly fashioned by
a broader constellation of contemporary concerns. The origins of inoculation
therapy (much like the roots of von Pirquet's initial formulation of allergy), for
example, lay principally in late nineteenth- and early twentieth-century clinical preoccupations with infectious diseases and vaccine therapy and in closely
related understandings of hay fever as a condition caused by the actions of a
pollen toxin, rather than in theoretical expositions or laboratory studies of
anaphylaxis and hypersensitivity in animals. The primary aim of this chapter
is to explore the context in which inoculation therapy was first devised as a
treatment for hay fever by two British physicians in the first decade of the

twentieth century and the manner in which, although its efficacy and safety were sometimes extensively criticized, desensitization was subsequently embraced by doctors across Europe and North America as the cornerstone of their allergy practice. In the process, I shall argue that the energetic adoption of desensitization and the expansion of clinical allergy as a speciality in the Western world was accompanied, and perhaps facilitated, by gradually widening professional, political and public awareness of the expanding scale of allergic diseases across continents, classes and cultures.

Hay fever, class and culture

In 1819 a British physician, John Bostock (1773–1846), published a detailed account of a 'periodical affection of the eyes and chest', from which he himself had suffered for many years. Appearing 'about the beginning or middle of June in every year' and lasting around two months, the condition was characterized by itchy eyes, a nasal discharge, paroxysmal sneezing, difficulty in breathing and a general malaise.[2] Although previous medical authors (including Rhazes in the tenth century, Jacobus Constant de Rebecque in the seventeenth century, and, as Bostock was aware, the prominent Enlightenment physician William Heberden) had occasionally noted the presence of similar symptoms during the summer, putatively provoked by the aroma of certain flowers, Bostock is generally credited with the first clear clinical description of a new disease, sometimes referred to in his honour as 'Bostock's catarrh'.[3]

As Bostock appreciated, the condition that he described was not common. Nine years later, however, he was able to present a more expansive account of the clinical features collected from a further twenty-eight cases of what he termed 'catarrhus aestivus or summer catarrh', but what was increasingly referred to by doctors and the public alike as 'hay fever'. According to Bostock, the symptoms were precipitated not by 'the effluvium of new hay' as was commonly supposed, but primarily by excessive heat and sunshine and by physical exertion. Accordingly, he advocated travelling to cooler, fresher coastal regions, such as Ramsgate in south-east England, during the summer months in order to avoid or alleviate the condition. Significantly, having noted that the condition had been recognized as a 'specific affection' only recently, Bostock suggested that hay fever occurred only 'in the middle and upper classes of society', being supposedly unheard of 'among the poor'.[4]

Hay fever soon began to attract medical attention. In the early 1830s John Elliotson (1791–1868), physician and founding President of the Phrenological Society, discussed the clinical features of hay fever in a series of lectures to medical students at St Thomas's Hospital in London. According to Elliotson, who had first heard about the condition from one of his patients, hay fever was caused not by heat and sunshine as Bostock had surmised but by exposure to 'the flower of grass'. In addition, he raised the possibility of hay fever being induced by contact with animals, in one case by 'the emanation from a rabbit'. More strikingly, however, Elliotson contested Bostock's assertions about the class distribution of the condition. Although he acknowledged that 'it seems so much among the higher orders', Elliotson nevertheless argued that hay fever was likely to be routinely misdiagnosed as a common cold in the 'poor people' who attended dispensaries, resulting in an under-estimation of its incidence 'among the lower orders'.[5]

Regarded by some medical authors as an 'exceedingly rare occurrence',[6] during the mid-nineteenth century hay fever appeared to be becoming increasingly common particularly in Britain and North America. According to Charles Blackley (1820–1900), a British general practitioner and homoeopath who published a comprehensive treatise on the subject in 1873, the rising prevalence of hay fever in England during the Victorian period could be accounted for either in terms of 'the increased attention, directed to the disease, having had the effect of bringing the cases, which do occur, much more distinctly under the notice of medical men', or alternatively 'by the greater prevalence of those conditions which act as predisposing and exciting causes'. Whatever the precise reasons, Blackley noted that the apparent rise in hay fever had excited increased interest both 'amongst the laity and amongst the members of the medical profession'.[7]

Greater attention to the clinical features and social distribution of hay fever was manifest in various ways. At one level, the gradual efflorescence of cases stimulated the growth of popular hay fever societies, particularly in North America. The United States Hay Fever Association, founded in 1874, was based in Bethlehem, a prestigious health resort in the White Mountains of New Hampshire, to which members of the Association flocked in order to escape the perils of summer and autumn pollen clouds. A similar Western society was established in Petosky, Michigan, in 1882. Both organizations boasted an elite membership drawn predominantly from the professional middle classes and were equally committed to promoting research, preserving the atmospheric purity of hay fever resorts frequented by the affluent and genteel classes, and proclaiming hay fever as a fashionable, even desirable, affliction.[8] When ragweed was indicted as the plant primarily responsible for provoking bouts of autumnal hay fever, the American hay fever associations, in conjunction with the Department of Agriculture and the Public Health Service, also campaigned for the eradication of what was regarded as a common weed.[9]

Hay fever also intrigued medical practitioners, not only in the United States but also in continental Europe and more particularly in Britain, which was regarded by some commentators as the 'haunt of hay fever'.[10] In 1859 the German physician Philipp Phoebus (1804–1880) initiated an extensive international survey of the pathology and treatment of hay fever, focusing particularly on the ethnographic and geographic distribution of the condition. Phoebus's enquiries, which prompted correspondence and accounts in medical journals in various countries, resulted in the publication of a major text on hay fever in 1862, in which he argued, like Bostock before him, that hay fever was caused by the 'first heat of summer' (and particularly by the impact of ozone) acting on a predisposed individual, and in which he offered evidence that those of Anglo-Saxon parentage were most susceptible to the condition.[11]

It was in the 1870s, however, at precisely the time when hay fever was emerging as a fashionable disease among the elite classes, that three medical authors independently published major monographs on the subject. In North America, both Morrill Wyman (1812–1903) and George Beard (1839–1883) pursued extensive studies of the disease. According to Wyman, who like many authors on the subject had suffered from hay fever since childhood and who took regular 'hay fever holidays' in the White Mountains, the appearance of his symptoms coincided neatly with (and more impressively were clearly provoked by exposure to) the flowering of ragweed (*Ambrosia artemesiaefolia*).[12] Although Beard's enquiries led him to support Wyman's conclusions about the pivotal role of ragweed, he also argued that hay fever was primarily a manifestation of 'American nervousness', that is, a form of nervous exhaustion precipitated by the peculiar stresses and strains of modern American civilization. For Beard, hay fever was 'essentially a neurosis' generated, like neurasthenia, by the diverse pernicious features of modern life: novel modes of transport and communication; the range of 'unrhythmical, unmelodious' noises accompanying modern industrialization; an increase in the amount of business and the pace of discovery; climate change; domestic and financial troubles; the increased education and mental activity of women; and even greater liberty.[13] 'Modern nervousness', argued Beard evocatively in 1881, 'is the cry of the system struggling with its environment.'[14]

In Britain, the careful studies of Wyman and Beard were mirrored by experiments conducted by Charles Blackley. Like many of his contemporaries,

Blackley was particularly concerned to clarify the precise cause of hay fever, from which he too had suffered for many years. Most writers acknowledged that predisposing constitutional factors, or what the British physician Walter Hayle Walshe (1812–1892) referred to in 1871 as an 'unalterable nervine idiosyncrasy',[15] played a crucial role. Nevertheless, there were considerable disputes about the relative contributions of a range of potential precipitating or exciting causes of individual attacks of hay fever. In 1859 Blackley embarked on a series of meticulous experiments to settle the issue. Using both himself and his patients as subjects, Blackley effectively dismissed previous accounts of hay fever that had prioritized the role of benzoic acid, coumarin, various odours, ozone, dust and the influence of heat and light. In addition, although he acknowledged that more research was needed, he questioned the role of emanations from animals. In an expansive monograph reporting his findings, first published in 1873, Blackley emphatically concluded that 'pollen of all kinds will give rise to some of the symptoms of hay-fever, and that all the other so-called causes have little or nothing to do with generating the disease'.[16]

Blackley's investigations were notable for the assiduity with which he assessed and eliminated competing causes of hay fever in turn and for his elaboration of novel apparatuses for collecting, measuring and charting the seasonal distribution of pollen in the atmosphere. However, although Blackley's publication was favourably reviewed in medical journals and although both his experiments and his theories were eagerly supported by some leading medical authorities, such as the ear, nose and throat specialist Morell Mackenzie (1837–1892),[17] Blackley's belief that pollen was the sole proximate cause of hay fever, in both its catarrhal and asthmatic forms, was not universally accepted by his contemporaries. Drawing on the explanatory power of germ theories of disease in this period, some authors (referred to dismissively by Mackenzie as 'zealous bacteriomaniacs')[18] emphasized the aetiological role of organisms in the nasal secretions of hay fever sufferers and accordingly advocated the local application of quinine and other agents.[19] In addition, writers such as George Beard and the British physician William Young (1843–1900), who linked hay fever to a diet rich in hydrocarbons, continued to place particular emphasis on the impact of modern lifestyles.[20] In 1903, however, Blackley's preoccupation with pollen as the causative agent found influential support from the researches of William P. Dunbar (1863–1922), an American physician who was Director of the State Hygienic Institute in Hamburg. Having dismissed the role of bacteria, and indeed a variety of other possible agents such as soot and dust, Dunbar's experiments led him to stress a combination of idiosyncratic constitutional and external exciting factors in his conclusion that 'a group of persons exist who show a specific susceptibility to irritation by the pollen of grasses'.[21] Significantly, Dunbar's belief that hay fever was the product of a pollen toxin, which led him to generate a specific antitoxin analogous to those raised against infectious diseases, provided a crucial context for the development of inoculation therapy in the first decade of the twentieth century.

In addition to attempting to elucidate the precise factor that triggered individual attacks of hay fever, Blackley, Beard and Dunbar also carefully considered the possible causes of modern trends in the prevalence of the disease. According to Blackley, the recent rise in cases could be traced in part to shifting agricultural practices and demographic transformations. During the eighteenth and nineteenth centuries, Blackley argued, not only had the area of land under cultivation gradually increased, but it had also become more common to grow hay-grass rather than buckwheat as food for cattle. The impact of greater production of hay, itself driven partly by the 'growth of commerce and the general increase of wealth and luxury', was exacerbated by migration to cities and towns. Apparently unprotected by early exposure to grass pollen, the modern urban dweller readily developed a vulnerability to hay fever. As Blackley pointed out in a critical passage that presaged the notion of specific desensitization developed by members of the Inoculation Department at St Mary's Hospital in London, evidence that farmers rarely experienced the condition could be explained partly in terms of 'the acquisition of a certain degree of insusceptibility', or 'immunity', to pollen generated by 'continued exposure to its influence'.[22]

Contemporary medical understandings of the emergence of hay fever as a product of exposure both to rising levels and to the shifting distribution of pollen in the modern environment clearly framed approaches to treatment. Although several practitioners advocated the nasal application, ingestion or inhalation of a variety of substances (including cocaine, quinine, arsenic, nux vomica and tobacco smoke) as a means of palliating attacks,[23] most late nineteenth-century writers emphasized avoidance, or 'climate therapy', as the most effective strategy for hay fever sufferers. While American writers advocated retreating to 'hay fever havens' in the mountains to evade the action of pollen, British authors preferred to send patients to the sea, particularly if the 'sea-side place has the form and character of a small island or a narrow peninsula' surrounded by the ocean and therefore more likely to be free from pollen-bearing land-breezes.[24] Such advice served to establish certain coastal and mountain regions on both sides of the Atlantic as fashionable hay fever resorts and to promote a form of health tourism.[25] If travel to the mountains or sea proved impossible, hay fever sufferers were advised to stay indoors or to travel to the centre of a large, densely populated town where the levels of pollen were expected to be minimal.[26]

However, while recognizing the importance of environmental factors in the appearance and blossoming of hay fever in the nineteenth century, Blackley, Beard and others also regarded the rise of hay fever in constitutional and cultural terms. When Bostock had first reviewed his experiences of a number of cases in 1828, he had suggested that hay fever occurred predominantly in the middle and upper classes. Over subsequent decades, medical writers and hay fever sufferers alike often reiterated the link between hay fever and class. According to Blackley, for example, hay fever was regularly regarded as 'an aristocratic disease', which was particularly prevalent among members of the learned professions, notably theology and medicine: 'there can be no doubt that, if it is not almost wholly confined to the upper classes of society, it is rarely, if ever, met with but among the educated'.[27] Similarly, from a study of what he termed 'Southern Negroes', George Beard concluded that 'nervous diseases do not exist, or exist but very rarely among savages or semi-savages, or even among barbarians', and that even to suggest 'hay-fever or nervous dyspepsia among these people, is but to joke'.[28]

In a lecture delivered to the West London Medico-Chirurgical Society in 1887, Sir Andrew Clark (1826–1893), consulting physician and Emeritus Professor of Clinical Medicine at the London Hospital, clearly spelled out hay fever's distinctive personality:

> And when once hay-fever appears it exhibits still further the closeness of its relationships to the nervous system by choosing the man before the woman, the educated before the ignorant, the gentle before the rude, the courtier before the clown ... It prefers the temperate to the torrid zone, it seeks the city before the country, and out of every climate which it visits it chooses for its subjects the Anglo-Saxon, or at least English-speaking, race.[29]

Clark's words suggest that, while the characteristic paroxysms of hay fever might be provoked by pollen, the condition was thought to occur only in those possessing the requisite 'nervous constitution', which was often inherited but which could also be acquired through education and civilization. As

Blackley, Beard and Dunbar all recognized, the ability of education (or what Blackley referred to as 'mental culture')[30] to generate a predisposition to nervous diseases such as hay fever could be used to explain not only the apparent geographic and ethnographic distribution of the condition tentatively identified by Phoebus in the 1860s and confirmed by Clark two decades later, but also its relatively recent appearance in human history. 'The fact of exemption from hay fever of savages and practically of the laboring classes in civilized countries,' wrote Dunbar in 1903, 'as well as other considerations, suggest that we must look upon hay fever as one of the consequences of higher civilization.'[31] In a similar vein, Blackley recognized that the lack of education and mental culture among the farming classes might, in conjunction with early exposure to pollen, contribute to the low prevalence of the condition in that occupational group. In addition, as Blackley presciently warned, the expansion of educational opportunities during the nineteenth century not only explained the appearance of the disease in that period but also raised the spectre of further escalations in the frequency of hay fever:

> Taking all these circumstances into account, it is highly probable that hay-fever was at one time altogether unknown, and it is tolerably certain that it has not only been much more frequent of late, but that, as population increases and as civilisation and education advance, the disorder will become more common than it is at the present time.[32]

Some commentators pushed the argument linking constitution, culture and disease even further. As Gregg Mitman has shown, members of the American hay fever associations were publicly proud of their infirmity, which served not only to distance them from the lower classes but also to define them positively as the possessors of sensitivity, wealth and leisure.[33] In England, this refrain was taken up most eagerly by Morell Mackenzie. Consulting physician to the Throat Hospital in London and founder of the *Journal of Laryngology and Rhinology* in 1887, Mackenzie became renowned initially for his expertise in laryngology but subsequently also for his disastrous failure to diagnose throat cancer when called in to advise the Crown Prince Frederick III of Prussia, a mistake for which he was expelled from the Royal College of Surgeons.[34] In a short treatise first published in 1884, Mackenzie reiterated what was by now becoming a popular motif in the medical literature by insisting that hay fever afflicted the British and American people far more frequently than the French, Germans, Russians, Italians, Spanish and Scandinavians. However, for Mackenzie this superficially disturbing fact 'in reality affords matter for self-congratulation as indicating our superiority to less favoured peoples in culture and civilisation'.[35] Similarly, individual hay fever sufferers should be mollified by the social geography of the disease.

> Sufferers from hay fever may, however, gather some crumbs of comfort from the fact that the disease is almost exclusively confined to persons of cultivation. As, therefore, summer sneezing goes hand-in-hand with culture, we may, perhaps, infer that the higher we rise in the intellectual scale, the more is the tendency developed. Hence, as already hinted, our national proclivity to hay fever may be taken as a proof of our superiority to other races.[36]

With pointed reference to contemporary disputes about the education and emancipation of women, Mackenzie explained the apparent gender, as well as class and racial, distribution of hay fever in equally hubristic terms. Although some authors disputed the male preponderance of the disease identified by Mackenzie and others,[37] Mackenzie himself was in no doubt about the increased prevalence of hay fever in men, a circumstance that he mockingly 'commended to the earnest attention of the advocates of the equality of the sexes'.[38] Echoing earlier formulations of certain diseases as fashionable, desirable and, most importantly, heritable conditions, Mackenzie insisted that when 'this idea of the intimate connexion between hay fever and culture has been firmly grasped by the public mind, the complaint will, perhaps, come to be looked on, like gout, as a sign of breeding'.[39] In a similar fashion to tuberculosis and gout before it, hay fever had thus become a badge of honour, to be worn only by the civilized, educated and cultured elite.

It was this pretentious public image of hay fever as a noble complaint that occasionally surfaced in contemporary literature. In *Howards End* (1910), in which E. M. Forster astutely dissected the intellectual and moral contours of early twentieth-century English class divisions as well as exposing the vulnerability of outmoded liberal-humanist values, hay fever appears as the embodiment of innate cultural refinement. From the opening passages of the novel, it is clear that both Tibby Schlegel and Charles Wilcox, members by birth of the landed and leisured elite, are afflicted with the condition: 'The hay fever had worried him a good deal all night. His head ached, his eyes were wet, his mucous membrane, he informed her, in a most unsatisfactory condition.'[40] By contrast, Leonard Bast, a lowly insurance clerk upon whom Tibby's sisters take pity and who dies when a bookcase falls on him during a struggle with Charles, is untouched by the complaint. Significantly, in Forster's rendition of the providential nature of hay fever, Bast remains consigned to his station, perpetually excluded from the ranks of the civilized 'hayfeverites' (as they were known in America), regardless of his efforts to improve himself through study; indeed, in some ways, his studies prove his downfall since he is literally killed by the human and material constituents of the culture in which he is so eager to participate. For Forster's elite protagonists, culture acquired through education could never bridge 'the gulf that stretches between the natural [that is, lower class] and the philosophic man'.[41] From this perspective, hay fever constituted both a symbol and a guardian of supposedly preordained class divisions, serving to naturalize in stark biological terms the social and political boundaries constructed and contested during the processes of industrialization. As Morell Mackenzie had conjectured several years earlier, 'soon, no doubt, the presence or absence of the tendency to sneeze at the sight of a rose will become a test, surer than the letter *h* for the separation of the elect from the common herd'.[42]

It is striking that, as most nineteenth-century medical writers made clear, hay fever was routinely associated with asthma long before the two conditions were regarded as parallel manifestations of allergy. The term asthma itself has a much longer history than hay fever, stretching back to ancient medical texts. In Hippocratic, Galenic and Chinese traditions, asthma constituted merely a generic form of dyspnoea, that is, difficulty breathing or shortness of breath. Typified by panting or wheezing, or what the Roman stoic philosopher Seneca referred to as 'a sort of continued "last gasp"', asthma was most commonly attributed to humoral imbalance.[43] Over subsequent centuries, occasional treatises by physicians tended to confirm this use of the term, but also began to challenge ancient understandings of the aetiology and pathology of asthma. During the seventeenth century, for example, studies by the Belgian Jan van Helmont (1577–1644), and two English doctors, Thomas Willis (1621–1675) and John Floyer (1649–1734), not only focused attention on the lungs as the organic seat of the disease but also identified particular environmental triggers of asthma attacks, such as dust, feathers, tobacco smoke, certain foods, exercise and emotions, and speculated on the significance of the appearance of asthma in several members of the same family.[44]

During the late eighteenth and early nineteenth centuries, a variety of novel tools and methods for examining patients and diagnosing disease were introduced to clinical practice: percussion of the chest by Leopold Auenbrugger in 1761; auscultation with a stethoscope by René-Théophile-Hyacinthe Laennec in 1819; and the spirometer in 1846. Together with the emergence of a more scrupulous pathological anatomy, these techniques facilitated the gradual differentiation not only between 'asthma' as a distinct condition of the lungs and the more general symptom of dyspnoea, but also between the renal, cardiac and bronchial forms of asthma regularly described in medical treatises.[45] As clinical confidence in locating asthmatic symptoms in the lungs grew during the nineteenth century, medical authors increasingly advocated restricting the use of the term asthma to the bronchial form, which could occur in either spasmodic or paralytic configurations and which was often found in conjunction with hay fever.[46]

Increased medical interest in bronchial asthma during the late nineteenth century, manifest particularly in major monographs and articles by the British physician Henry Hyde Salter (1823–1871),[47] generated new understandings of aetiology and pathogenesis that were clearly shaped by contemporary theories of disease. In particular, asthma came to be regarded, much like hay fever, as a form of hereditary neurosis in which 'tonic contraction of the circular fibres' resulted in obstruction of the smaller bronchi.[48] More extensive pathological studies in the laboratories of European scientists and clinicians also revealed what were thought to be characteristic histological findings, namely the colourless crystals identified by Jean Charcot (1825–1893) and Ernst von Leyden (1832–1910) and the spiral casts first noticed by Heinrich Curschmann (1846–1910), both present in the sputum of many asthmatic patients.[49] More significantly, the social characteristics of the disease were also transformed. As John Gabbay has suggested, some eighteenth-century writers, such as the Scottish physician John Millar (1733–1805), had considered asthma to be primarily a disease of artisans. By contrast, although the English surgeon Thomas King (1809–1847) and others continued to dismiss arguments indicting social class and fashionable lifestyles, during the nineteenth century, asthma, like hay fever, became predominantly a disease of the upper classes, rarely found in either municipal or charitable hospital wards but regularly diagnosed and treated by physicians privately attending the educated, intelligent elite.[50]

As in the case of hay fever, the social contours of asthma may well have dictated therapeutic preoccupations with climate therapy in seaside resorts or continental mountain retreats, affordable only by the rich.[51] However, while the pursuit of fresh, clean air proved popular both in Europe and America during the late nineteenth and early twentieth centuries, doctors also advocated a range of familiar and novel local and systemic treatments, designed to reduce nervous tone and to reverse bronchial irritation. Although Henry Hyde Salter, for example, was opposed to the common use of opium because of its potential 'to excite involuntary muscular action, and induce a tendency to spasm',[52] he nevertheless recommended a variety of popular commercial remedies, classified according to whether they acted as depressants, stimulants or sedatives: tobacco; tartar-emetic; ipecacuanha; coffee; chloroform; medicated cigarettes, particularly those containing stramonium or belladonna; Indian hemp or cannabis; ether; and lobelia.[53] Subsequently, other writers, such as Walter Walshe, William Osler and John Thorowgood (1833–1919), added their own favourite preparations to this list, but Salter's general approach to treatment as well as his choice of particular preparations continued to dominate asthma therapies in most Western countries, and to generate revenue for the manufacturers of proprietary medicines, deep into the twentieth century.[54]

The impact of asthma on the lives of sufferers, and the range of remedies that were consumed in order to relieve the condition during that period, are both evident in the life and letters of the French author Marcel Proust (1871–1922), whose seven volume cycle of novels, *A la recherche du temps perdu*, published between 1913 and 1927, rapidly became a literary classic. The son of a Roman Catholic doctor and a Jewish mother, Proust experienced his first severe attack of asthma at the age of nine and was regularly troubled by the condition throughout his life. In 1919, for example, he wrote of the manner in which 'a prolonged attack of asthma had ... rendered me incapable of making the slightest move these last few days'. The following year, in a letter to a fellow author, Marcel Boulenger, Proust explained that he had been 'gasping for breath so continuously' for several days that writing had become difficult.[55] In addition to making curative trips to the coast, Proust attempted to relieve his symptoms with a miscellany of treatments, many of which were administered in a special smoking room set aside for his 'fumigations'. In particular, he used stramonium or Espic cigarettes, Legras or Escouflaire powders, ephinephrine, caffeine, carbolic acid fumigants, isolation, autosuggestion, morphine, and opium, which was also used by Charles Dickens (1812–1870) for the same purpose in the mid-nineteenth century. While these preparations and psychological strategies may have ameliorated Proust's condition, which has generally been ascribed, like many of his illnesses, to his close dependency on

STRAMONIUM CIGARETTES HELPFUL IN

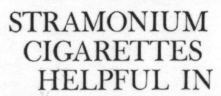

ASTHMA

**as reported in the British
Medical Journal, August 15, 1959**

Noted allergist reinvestigates
an old treatment for bronchial asthma

For about 150 years Europeans have inhaled smoke from burning stramonium leaves to relieve asthmatic attacks.

Now a noted allergist reports in the British Medical Journal that results of controlled studies leave no doubt that inhaling stramonium (atropine*) smoke has a beneficial effect on the function of the lungs in bronchial obstruction.

The results indicate that smoking stramonium cigarettes has a definite place in the treatment of asthma, increasing the vital capacity and giving a feeling of relief, without unpleasant side effects. In many cases during the controlled study the patients voluntarily commented on their increased ease of breathing.

Stramonium cigarettes have been manufactured by R. Schiffmann Co. for more than 80 years and have been *available without prescription in every drug store* throughout the U. S. and Canada under the name of ASTHMADOR. These cigarettes contain no tobacco and are not habit forming.

ASTHMADOR is also sold in pipe mixture or as aromatic incense powder. Sufferers from bronchial asthma will almost invariably find relief, as indicated in this report.

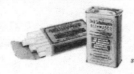

*Atropine
is the
alkaloid of
stramonium.*

A US magazine advertisement of *c.* 1959.

his mother, they failed to provide a cure and Proust remained chronically incapacitated by both asthma and hay fever.[56]

Significantly, the knowledge that leading literary figures such as Dickens and Proust suffered from asthma and hay fever served to substantiate contemporary perceptions of those maladies as closely related diseases that occurred most frequently in the civilized and educated classes of the Western world. While Clemens von Pirquet's notion of allergy immediately provided fresh insights into the aetiology of these established conditions in the early twentieth century, its emphasis on a common pathology also served to consolidate traditional links between hay fever, asthma and a miscellany of idiosyncrasies such as urticaria, eczema and food intolerance. By establishing a neat explanatory framework, as well as a convenient terminology, for this seemingly distinct group of conditions, Clemens von Pirquet thus sowed the seeds for the emergence of a new medical speciality of clinical allergy.

However, the growth of allergy as a distinct medical discipline and the creation of allergy clinics during the first half of the twentieth century in both Europe and North America were also driven and moulded by other factors. In the first place, interest in allergic disorders may have been stimulated by burgeoning clinical and physiological studies of idiosyncrasies and, more particularly, by reports of rising trends in hay fever.[57] In addition, closer clinical interest in hay fever and asthma may have reflected mounting concerns about the economic and social impact of chronic, rather than acute, diseases and a growing commitment to more accurately charting levels of morbidity as well as mortality.[58] In this context, it is significant that, by the 1930s, hay fever had become the fourth most common form of chronic disease and a major public health concern in the United States.[59]

More immediately, however, the emergence of clinical allergy was promoted by the invention and dissemination of a novel form of treatment, born, like the notion of allergy itself, from contemporary fixations with the application of vaccine therapy and serotherapy in the struggle against infectious diseases. Specific desensitization or therapeutic inoculation with extracts of pollen and other allergens, initially developed in the Inoculation Department at St Mary's Hospital in London, dominated approaches to allergy on both sides of the Atlantic for much of the twentieth century, rapidly displacing climate therapy as the treatment of choice in hay fever and asthma, and surviving intense competition from the industrial manufacture and promotion of a wide range of pharmaceutical agents, such as the antihistamines. From 1911, when Leonard Noon first published early results from his clinical studies, therapeutic approaches to hay fever, asthma and associated allergic disorders focused primarily on manipulating the patient's specific biological reactivity rather than altering the environment in which they lived and worked.

Prophylactic inoculation and the origins of clinical allergy

The emergence of clinical allergy as a medical speciality can be traced to critical developments in biomedical science and clinical practice in British laboratories and hospitals around the turn of the nineteenth into the twentieth century. The earliest and indeed for several decades the largest clinic for allergic diseases in England was situated in the Inoculation Department at St Mary's Hospital in London, which had been created, and for many years was directed, by Sir Almroth Wright (1861–1947). Having obtained his medical qualifications from Trinity College Dublin in 1883, Wright embarked on a full-time research career in pathology, working first in Germany and then in London, Cambridge and Sydney before being appointed to the Chair of Pathology at the Army Medical School at Netley in 1892. Wright's early work focused particularly on developing vaccines designed to stimulate active, rather than passive, immunity against a range of infectious diseases, such as typhoid, cholera, tuberculosis and staphylococcal skin infections. In 1902 Wright left Netley to become the head of pathology at St Mary's Hospital, where he continued his influential studies of immunization both in the laboratory and the clinic.[60] Encouraged by the enthusiastic reception of his work on 'vaccine therapy' (in which vaccines were used to treat ongoing infections), Wright established the Department of Therapeutic Inoculation at St Mary's. Crucially, in 1908, Wright secured a lucrative contract for vaccine production with an American pharmaceutical firm, Parke, Davis & Company, an association that clearly shaped the nature and direction of research in the Department for many years.[61] Although some colleagues were critical of Wright's association with industry, fearful that it might compromise scientific freedom,[62] the contract with Parke, Davis & Company effectively guaranteed the Department's survival and eventually also subsidized research on the treatment of allergic diseases.

Immortalized in contemporary literature, knighted in 1906 and renowned as the 'British Pasteur', Wright inevitably attracted many promising clinicians and scientists to the Department.[63] In 1904 Wright was joined by John Freeman (1876–1962), a young medical student at St Mary's. After qualifying in medicine in 1905 and having spent some time studying at the Pasteur Institute in Paris, Freeman returned to take up a research position in Wright's department, contributing especially to Wright's studies of vaccine therapy.[64] In 1907 Freeman persuaded an old school friend, Leonard Noon (1877–1913), to join him at St Mary's. Having trained in medicine at Cambridge and St Bartholomew's and having studied with Freeman in Paris, at that time Noon

John Freeman.

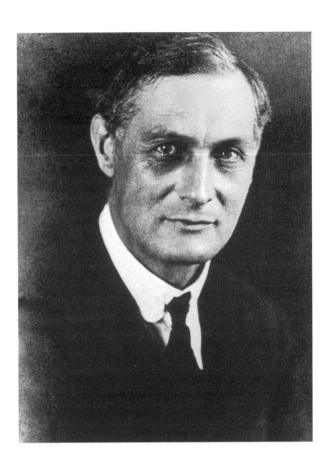

was working at the Lister Institute, evaluating the potency of diverse anti-septic agents in the treatment of wound infections.[65] Initially seconded to study the digestive, opsonic and bactericidal properties of pus, in 1908 he began to expand his clinical interest in immunization to the development of vaccines against hay fever. Although this clearly constituted only one of a number of avenues that were being explored in Wright's department, where ideas for 'researches on immunisation were as thick as blackberries',[66] the study of hay fever was to occupy Noon until his premature death from tuber-culosis in 1913 and came to dominate the whole of Freeman's professional life, both in the laboratory and the clinic, until his death in 1962.

The central features of Noon's and Freeman's approach to hay fever first appeared in two seminal publications in the *Lancet* in 1911. In the first article,

Noon provided preliminary details of the diagnostic and therapeutic protocol that he and Freeman had devised for hay fever sufferers. According to Noon, hay fever constituted 'a form of recurrent catarrh affecting certain individuals during the months of May, June, and July'. Arguing that the condition was caused by an idiosyncratic sensitivity to 'a soluble toxin found in the pollen of grasses', Noon explained that diagnosis could be readily achieved by 'dropping a little of an extract of grass pollen into the eye of the suspected individual' and observing the reaction. The same technique also served as a means of monitoring the efficacy of treatment. Convinced that passive immunization with a specific serum, such as 'pollantin' (which had been produced and marketed by William Dunbar),[67] was not only 'difficult and laborious' but also 'not calculated to bring about a permanent cure', Noon suggested that 'the induction of an active immunity' to the pollen toxin might offer a more satisfactory outcome. To this end, he embarked on a series of experiments with the aim of determining 'what degree of immunity can be induced in hay fever patients by inoculations of pollen toxin, how these inoculations may be best regulated, and whether the affection can by this means be permanently cured'.[68]

Between autumn 1910 and spring 1911 a small number of hay fever sufferers were inoculated subcutaneously with increasing doses of an extract of pollen from *Phleum pratense* or Timothy grass, which had been collected by Noon's sister, Dorothy, and which had been discovered to generate the most active extract. Recognizing the need for further studies, Noon was nevertheless cautiously optimistic about the initial results of inoculating his patients:

> The result of these experiments so far is to show that the sensibility of hay fever patients may be decreased, by properly directed dosage, at least a hundredfold, while excessive or too frequent inoculations only serve to increase the sensibility. It still remains to be seen whether the immunity thus attained is sufficient to carry the patients through a season without suffering from their annual attacks of hay fever.[69]

Noon's preliminary report was followed later the same year by Freeman's more detailed account of the treatment of their first twenty patients at St Mary's. In addition to setting out the protocol that was employed in preparing, quantifying and administering the various pollen extracts, Freeman carefully charted the dosage and timing of inoculations, clinical estimates of the patients' growing resistance to pollen as measured by the 'ophthalmo-reaction', and the patients' own assessments of the efficacy of treatment. During the course of the experiments, Freeman also established, at least provisionally, the cross-reactivity of different grass pollens, that is the ability of inoculations with one type of pollen to immunize against sensitivity to other pollens. Having dismissed possible sources of error in his results (such as observer bias, the psychological expectations of cure on the part of patients, and the possibility that the pollen season that year had been particularly mild), Freeman was enthusiastic about the impact of inoculation:

> Considering all the cases generally, there seems little doubt that there has been a distinct amelioration of symptoms. This improvement took several forms; a greater freedom from attack, the attack not so bad as in former years, and the attack sooner over, the constitutional disturbance not so great, less asthma. The people who had already developed hay fever when they commenced treatment were, perhaps, the most generous in their comments, possibly because they had recently had a reminder of what hay fever was like.[70]

Apparently unconcerned by the absence of a clear explanation for the clinical effects of inoculation, Freeman claimed that the 'increase in immunity produced by pollen vaccine is in itself the best proof of the soundness of this line of treatment, whether prophylactic or phylactic'.[71]

Three years later, shortly after Noon's death, Freeman published an update in which he attempted to determine for how long a course of inoculation might offer relief from the symptoms of hay fever. From a survey of 84 patients, he concluded that a complete course of injections protected hay fever sufferers not only for that year but also generally for at least one more hay fever season. In addition to discussing some of the possible reasons why either prophylactic or therapeutic inoculations might fail in some patients, Freeman also introduced what became a longstanding personal preoccupation with the superiority of 'experiential' over 'statistical' methods of judging the results of treatment: 'But few people, and these only in rare circumstances, act on statistics. They act instead on experience, either of themselves or others; and it seems desirable to consider, what in my experience, makes me convinced that this line of inoculation treatment is emphatically successful.'[72] As Christopher Lawrence and George Weisz have argued, a preference for clinical experience over statistical evaluation of data, and for clinical holism over specialization, was not unusual amongst a certain breed of clinicians in this period, and it became a characteristic feature of the work of Freeman and his colleagues in the allergy clinic at St Mary's during the inter-war years.[73]

Noon's and Freeman's efforts to reduce sensitivity to pollen did not constitute the first attempt to immunize patients actively against foreign substances in this way. In 1900 H. Holbrook Curtis, a New York physician, had reported what he termed the 'immunizing cure of hay-fever'. Prompted by his recollections of a patient who had rendered herself tolerant to certain substances by taking 'a tincture or syrup in drops for several days', Curtis employed the same technique in his treatment of hay fever in an unmarried 35-year-old woman, who characteristically was 'neurasthenic' and came from 'one of the best known families in St Louis'. By administering 'internally the watery extract of certain flowers and their pollen, as well as in small doses by hypodermic injection', Curtis successfully induced tolerance to roses, violets and lily of the valley. Encouraged by the outcome, and preferring the practical advantages of tinctures over hypodermic medication, Curtis attempted to treat what he termed 'rag-weed corasthma' using supplies of ragweed pollen obtained from a botanist working for a pharmaceutical firm. The remarkable clinical results led Curtis to speculate that his efforts, if verified by others, constituted 'a great discovery'.[74]

In England, a similar technique was employed in 1908 by a London physician, Alfred T. Schofield, who recorded a successful attempt to prevent the urticaria and asthma caused by an idiosyncratic intolerance of eggs by administering pills containing gradually increasing amounts of raw egg to a 13-year-old boy.[75] In devising their approach to treatment, however, Noon and Freeman did not appear to draw on Curtis's and Schofield's earlier attempts to immunize against hay fever and food intolerance, or indeed to relate their clinical studies to either the growing physiological literature on anaphylaxis or the speculative pathology that linked experimental anaphylaxis and allergic reactivity with human hypersensitivities. On the contrary, it is noticeable that, while other contemporary authors (such as Humphry Rolleston) rapidly assimilated older notions of idiosyncrasy and intolerance into the new language of allergy and anaphylaxis, Noon and Freeman appeared to pay scant attention to this trend. Apart from an occasional reference to Besredka's work on 'anti-anaphylaxis',[76] and the eventual (but rather reluctant) adoption of the word 'allergy', Freeman's published writings demonstrate a distinct disregard for the blossoming physiological and pathological fascination with the mechanisms and meanings of allergy and anaphylaxis initiated by Richet and von Pirquet. Instead, the specific approach to hay fever (and ultimately other allergies) adopted by Noon and Freeman evolved from quite distinct research and therapeutic traditions, relating especially to Almroth Wright's studies of infectious diseases at St Mary's.

At one level, Noon and Freeman were clearly aware of, and duly acknowledged, the seminal contributions to understandings of the aetiology of hay fever made by Blackley and Dunbar. In particular, they adopted earlier theories about the pivotal role of a pollen toxin and pursued Dunbar's interest in immunization. However, the precise strategy introduced by Noon and Freeman was heavily influenced by trends in bacteriology, in which many investigators were attempting to develop not only passive vaccination with specific antitoxins (in the manner of Dunbar's 'pollantin') but also active prophylactic and therapeutic bacterial vaccines. Studying under Wright, both Freeman and Noon were well acquainted with the fashionable vaccine therapy for infectious diseases. Indeed, Freeman's early research in the Inoculation Department had focused on the use of the opsonic index as a test of immunity and on the development of therapeutic immunization. Noon's and Freeman's insistence on stimulating active immunity to pollen constituted a logical extension of Wright's preoccupations with active, rather than passive, immunization against bacterial infections. As Freeman commented in his paper of 1911, their studies of the effects of vaccination in hay fever neatly brought 'the pollen inoculation work into line with the bacterial inoculation work of Wright and his school'.[77] Reflecting on the work of Freeman and Noon many years later, Wright himself not only stressed the prominence of their research on hay fever in the history of the Department but also endorsed Freeman's opinion of the intellectual and pragmatic roots of pollen desensitization:

> This method which makes use of inoculations of Grass Pollen Extract may be regarded as an offshoot of Anti-Typhoid Inoculation and Vaccine Therapy. It was afterwards followed up by Dr Freeman with a similar method of treatment for cases of Asthma produced by other causes.[78]

Noon's method of treating hay fever by actively inducing immunity to pollen was rapidly assimilated into clinical practice on both sides of the Atlantic. In Britain, contributors to the *Lancet* reported the outcome of cases treated by Noon's method, debated the most appropriate means of preparing, quantifying and administering pollen, discussed the possibility of similarly vaccinating against asthma, and advertised the availability of commercial 'hay fever reaction outfits' containing pollen extracts prepared at St Mary's and marketed and sold by Parke, Davis & Company.[79] In addition, the technique was adopted and adapted by clinicians in the United States, who devised their own diagnosis and treatment protocols, and who were assisted in the production and distribution of pollen extracts by pharmaceutical companies such as Lederle and Abbott Laboratories.[80] In particular, the technique was evaluated and developed by Karl Koessler (1880–1925) and Robert A. Cooke. Koessler, a Viennese-trained physician practising in Chicago and later President of the American Association for the Study of Allergy, had worked with Almroth Wright at St Mary's before emigrating to America, where he first began work on active immunization for hay fever in 1910.[81] Cooke, a founding member of the Society for the Study of Asthma and Allied Conditions, cited the contributions of both Koessler and Freeman in his first publication in 1915, and continued to explore the efficacy, safety and mechanism of active immunization throughout his professional life.[82]

Although American clinicians and scientists developed their own approaches to vaccinating with pollen, commentators on both sides of the Atlantic generally acknowledged that the papers published by Noon and Freeman between 1911 and 1914 constituted the first systematic account of therapeutic and prophylactic inoculation against hay fever and, in the process, ostensibly signalled the birth of clinical allergy in Britain and elsewhere. By providing what appeared to be a viable alternative to climate therapy and to the wide range of commercial preparations available for asthma and hay fever, the form of inoculation or desensitization developed at St Mary's became the cornerstone of treatment for allergic disorders worldwide until well after the Second World War. As the prominent German-born American allergist Max Samter (1908–1999) put it in 1979, 'the practice of allergy is virtually synonymous with immunotherapy'.[83]

The expansion of clinical allergy

During the inter-war years, the scope and nature of clinical allergy shifted substantially particularly in Western industrialized countries. In 1920, in an extensive overview of contemporary knowledge about hay fever, asthma, food idiosyncrasies and a miscellany of related conditions, delivered to the Royal Society of Medicine in London, John Freeman concluded that it 'might be an exaggeration to say that the study of these toxic idiopathies will open a new field of medicine, but I feel confident that they throw light from a new angle across a very large field of the old medicine'.[84] In some ways, Freeman's comments can be read as a prescient warning of the difficulties that allergists were soon to face in their attempts to gain recognition and speciality status for their nascent discipline, and more particularly in their struggles with practitioners of paediatrics, dermatology and internal medicine for jurisdiction over a range of non-organ-specific immunological diseases. In other ways, however, Freeman seems to have misjudged the moment. For it was precisely at that time that allergy did indeed appear to constitute a new field of medicine, coalescing around a discrete form of therapy and concentrating on a set of conditions that were emerging as a distinct focus of public and professional interest on both sides of the Atlantic.

In North America the hay fever societies established in the late nineteenth century were followed in the early twentieth century by the creation of allergy clinics, the first of which were opened by Isaac Chandler Walker in Boston in 1916 and by Robert Cooke in New York two years later. By 1935, 35 clinics dedicated to the treatment of allergic diseases, and in some cases to educating medical students, had been approved by a joint committee comprising members of the two American professional allergy assocations.[85] These associations had been formed in the 1920s in response to growing demands for a suitable forum in which allergists could discuss their clinical interests. The Western Society for the Study of Hay Fever, Asthma and Allergic Diseases was founded by Grant I. Selfridge (1864–1951), Albert H. Rowe (1889–1970) and George Piness (1891–1970) in 1923. Dominated by clinicians with a commitment to popularizing the speciality, the Western Society convened its first conference in San Francisco in June the same year.[86] Two years later, the (Eastern) Society for the Study of Asthma and Allied Conditions held its inaugural annual meeting in Washington, DC. The Eastern Society, boasting a more academic and elite membership than its Western counterpart, had been formally established in 1924 by a small group of New York physicians, including Robert Cooke, Francis M. Rackemann (1887–1973), George M. MacKenzie (1895–1952) and Harry L. Alexander (1888–1969).[87]

During the 1930s a number of factors conspired to encourage members of the two associations to consider joining forces. First, as both societies gradually gained national, rather than merely regional, reputations, many clinicians and scientists held dual membership, rendering separate meetings excessive and expensive. Second, leading allergists in both societies recognized the benefits to be obtained from concerted action on matters relating to the development of the discipline, the monitoring and maintenance of professional standards, and the need to defend themselves against occasional charges of quackery and profiteering, driven especially by doubts about the safety and efficacy of allergen immunotherapy. In 1943, after a series of lengthy negotiations, the two associations merged to form the American Academy of Allergy with an initial membership of 272.[88]

The two parent organizations, as well as the Academy, provided an authoritative administrative framework for the effective expansion of clinical allergy in North America. The societies developed training schemes for American physicians and medical students interested in allergy, generated financial support for research, particularly through the activities of the Allergy Research Council established in 1929, and facilitated the emergence of a global network of allergists by inviting leading international clinicians and scientists, such as Maurice Arthus, Charles Richet, Carl Prausnitz, Willem Storm van Leeuwen (1882–1933) and John Freeman, to become society members and to speak at conferences. In the 1940s the Academy also stepped up its campaign for professional recognition of allergy as a distinct sub-speciality. Plagued by intense political disputes, particularly about the relationship between allergy, on the one hand, and internal medicine and paediatrics, on the other hand, and to some extent divided by the creation of splinter organizations, such as the American College of Allergists (which published its own journal, *Annals of Allergy*), the Academy's efforts to gain speciality status by setting up an autonomous Board of Allergy with the power to provide certification for clinical allergists floundered. Although the importance of allergy was recognized in the creation of the National Institute of Allergy and Infectious Diseases in 1955 and although the American Medical Association established a separate Section on Allergy in 1964, it was not until the 1970s that the American Board of Allergy and Immunology, including representatives from paediatrics and internal medicine as well as from the various allergy organizations, was founded.[89]

During the inter-war years, members of the American allergy societies helped to define the clinical and scientific contours of the subject for allergists worldwide, not only through the publication of influential monographs and journal articles but also through the founding of an academic journal, the *Journal of Allergy*, dedicated to the subject in 1929.[90] For some years, leading American allergists had successfully published their studies in the *Journal of Immunology*, which had been founded, and was edited for 25 years, by Arthur Coca, who was Professor of Immunology at New York Hospital and who, with Robert Cooke, had introduced both the specific notion of 'atopy' to describe the hereditary predisposition to hay fever and asthma and a general scheme for classifying hypersensitivity in 1923.[91] Impetus for a separate allergy journal came from Harry Alexander, a founder member of the Eastern Society, and French K. Hansel (1893–1981), an ear, nose and throat specialist in St Louis who set up allergy clinics and training courses in otolaryngological allergy from the late 1920s, published extensively on the role of allergy in diseases of the nose and sinuses, and provided inspiration for the establishment of the American Society of Ophthalmalogic and Otolaryngic Allergy in Chicago in 1941.[92]

Early issues of the *Journal of Allergy* carried an eclectic mix of articles that both reflected and helped to shape the initially fragmented field of clinical allergy in the inter-war years. Contributions included discursive pieces on theoretical and semantic issues and on the classification of allergies, papers on training requirements and professional standards, reviews of leading monographs as publications blossomed in the 1930s, summaries of society proceedings, focused accounts of laboratory and clinical studies of crucial allergic conditions (hay fever, asthma, food allergies, eczema and bee stings), reports of the efficacy of different treatments, and abstracts of articles published elsewhere, including the incorporation of *Allergy Abstracts* into the journal from 1944.[93] Although the notion of 'minor allergy' was itself contested by some contributors, a number of articles also served to widen the scope of clinical allergy by claiming that a miscellany of supposedly trivial conditions, such as headaches, migraine, epilepsy, diarrhoea and heartburn, were essentially allergic in nature.[94]

The *Journal of Allergy* also included results from botanical studies pursued by allergists, botanists and plant physiologists often working together. As Gregg Mitman has argued, although attempts by pharmaceutical companies like Lederle to standardize pollen vaccines for national use were hampered by evidence of striking geographical and meteorological variations, growing clinical interest in charting the specific types and distribution of pollen locally and nationally provided botanists such as Oren C. Durham (1889–1967) and the Canadian-born Roger P. Wodehouse (1889–1978) with lucrative career opportunities and, by focusing attention on particular species of pollen, served to broaden the scope of their ecological studies. At the same time, natural history changed the face of clinical allergy by introducing 'a taxonomic and geographic perspective' on allergic diseases.[95] In practice, collaboration between America clinicians, botanists and pharmaceutical companies found expression in efforts to measure and broadcast levels of pollen. Although there were disputes about the accuracy of measurements in the face of meteorological shifts and the uneven distribution of pollen in the atmosphere, pollen counts, initially recorded by Durham in conjunction with the

United States Weather Bureau during the 1920s, first appeared in the weather section of a daily New York newspaper in 1937.[96] By the 1950s, pollen forecasts had become an international venture, 'integral to the very ecological, institutional, and therapeutic infrastructure upon which allergy as a medical specialty within the United States was built'.[97]

In Europe, the development of clinical allergy was more gradual and more piecemeal. In mainland Europe, as in the United States, early public interest in hay fever was evident in the establishment in the late nineteenth century of a Hay Fever League, which included sufferers from Germany, Austria, the Netherlands and Switzerland who met every year in Heligoland not only to escape rising levels of pollen during the early summer months but also to promote 'research into the etiology and therapy of the disease'.[98] Interest in allergic diseases also blossomed among Continental doctors and scientists in the early decades of the twentieth century, prompted partly by physiological and clinical studies of the mechanisms and meanings of anaphylaxis and allergy but also perhaps by rising trends in hay fever and asthma. During the 1920s, '30s and '40s Continental clinicians, like their American counterparts, began to establish clinics and lecture courses, to present academic papers to an expanding international community of scholars, and to publish monographs, edited collections and journals, such as *Progress in Allergy*, founded by the Hungarian physician and biologist Paul Kallós (1902–1988) in 1939, or *Acta Allergologica* (which later became known simply as *Allergy*), first published in 1948.[99]

Developments in Europe and North America were often reported in the British medical press and there is evidence, in some cases, of significant cross-fertilization of ideas. John Freeman's decision to study the role of moulds in allergic diseases and to appoint a mycologist to the staff of the Inoculation Department at St Mary's, for example, was supposedly stimulated by a visit to London by the Dutch allergist Willem Storm van Leeuwen, whose use of the 'allergen-proof' chamber to treat asthma was also well known to British clinicians. Interestingly, the study of moulds in the Department may in turn have contributed to the discovery of penicillin.[100] As close study of Freeman's work at St Mary's demonstrates, however, both the growth of clinical allergy in Britain and the directions in which British allergists pursued laboratory and clinical research also had their own dynamic and trajectory, shaped by local institutional and economic factors as well as broader epidemiological and intellectual trends.

During the 1920s and '30s, interest in allergic disorders among British clinicians clearly expanded. Although the Allergy Clinic set up by John

Freeman at St Mary's continued to operate as the largest specialist centre of its type, other clinics were established throughout the country during these decades, particularly after the founding of the Asthma Research Council (known since the 1980s as the National Asthma Campaign and more recently as Asthma UK). The Council was formed to much public and professional acclaim in 1927, following a preliminary meeting of a group of asthma sufferers (including clinicians, scientists and philanthropists) at the Royal United Service Institution in London.[101] Motivated partly by the 'vast amount of suffering and unemployment' experienced by more than 200,000 children and adults with asthma, the Council was dedicated to raising and distributing funds for the purpose of promoting 'intensive research into the cause and treatment of asthma and allied diseases'.[102] Endorsed by the Ministry of Health and coordinated by a medical advisory committee that included John Freeman, Humphry Rolleston and the founder of the British Society of Gastroenterology, Sir Arthur Hurst (1879–1944), the Council's fund-raising, educational and clinical work received extensive coverage in the pages of the daily press, particularly The Times.

Under the auspices of the Council, a number of hospitals established centres for research and treatment. Clinics and laboratories in Liverpool, Edinburgh, Manchester, Glasgow, Birmingham, Belfast and London (at King's College, St Mary's, Guy's and Great Ormond Street hospitals), for example, were all planned to contribute to 'a well-designed network of small centres throughout the British Isles', ideally placed to gather information not only about the geographical and climatic distribution of allergic disorders but also about 'the influence of heredity on the whole asthma syndrome'.[103] Both the medical and the popular press released regular accounts of significant therapeutic initiatives. In 1936, for example, The Times reported the opening of a new clinic at St George's Hospital in London offering patients a novel treatment for hay fever with a supposedly guaranteed cure rate of 98 per cent. The treatment, which had been the subject of an extensive five-year trial conducted in the hospital's physiotherapy department, consisted of 'the application, by electricity, of a coating of ionized zinc to the inside of the nostrils'.[104]

While allergy clinics across the country developed and promoted their own styles of treatment for hay fever and asthma, during the inter-war years British approaches to allergy were dominated by John Freeman's studies of hay fever and desensitization at St Mary's. Freeman was a regular contributor to leading medical journals, helped to establish an Allergy Club which met for informal discussions in West End pubs, and attracted a number of crucial researchers to St Mary's, often supported by funds from the Asthma Research Council.[105] Many of his colleagues (such as David Harley, W. Howard Hughes, Rosa Augustin, Jack Pepys, and Jonathan Brostoff) made substantial contributions to the development of the field and continued to promote the study and treatment of allergic diseases after Freeman's death. In 1962 A. W. Frankland, who had become a full-time member of the department in 1947 and after whom the Allergy Clinic at St Mary's Hospital was subsequently named, replaced Freeman as Director of the Department of Allergy.[106]

As Freeman made clear in his idiosyncratic monograph on allergic diseases, published in 1950 and dedicated to Leonard Noon, laboratory and clinical studies at St Mary's relied heavily on the availability of regular supplies of pollen. Noon and his sister, Dorothy, had started collecting pollen for clinical research in 1907 and had developed effective means of planting, picking the grass heads, collecting, drying and extracting the pollen, and standardizing those extracts. Obtaining the maximum yield from Noon's approach, which remained largely unchanged over the years and which was successfully extended in critical respects to the preparation of other allergens, was facilitated in 1936 by the establishment of the Pollenarium, built on three acres of land at Pyrford near Woking in Surrey, which had been supplied by the 1st Earl of Iveagh, a friend of Almroth Wright and chairman of (and regular benefactor to) the St Mary's Inoculation Department Committee for more than three decades from his appointment in 1921. Managed for many years by Dorothy Noon and extended in 1955 to 'allow research with new types of pollen',[107] the Pollenarium continued to produce the large quantities of pollen required for the production of therapeutic and prophylactic vaccines and diagnostic solutions until it closed in 1971.[108]

Clinical practice and research in the Allergy Department at St Mary's focused on a range of diseases. While hay fever constituted the archetypal allergic disease, Freeman and his colleagues, much like allergists in North America and Europe, also studied a variety of seemingly related conditions: asthma, eczema, prurigo, urticaria, angioneurotic oedema, ichthyosis, dermographia, bites and stings of insects and nettles, idiotoxic albuminuria, paroxysmal hydrarthrosis, food and drug idiosyncrasies, idiotoxic enteritis, migraine and epilepsy.[109] However, much of the research was shaped largely by the pragmatic concerns of clinical practice rather than by the need to elucidate theoretical issues. Freeman was particularly keen to improve the diagnosis of allergic disorders through the modification of conjunctival and skin tests and to generate better treatment protocols for pollen desensitization.

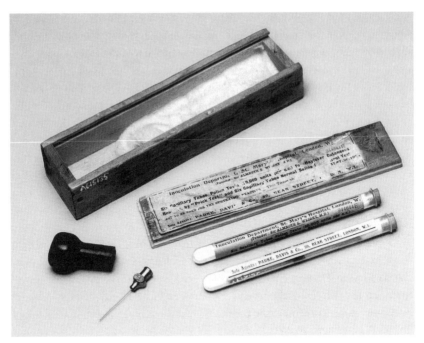

Hay fever allergy kit, *c.* 1925–35.

To this end, he experimented not only with the 'leisurely desensitization' that he and Noon had introduced in 1911, but also with 'intensive desensitization' (comprising inoculations every day for a week or so), 'rush inoculation' (with a series of injections given during a single day) and self-inoculation, in which suitably selected hay fever sufferers (invariably men from the educated classes) learned to inoculate themselves.[110] Significantly, these concentrated and self-administered courses of desensitization appear to have been designed to accommodate the hectic professional and social lifestyles of his patients (particularly perhaps those seen in his private practice) rather than being driven by any clear conceptual rationale for the varying treatment regimes.[111]

In spite of a general decline in interest in vaccine therapy from the 1910s,[112] and in spite of competition from a range of novel pharmaceutical agents introduced for the treatment of allergic disorders during the middle decades of the century, desensitization remained at the therapeutic heart of clinical practice at St Mary's. Like other laboratory and clinical research in the Inoculation Department, work on allergy was supported financially by a contract with the

American pharmaceutical firm, Parke, Davis & Company, which although based in Detroit also manufactured products at a factory built in Hounslow in 1907. The company purchased pollen preparations from the Allergy Department and marketed them commercially as 'Pollaccine'. Available in the form of kits containing graded dilutions of pollen extracts together with appropriate syringes, Pollaccine was sold to other hospital centres and general practitioners for use in both dermal testing and prophylactic or therapeutic inoculation. The company also published advice booklets for doctors, written by staff in the Inoculation Department and detailing the range of vaccines that could be purchased not only for combating hay fever and other allergies but also for the treatment of infections.[113] The deal with Parke, Davis & Company continued to subsidize research and clinical work in the Inoculation Department until 1960, when commercial production was taken over by Beecham Research Laboratories Ltd, under the terms of a seven-year covenant which promised substantial grants for research at what by that time had become the Wright-Fleming Institute of Microbiology.[114] The Beecham group included the allergy division of C. L. Bencard Ltd, one of Parke, Davis & Company's competitors in the production of diagnostic and therapeutic kits for allergies.[115]

Although Freeman's clinical curiosity, both at St Mary's and in his private practice, was largely absorbed by the challenge of perfecting desensitization, he was not immune to fostering other research initiatives. Throughout the 1930s and '40s research fellows and visiting scholars affiliated to the Allergy Department not only contributed to Freeman's ongoing clinical research projects but also pursued their own interests, some of which served significantly to reshape the field of allergy studies. During the 1930s David Harley, a research fellow in the Department funded by the Asthma Research Council, published the results of a number of experiments exploring the nature of antibody-antigen (or more specifically reagin-allergen) mixtures. In addition, Freeman also encouraged research into the biological polyvalency of antigens in relation to the pollens responsible for causing hay fever, publishing papers with W. Howard Hughes, a medical graduate from St Mary's Hospital and an assistant in the Department.[116] Some years later, when Rosa Augustin (née Friedmann) was appointed to the Department in 1952 with the help of a grant from the Asthma Research Council, she not only carried out, with A. W. Frankland, probably the first controlled trial of desensitization, comparing the efficacy of various pollen preparations with that of phenol saline, but also published the results of a series of internationally acclaimed studies of the chemical structure and standardization of allergens.[117] In addition to collaborating with Augustin in the desensitization trial and to carrying out early clinical trials of antihistamines in the 1950s, Frankland published extensively on a range of topics within the broad field of allergy, arguably taking over Freeman's mantle as the country's leading allergist.[118]

During the inter-war years, researchers at St Mary's also investigated the psychogenic aspects of allergies, thereby resurrecting clinical interest in earlier theories of asthma and hay fever that had recognized the role of emotions in triggering symptoms. In 1938, for example, Erich Wittkower (1899–1983), a German physician who was at that time working at the Tavistock Clinic in London and who later became professor of psychiatry at McGill University in Canada and president of the American Psychosomatic Society, published the results of a study into 'the allergic personality' in relation to hay fever, which he had pursued with Freeman's support at St Mary's. Wittkower concluded that the typical hay fever patient was a delicate, upper-class, only child who subsequently developed into an emotionally and socially maladjusted adult.[119] Wittkower's work on hay fever, together with his reflections on eczema as the product of emotional insecurity, fitted neatly with, and may well have been driven by, a growing clinical interest in psychosomatic diseases and psychosocial medicine during the 1930s, but they also coincided with specific debates about the possible psychological and constitutional determinants of allergic diseases.[120] Echoing Richet's earlier formulations of the continuum between physiological reactions and expressions of the mind and his portrayal of the parallel phenomena of humoral and psychological personalities, preoccupations with psychogenic causes of allergy were especially evident in accounts that stressed the links between hormones, the autonomic nervous system and the environment in the pathogenesis of allergy and in neo-Freudian interpretations of the role of maternal love in the aetiology of asthma that emerged during the 1940s.

In his study of 'allergic man', originally published in German in 1936 and translated into English in the 1940s, for example, the Austrian physician Erwin Pulay (b. 1889) echoed contemporary physiological interest in homoeostasis by arguing that hypersensitivity should be regarded primarily as a 'disorder of the regulatory apparatus of our organism'. At one level, the constitutional predisposition to allergy, he suggested, was the product of hormonal abnormalities, particularly imbalances in the sex hormones. Indeed, he insisted that patients with allergic diseases should be classified as belonging to the 'intersexual state', and that they were consequently amenable to treatment with 'sexual hormones'. At another level, individual allergic attacks were supposedly precipitated by 'faulty oxidisation' and the subsequent accumulation of toxic waste products. At both levels, the crucial pathology consisted of an inability to maintain 'functional unity' and stability in the face of environmental challenge.[121]

Although Pulay's formulation of hypersensitivity lay beyond the boundaries of mainstream allergy studies in this period, the biological and neo-Hippocratic tenor of his writing and his creation of a link between constitutional medicine, endocrinology and allergy resonated not only with Freeman's brand of clinical individualism evident at St Mary's but also with parallel social struggles to maintain political stability in an increasingly volatile and insecure world and with broader ecological approaches to human disease being developed elsewhere. In particular, Pulay's preoccupation with hormonal imbalance as the physiological basis for a spectrum of clinical conditions echoed the work of Hans Selye (1907–1982) on stress and disease. Born in Vienna and raised in Hungary, Selye qualified in medicine and completed a doctorate in organic chemistry at the German University of Prague before accepting a Rockefeller Research Fellowship to study at The Johns Hopkins University. In 1933 Selye was appointed as a lecturer at McGill University before moving to the University of Montreal, where he founded and directed the Institute of Experimental Medicine and Surgery. In 1936, while attempting to identify new hormones from ovarian and placental extracts, Selye formulated his central notion of a 'general adaptation syndrome', in which certain disorders (including allergy, gastric ulcers, high blood pressure, rheumatic diseases, and nervous and emotional conditions) could be explained in terms of 'errors in our adaptive response to stress', mediated through the endocrine system.[122]

In addition to drawing on contemporary biological formulations of stress and disease, Erwin Pulay also raised the possibility of 'mental allergy', that is a mental intolerance to certain emotional and psychological stimuli. In its extreme form, this could lead to a sudden shock reaction (what he termed 'anaphylaxis of the soul') that could be sufficiently profound to lead to suicide.[123] However, in developing the links between body and mind emerging in the field of psychosomatic medicine, a number of authors also stressed the explicit role of psychological factors in precipitating clearly defined organic allergic symptoms. According to the American psychoanalyst Helen Flanders Dunbar (1902–1959), for example, asthma could be triggered both by external factors (dust, pollen, food, and animal hair) and also by internal causes, including disturbances of the endocrine and emotional systems or faulty metabolism. Dunbar was the first chief editor of the journal *Psychosomatic Medicine* established in 1939, a co-founder of the American Psychosomatic Society in 1942, and one of the leading intellectual forces behind the emergence of psychosomatic medicine and clinical holism in the United States. In a stream of academic and popular publications during the 1930s and '40s, Dunbar argued that a predisposition to asthma (and various other diseases) could be traced particularly to 'a conflict about longing for mother love and mother care', a psychological situation that she referred to broadly as 'allergy *con amore*'. In some children, Dunbar suggested, asthma could be the result of frustration borne out of insufficient motherly love, a phenomenon that was also explored by John Bowlby (1907–1990) in his influential studies of the impact of maternal deprivation on children's behaviour and the generation of juvenile delinquency.[124] In other children, asthma could be triggered by the 'fear of being smothered by too much' maternal love, or what Dunbar termed 'smother love'. Although like Pulay, Dunbar interpreted this as a problem of sexuality, she preferred to couch her assessment in Freudian terms of suppressed libido rather than in terms of a constitutionally determined hormonal imbalance:

> In fact, one of their most common difficulties is a sexual problem, often very closely related to the maternal. In general the allergic have had a strong sexual curiosity and temptation – not necessarily a strong sexual desire – and they tend to be afraid of it.[125]

Psychodynamic approaches to allergic diseases became increasingly prominent during the post-war period, perhaps because they served not only to consolidate radical liberal critiques of biomedical reductionism but also, paradoxically, to reinforce both contemporary fantasies of the good mother and reactionary pressures to condemn women to the domestic sphere in the aftermath of the Second World War. A putative, moralizing association between emotions and allergy was also evident in popular culture during the middle decades of the twentieth century. In a play simply entitled *Allergy* and first performed in 1966, for example, the Scottish playwright C. P. Taylor (1929–1981) explored the manner in which emotional stress could precipitate allergic skin complaints. One of the play's central characters, Christopher, develops a 'very nasty, ugly red rash' whenever he contemplates committing adultery with Barbara; in response to concerns that the rash might be infectious, he insists that it is merely an allergy. At around the same time, the American confessional poet Anne Sexton (1928–1974) captured the emotional desolation of suburban marriage by referring to a married couple as 'two asthmatics whose breath sobs in and out through a small fuzzy pipe'.[126] Links between asthma and sexual passion also appeared in newspaper cartoons from this period. Reg Smythe's *Andy Capp* cartoon from 1958, for example, not only suggested symptomatic similarities between certain emotions and asthma but also hinted at a possible causative relationship between the two states.[127]

Psychological theories of asthma and other allergic conditions were not without research and therapeutic implications. Interest in the psychogenic causes of allergy served to stimulate studies of the possible role of hypnosis in modifying allergic manifestations. In the 1950s and '60s, for example, a number of clinical trials in Britain examined the efficacy of hypnosis especially in children with asthma.[128] Supported by grants from the Medical Research Council (which had funded investigations into the psychological profiles of asthmatic children in the 1930s),[129] Stephen Black also published a series of papers in the 1960s indicating the potential for direct suggestion under hypnosis to moderate both immediate and delayed type hypersensitivity

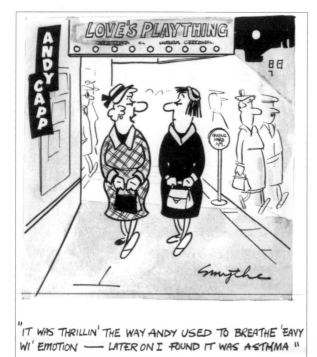

" IT WAS THRILLIN' THE WAY ANDY USED TO BREATHE 'EAVY WI' EMOTION —— LATER ON I FOUND IT WAS ASTHMA "

An *Andy Capp* cartoon, March 1958.

reactions.[130] Medical reports on the use of hypnosis were often covered in the national press: in 1968 *The Times* highlighted the ability of hypnosis both to reduce wheezing and to diminish reliance on bronchodilator drugs, particularly in the case of women who were portrayed as incapable of mastering therapeutic relaxation and breathing exercises.[131]

In addition, recognition of the emotional triggers of asthma may well have encouraged the use of open-air schools for young asthmatics. Such schools had been established in English rural and coastal areas in the early twentieth century in order to provide pre-tuberculous children living in cities with a more healthy environment of fresh air, simple food and regular exercise.[132] As mortality from tuberculosis declined as the result of improved standards of living and the introduction of antibiotics, open-air schools were increasingly used for children with asthma and bronchitis, and eventually also for 'maladjusted' children. In a parallel development, organizations such as the British Red Cross and International Help for Children also provided financial support for some asthmatic children to benefit from the clean air and 'optimistic atmosphere' of Continental spas and high altitude retreats, such as Davos in Switzerland and Font Remeu in the Pyrenees.[133] Although avoidance of pollutants in the domestic and urban environment constituted a crucial rationale for removal to an open-air school or mountain retreat, it was suggested that asthmatic children also benefited from what American physicians termed 'parentectomy', that is being separated from a suffocating emotional environment at home. As leading American proponents of this approach put it in 1956:

> However, it must be stressed that climate plays only a small role in the eventual results achieved ... Environmental tension, which is a product of the reaction of the child to his parents, seems to be the dominating factor in most of our cases.[134]

While British doctors acknowledged the emotional component of allergic diseases, they were often opposed to 'parentectomy', partly because it was thought to over-simplify the factors involved in intractable asthma and partly because it could lead to the 'indiscriminate separation of children from their homes, which is a potentially harmful practice'.[135] Moreover, although John Freeman was clearly intrigued by psychological studies and included a substantial discussion of emotive factors in his 1950 monograph, his attention, like those of many other allergists, remained steadfastly focused either on desensitization or on the elaboration of novel pharmacological agents as the most effective forms of treatment available for allergies. Although the breadth of allergy studies had expanded dramatically during the first half of the twentieth century to include biochemical and immunological analyses of allergens as well as psychological and hormonal approaches to diagnosis and treatment, allergists were largely defined, and to some extent plagued, by their persistent preoccupations with allergen immunotherapy.

The golden calf

As the struggles of American allergists to achieve professional recognition adequately demonstrate, the rapid growth of clinical allergy in the early twentieth century was not unproblematic or uncontested. Indeed, the early history of clinical allergy in Britain in particular highlights the extent to which the emergent speciality was troubled by anxieties about the style of clinical medicine practised by allergists, about the safety and efficacy of desensitization, and about the potential for profiteering. At one level, Freeman's unconventional blend of clinical practice and laboratory research did not always sit comfortably with growing state and professional interest in more extensive testing and greater regulation of new medicines. Throughout his life, Freeman remained an ardent empiricist, emphasizing the centrality of clinical experience (or the 'experiental method') over either theory or statistical evidence.[136] This feature of his work is apparent not only in his flexible approach to establishing therapeutic doses in particular patients, but also in his close descriptions of the cardinal clinical features of patients with allergy (such as the 'allergic nose') and in his writings, which are illustrated with individual case studies and anecdotes, rather than tables and figures.[137] Revealing the holism characteristic of a certain breed of British physicians in this period, and self-consciously pursuing an appreciation of individuality that was increasingly absent from immunological studies, Freeman warned against basing clinical decisions merely on an accumulation of cases:

> It all boils down to this: you must not treat human beings as mere cases – of hay-fever or whatever it may be. You must observe the traditional medical maxim of 'treat the individual man' and all his special commitments at the moment; this is as true for us doctors who work in laboratories as for doctors who never go into them. It is especially important when you are deciding whether the patient, though undoubtedly sensitive to grass pollen, is really suitable for a desensitization treatment.[138]

Like his mentor, Sir Almroth Wright, Freeman was a great advocate of close cooperation between the laboratory and the clinic, regarding the two as 'symbiotic'.[139] In 1948, when administrative changes following the National Health Service Act threatened the autonomy of the Department, Freeman stressed to his colleagues on the Department's council 'the importance of not divorcing the Clinic from the laboratories'.[140] However, Freeman also followed Wright in being deeply suspicious of the increasing state control of medicine. Reflecting nostalgically on the intellectual freedom that he had enjoyed at St Mary's during his career and clearly displaying his devotion to Wright, Freeman questioned the impact of the National Health Service:

> Can the conditions Wright won for us ever be repeated? The nearer I come to the launching of this book, the more I doubt if such unhampered and undirected researches as I here describe can find a place in a planned, and therefore stereotyped, society. Is there any place for an unconventional Almroth Wright in the Brave New World?[141]

Perhaps coloured by an awareness of the often troubled relationship between Almroth Wright and the Medical Research Council, Freeman's fears of the perils of pursuing independent research within the regulated confines of the modern world may well have been justified. Although the British government, under the auspices of the Council, did support a variety of research projects on allergic diseases during the middle decades of the twentieth century, there is evidence to suggest that the Council was indeed reluctant to sanction studies that did not promise to deliver quantifiable scientific results.[142] In this context, the major threat to Freeman's style of clinical practice at St Mary's came from the introduction of official procedures for accurately evaluating the efficacy, mode of action and safety of different types of treatment. From its origins in Noon's and Freeman's studies in the first decade of the twentieth century, desensitization was clearly plagued by vigorous debates about such issues, thereby exposing allergists to increasingly strident charges of quackery and profiteering.

In the first place, it is clear that even advocates of prophylactic and therapeutic inoculation frequently disagreed about many practical aspects of the treatment. Shortly after Noon and Freeman's initial communications, B. P. Sormani, a lecturer in serology at the University of Amsterdam, manipulated some of Almroth Wright's principles as well as citing his own experimental experiences both to discredit 'Noon's dosage method' and to suggest an alternative means of preparing the pollen extract to be used in the treatment of hay fever. Sormani's article in the *Lancet* prompted a swift and dismissive letter from Freeman who, while claiming to be in 'considerable agreement' with Sormani's general advice, nevertheless rejected his particular methodological points emphatically and continued to employ a pragmatic, but vague, approach to dosage based upon clinical examination.[143]

Debates about dosage were compounded by differences in the standardization of specific pollen extracts. For many years, Freeman and his protégées employed the Noon Unit, 'equal to the amount of extract that can be obtained from one-millionth of a gramme of *Phleum pratense* pollen'.[144] Without entirely condemning the British method, American allergists, such as Robert Cooke, preferred to standardize extracts according to their nitrogen content, an approach that appeared 'to give preparations of equal and regular toxicity'.[145] Significantly, the advent of commercially prepared allergen extracts may have accentuated, rather than obviated, this problem. In 1930 Freeman complained that sets of 'protein reagents' provided by 'several first-class firms' for diagnostic tests could easily 'become denatured and so give only a poor reaction or none at all'.[146] As recent debates indicate, this concern did not evaporate. The variable standard of commercial allergen extracts for diagnosis and treatment not only continued to cause anxiety amongst allergists, but also became one of the central concerns of the Committee on Safety of Medicines, which pointed out in 1986 that a 'confusing number of different units are used to express the allergen content of the products currently marketed' and warned that the 'absence of a standard unit means that products containing the same allergens are not interchangeable'.[147]

The absence of standardized allergen extracts coincided with inconsistencies in the diagnostic process. While most authors routinely agreed on the need for the accurate identification of specific allergic sensitivity, in practice a variety of diagnostic tests were employed. According to Freeman, surveying the field in 1930, diagnosis could be achieved by applying allergens to the eye, the lips and the skin (either by a scratch or prick test or by intradermal injection), or by demonstrating the presence of specific antibodies by passive transfer, the Prausnitz-Küstner reaction. The relative merits of these diagnostic procedures, and the precise clinical implications of the results, were assessed only rarely, and when they were considered their clinical value was frequently questioned. Although Freeman advocated skin tests both as a diagnostic tool and as a means of monitoring the progress and efficacy of treatment, even he acknowledged that they had 'had too much medicinal virtue ascribed to them;

in their clinical use they have almost developed into one of the pathological rituals designed towards magical healing'.[148]

Inconsistencies in diagnostic procedures and allergen preparations were mirrored by vast differences in treatment protocols and by the absence of standard tests of efficacy. When Noon and Freeman first introduced prophylactic inoculations for hay fever in 1911, they employed what Freeman later referred to as 'leisurely desensitization', that is, a series of injections spread over a few weeks or months prior to the pollen season. A few years later, Freeman adopted a procedure referred to as 'intensive desensitization', comprising daily injections of gradually increasing doses, particularly for patients sensitive to animals. Significantly, Freeman offered no conceptual rationale for this modification, pointing out simply that he 'fell into the way of inoculating these patients every day' because such patients 'were usually in a great hurry to go and hunt, or look after their dogs, or retrieve their cats from quarantine with the veterinary surgeon'.[149] The apparent success of intensive courses of immunotherapy in animal allergies encouraged Freeman to extend this approach to hay fever sufferers.

Freeman's sensitivity to the dictates of his patients is further evidenced both by his elaboration of an even more rapid treatment protocol, referred to as 'rush desensitization', and by his support for self-inoculation, the advantages of which were clearly located in the practical interests of the patient (and indeed the doctor) rather than in any concern for conceptual elegance. Interestingly, Freeman did not insist that it was necessary to 'adhere rigidly to the leisurely, intensive, or "rush" methods', but accepted that 'an intelligent blend may serve one's turn better'.[150] Clinicians treating allergies followed Freeman's advice, devising their own protocols and preparing their own allergen extracts to suit the demands of their own time and that of their patients. Freeman's flexibility and his professed preference for clinical experience over statistics in judging dosage and efficacy may have suited the idiosyncrasies of his own character and the particular demands of the Inoculation Department at St Mary's in the inter-war years. However, it was, ironically, this flexibility that became a burden to the next generation of allergists. The multiplicity of approaches to desensitization made comparison of results difficult. As the need for establishing the therapeutic efficacy and safety of pharmaceutical products became more urgent in the post-war period, allergists who failed to standardize their extracts or to perform randomized control trials were accused increasingly of relying on anecdotal, rather than scientific, evidence. Although the first controlled trial of immunotherapy was carried out by

Frankland and Augustin under Freeman's supervision in 1954, the reluctance of allergists to test their theories and practices in this way became a source of increasing anxiety amongst both proponents and critics of desensitization.

Wide variations in diagnostic and treatment programmes highlighted, and in part stemmed from, the absence of a coherent explanation of precisely how desensitization might work. Noon's and Freeman's understanding of the pathogenesis of hay fever as the product of a toxin was soon discarded and replaced by explanations that emphasized the role of allergy, in which the clinical symptoms and tissue damage were thought to be caused by a reaction between allergen and tissue-fixed antibody (or reagin) with the subsequent release of inflammatory mediators such as histamine. While more sophisticated explanations of the pathogenesis of allergic disorders gave the emerging field of allergy some degree of intellectual and experimental focus, their incompatibility with the toxin hypothesis proved frustrating for allergists attempting to establish the immunological mechanism of desensitization. One of the earliest, and most enduring, alternative explanations was provided in 1935 by Robert Cooke and his colleagues in New York, who suggested that injections of allergen promoted the production of 'a peculiar blocking or inhibiting type of immune antibody that prevented the action of allergen on the sensitizing antibody'.[151] This hypothesis was subsequently explored by many allergists but it remained contested. In particular, reports of the lack of correlation between levels of 'blocking antibody' (later identified as IgG) and clinical improvement prompted allergists to postulate a variety of alternative, or additional, mechanisms for desensitization.[152]

Proponents of prophylactic desensitization were also troubled by fears about its safety, especially in asthmatics. In 1915 Robert Cooke warned that 'liberal use' of desensitization in patients with hay-asthma 'could conceivably induce death by anaphylactic shock'.[153] Cooke's caution was repeated regularly in the British medical press throughout the next few decades and was increasingly accompanied by case reports of serious adverse reactions and death during treatment and by suggestions for preventing fatalities, such as the inclusion of adrenaline in the syringe. In 1933, for example, David Harley warned that desensitization was difficult and that severe reactions and fatalities had occurred. The following year an editorial in the *Lancet* highlighted the tendency of asthmatics in particular to suffer potentially fatal attacks of asthma during desensitization. In 1942, at a meeting of the Association of Clinical Pathologists, D. N. Nabarro described 'alarming and almost fatal anaphylaxis' after intradermal injection of mixed antigen into an asthmatic patient, a reaction that was successfully treated only after multiple doses of adrenaline and oxygen inhalation. And in 1954, the death of a patient undergoing desensitization for asthma at Guy's Hospital not only led Parke, Davis & Company to recall stocks of Pollaccine but also prompted an informal coroner's inquiry and discussion in parliament.[154]

Concerns about the safety of immunotherapy were closely linked to questions about professional competence. In 1914, Freeman had warned of the problems that could be caused by inexperienced local doctors continuing the treatment that had been started in his clinics. Some years later, David Harley pointedly referred to the ability of 'advanced allergists' to produce 'brilliant cures' in certain cases.[155] In drawing a boundary between themselves and less experienced practitioners, Freeman and Harley were endeavouring to establish their superiority over other clinicians in the diagnosis and treatment of patients with allergic disorders and to distance themselves from persistent, if occasionally self-mocking, depictions of allergists as torturers.[156] In addition to promoting their own speciality, however, they may also have been protecting their economic interests. The treatment of allergic disorders was becoming an increasingly profitable business both for pharmaceutical companies producing diagnostic sets and vaccine kits (and later a vast array of anti-allergy drugs) and for clinical allergists, such as Freeman, who benefited from extensive private practices. The extent to which the prophylactic treatment of allergies and other diseases was influenced by commercial considerations did not pass unnoticed. In The Golden Calf, published in 1933, Charles W. Forward, an ardent advocate of vegetarianism, criticized the manner in which 'in this age of commercialism and bureaucracy, the doctor has been manoeuvred into a false position and made somewhat of a "catspaw" of by the manufacturing chemists and the so-called "Institutes" which make huge profits from the sale of vaccines and similar products'.[157] Five years later, the Scottish doctor and novelist A. J. Cronin (1896–1981) echoed Forward's reservations in his description of the manner in which Andrew Manson, the central character in The Citadel, was prepared to charge a rich female patient for pollen inoculations even though he considered the remedy to be worthless and had only 'achieved its popularity through skilful advertising on the part of the firm who produced it and the absence of pollen in most English summers'.[158]

While preoccupations with a novel form of treatment created new challenges for the nascent speciality of clinical allergy on both sides of the Atlantic, the field was also divided by familiar debates about terminology and teleology. As Freeman was the first to acknowledge, the definition of allergy remained problematic. In the preface to his monograph, he complained that 'the word allergy is in such a linguistic mess' that it 'obscures more than it illumines in medicine'. Agreeing with other commentators who considered that 'the net of allergy' had been cast too widely,[159] Freeman preferred the term 'toxic idiopathies' to describe the spectrum of conditions encompassing hay fever, asthma, food intolerance, eczema and urticaria, since this term could at least 'only mean what I mean it to mean'. However, Freeman recognized that 'Canute-like' resistance to the tide of professional and public opinion was futile and that allergy had already become generally accepted as a melodious, if ambiguous, clinical term.[160]

As the American pathologist Arnold Rice Rich pointed out in his sweeping study of the pathogenesis of tuberculosis, first published in 1944, the precise definition of allergy was not merely a semantic issue but, on the contrary, carried important implications for medical understandings of the aetiology and pathology of the condition and, more broadly, for the role of immunological studies in clinical accounts of disease. One of the enduring conundrums facing immunologists and allergists in the early twentieth century concerned the specific question that von Pirquet had attempted to answer with his formulation of allergy in 1906, namely the precise relationship between immunity and hypersensitivity and, by implication, the evolutionary role of hypersensitivity reactions in protecting against infectious diseases such as tuberculosis. Rich did not subscribe to a prevailing belief that hypersensitivity was a central defence mechanism, arguing instead that immunity and hypersensitivity could be effectively de-coupled and that there was no 'essential parallelism between the two states'. In the process, however, he suggested that much of the confusion on this issue was the product of 'the ambiguous use of the terms "allergy" and "immunity"'. In particular, he complained that the word allergy had 'become so debauched by indiscriminate usage that it would be fortunate, indeed, if it could be dropped completely from the vocabulary of science'.[161] Like those of Freeman and others, Rich's pleas to reject the word allergy, or at least to define it more carefully, generally fell on deaf ears. It is clear that by the 1940s and '50s the terms allergy and allergist were deeply embedded in modern Western medical minds, regularly appearing in the titles of journal and books and in the official names of institutions, societies and clinics. In conjunction with the adoption of allergen desensitization as a primary therapeutic strategy, widespread acceptance of the term allergy served to define a new clinical speciality.

The scale of allergy

When John Freeman published what he and his family referred to sardonically as the 'Bloody Book' in 1950, in which he candidly expressed his fears for the future of biomedical research into allergic diseases, he had already done much not only to establish clinical allergy as a distinct branch of medicine in Britain but also to situate St Mary's as a prominent centre of excellence in the field. By that time, Freeman's empire, the Allergy Department at St Mary's, housed probably the largest allergy clinic in the world. In 1952, for example, Freeman and his colleagues conducted 7,495 consultations (including 1,140 new patients) in the seasonal hay fever clinic, and 4,880 consultations (including 2,957 new patients) in the Clinic for Allergic Diseases, figures that far outnumbered the patients seen in the Institute's out-patient clinics for infectious diseases.[162] In that year, the *Annual Report* boasted: 'The Allergy Out Patient Department constitutes the only place in Great Britain where extensive trials on new or untried anti-allergic drugs can be carried out. Various drugs have been used in controlled trials and the results of some of these trials are to be published.'[163]

At the same time, the Allergy Department at St Mary's had become a focal point for students and practitioners of allergy, attracting visiting researchers from around the world, generating media interest, producing its own educational films for medical students, and training young allergists through programmes of postgraduate lectures and research fellowships.[164] Indeed, such was the reputation of the allergy clinic that in 1976 a feature article in *The Times* referred to the extent to which St Mary's 'is to allergies what the Pasteur Institute is to viruses'.[165]

From the 1950s, under the direction of A. W. Frankland and in a manner analogous to previous developments in charting the seasonal distribution of pollen in North America, the department also began to furnish British allergists with regular pollen counts. The following decade, daily pollen counts were made available first to the local London press and subsequently to the national press, as a 'warning service for hay fever sufferers during June and July'.[166] Significantly, at the end of the twentieth century, the daily grass pollen counts recorded at St Mary's Hospital since 1961 constituted 'the longest data set for any pollen monitoring site in Europe', providing modern aerobiologists with opportunities to examine trends in pollen concentration and distribution and to speculate about the impact of climatic fluctuations, shifting patterns of land use, and levels of air pollution on long-term trends in hay fever.[167]

Staff at St Mary's also provided early core membership of the British Association of Allergists, the first meeting of which was held at St Mary's Hospital on 24 January 1948, with A. W. Frankland as Secretary and with John Freeman and Henry Dale leading an extended discussion on the nature and meaning of allergy. Attracting members from a range of clinical and scientific specialities, the Association became an important forum for both national and international speakers to present the results of research, and in 1959 hosted the 4th European Congress of Allergy in London. Changing its name in 1964 to the British Allergy Society, and subsequently to the British Society for Allergy and Clinical Immunology, in 1971 the Society founded a new journal, Clinical Allergy (later Clinical and Experimental Allergy), dedicated to disseminating the fruits of both laboratory and clinical research, and edited by Jack Pepys (1914–1996), who had joined the Allergy Department at St Mary's in 1953 and who later became the first Professor of Clinical Immunology in Britain.[168]

In the post-Second World War period, studies of allergy also began to attract the interest of immunologists, who had previously been largely preoccupied with elucidating the biochemistry of antibodies and antigens. When the British Society for Immunology was founded in the early 1950s, for example, allergy (along with serological reactions, biological aspects of immunity, protection against disease and routine diagnosis) was thought to constitute one of the five major areas for immunological research, and a number of prominent scientists and clinicians working in the field of allergy (such as John Freeman, Carl Prausnitz, Henry Dale, Jack Pepys and A. W. Frankland) were elected as members or honorary members of the Society.[169] In 1966, in recognition of the clinical relevance of immunology, the Society founded Clinical and Experimental Immunology as the sister journal to Immunology, which had been first published in 1958. In addition, leading immunologists, such as John Humphrey (1915–1987), who was appointed head of the new Immunology Division at the National Institute for Medical Research in 1957 and who published a major textbook of immunology for medical students in 1963, dedicated much of their professional life to investigating the mechanisms of allergic reactions.[170] Indeed, as founding editor of Advances in Immunology, Humphrey also personally encouraged international interest in immunological studies of hypersensitivity.[171] Growing immunological interest in allergy reflected not only the blossoming of clinical and laboratory studies of allergic diseases in this period but also a general resurgence of interest in biological, rather than chemical, aspects of immunity. Like research on autoimmunity, tumour biology and the immunology of transplant rejection, studies of allergy both contributed to, and benefited from, the renewed focus on the cellular determinants of immunological reactivity that emerged in the 1950s.[172]

Significantly, British allergists were not alone in expanding and promoting their discipline during the middle decades of the twentieth century. National developments in North America and continental Europe, as well as Britain, facilitated greater international collaboration, not only in the form of academic meetings such as the European congresses on allergy held every three years but also in the shape of new societies and global health initiatives. The International Association of Allergology, shaped largely by the vision and enthusiasm of leading American allergists, was established in 1951 following the first International Congress of Allergists held in Zurich that year. Five years later, the European Academy of Allergology and Clinical Immunology was founded in Florence in order to promote basic and clinical research and to disseminate scientific information.[173] In addition, in the early 1960s allergic diseases emerged as a target for novel global research and training strategies in immunopathology coordinated by the World Health Organization.[174]

However, it is striking that although global interest in allergic diseases was rising, the growth of clinical allergy in this period was largely confined to the temperate Western world. While modern industrial nations often boasted an array of private and state-funded allergy services as well as lecture courses in allergy for doctors and medical students, both the range and availability of clinical and educational provisions were measurably poorer in the developing tropical world. As several post-war surveys conducted by the World Health Organization demonstrated, although clinics and societies had been established in some South American countries by the 1960s, there were no allergy clinics in Kuwait until 1964, none in Indonesia until 1972, and few allergy services in most African states until well into the 1970s. Moreover, when allergy clinics did exist in developing countries, they tended to be located only in major cities, leaving vast sections of the population without access to clinical facilities. Of course, this pattern of provision was partly dictated by stringent restrictions on local resources to fund health initiatives. In addition, it was also shaped by widespread professional and public perceptions that, in comparison to the hazards of acute infectious diseases, allergies constituted only 'minor ailments' in developing countries, and that hay fever and asthma were largely confined to the civilized, educated classes of the industrialized world.[175]

Crucially, however, these presumptions about the scale and social distribution of allergy were increasingly challenged both by growing public interest in allergic diseases, most evident initially in America, and by creeping convictions that the burden of allergic diseases was changing worldwide. As Milton and June Cohen pointed out in the preface to a popular book on allergies published in 1942, the 'American people have become intrigued with allergy'.[176] The extent of public curiosity and concern on both sides of the Atlantic is apparent in the increasing newspaper coverage of allergic diseases and in the occasional appearance of such diseases as standard motifs in plays and novels, most notably in *Hay Fever*, Noël Coward's portrayal of upper-class eccentricity written in 1924.[177] In addition, public interest is manifested by the proliferation of magazine advertisements for allergy products and services during the middle decades of the twentieth century, and by the growth of advice books written by allergists for the general public from the 1930s and '40s onwards. In 1939, for example, Warren Vaughan, author of specialist texts on the practice of allergy, published what he hoped would be 'a reasonably good bedtime story' for general readers anxious to understand their own allergies. Two years later he wrote a further account of this 'strange malady' aimed specifically at a general, rather than professional, audience and published in a series of non-technical books produced by the American Association for the Advancement of Science.[178]

As Vaughan was at pains to make clear, the importance of the subject lay in evidence that the incidence and prevalence of allergic manifestations were on the increase. In 1916, in their seminal paper on the inheritance of hypersensitivity, Robert Cooke and Albert Vander Veer (1880–1959) had estimated that approximately 7 per cent of the American population demonstrated some form of hypersensitivity.[179] By the 1930s estimates of the proportion of the population in which specific sensitization could be established by careful elicitation of patient and family histories ranged from 22.6 per cent, if only major allergic diseases were included, to approximately 60 per cent, if minor allergies were also counted.[180] In 1941 Vaughan suggested that in the United States there were 6 million hay fever sufferers, between 600,000 and 3.5 million people with asthma, and in the region of 12 million people who would at some stage require medical care for an allergic condition.[181]

According to Vaughan, such figures, together with evidence that allergies were beginning to plague developing nations, forced contemporary clinicians to reconstruct their understanding of allergy: 'The question will then be no longer "why do some of the population become allergic?" but rather "why are not all persons allergic at one time or another?"'[182] From this perspective, although some writers reiterated traditional beliefs that allergy was 'an

What you can do about
ALLERGIES

MILLIONS OF PEOPLE in our country are affected by some form of allergy. It is estimated that about four million people suffer each year from hay fever alone.

An allergy is a disorder or a *sensitivity* which some persons develop to normally harmless things like pollens, foods and dust. Many other factors may also be involved, such as chemicals, bacteria, etc.

The discomforts that occur when these trouble-makers come in contact with sensitive tissues are believed to be caused by a chemical called histamine.

This chemical is apparently released by the body's cells in such large amounts that the tissues themselves are affected and their normal functions upset. This results in sneezing, skin rashes, digestive upsets, and a variety of other discomforts.

Today, treatment for all types of allergy is becoming increasingly effective. There are diagnostic tests which help doctors identify even quite obscure causes. In addition, there are also new drugs which aid in controlling many allergic symptoms.

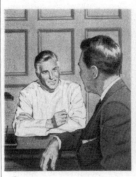

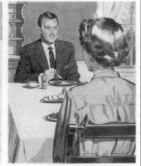

1. If you have an allergy, ask your doctor about *the antihistamines.* When administered under a physician's advice—as they must be, since they are toxic to some degree—they often give rapid, though *temporary,* relief.

The antihistamines are especially beneficial in those allergies—such as hay fever—which are caused by substances that are inhaled. For best results, however, these drugs should be used along with other measures designed to give more lasting relief.

2. If you have hay fever, the doctor may recommend that desensitizing treatments be given early in the year, long in advance of "the hay fever season."

This helps build up protection and enables many patients to go through the season with little or no discomfort. Prompt and proper treatment is desirable, as studies show that persons with untreated hay fever often develop asthma.

3. If you suspect a food allergy, consult your doctor about diagnostic tests which reveal foods that should be avoided.

Authorities caution against self-prescribed diets to relieve food allergies, because essential foods may be unnecessarily omitted.

It is especially important to follow this safeguard in infants and children who have digestive upsets or skin rashes thought to result from eating certain foods.

Emotional difficulties have been found to play a part in allergy disorders. Consequently, doctors may study the patient's background in an attempt to find and clear up emotional situations that may lead to more frequent or more severe attacks.

Today, through prompt and proper treatment—and *complete* cooperation between the doctor and the patient—most allergy victims can be greatly helped.

COPYRIGHT 1951 METROPOLITAN LIFE INSURANCE CO.

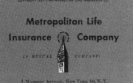

Metropolitan Life
Insurance ⚱ **Company**

(A MUTUAL COMPANY)

1 MADISON AVENUE, NEW YORK 10, N. Y.

Metropolitan Life Insurance Co.
1 Madison Avenue
New York 10, N. Y.

Please send me a copy of your booklet, 851-E, "Allergic to What?"

Name

Street

City   State

A US magazine advertisement of the 1950s.

aristocrat among diseases . . . limited to the chosen few',[183] hay fever and asthma could not be regarded as relatively rare diseases confined to the elite classes of the Western world. On the contrary, many clinicians were increasingly keen to emphasize that all 'individuals are potentially capable of developing allergy'.[184] As Vaughan himself put it in 1932, allergy 'is no longer exceptional; it is the rule'.[185] On the eve of the Second World War, allergy was on the verge of erupting as a public health and socio-economic problem of global proportions.

4

THE GLOBAL ECONOMY OF ALLERGY

> Allergic diseases represent a very serious problem in developed
> countries. With the progress of industrialization and the increased
> use of chemicals in everyday life, the incidence of allergic diseases
> in developing countries is increasing.
>
> World Health Organization, 1980[1]

In the aftermath of the Second World War, a variety of forces and events
conspired to substantially transform medical and popular understandings and
experiences of allergies. An epidemic of asthma in children living in impover-
ished conditions in many major American cities, a sudden surge in deaths
from asthma particularly in Britain and New Zealand, steeply rising levels of
hay fever, asthma and eczema in most modern industrialized countries, the
emergence of new forms of allergic reaction, and the dramatic eruption of
allergies in the developing world collectively suggested that pre-war perceptions of allergic diseases as mild and relatively uncommon conditions needed
urgent revision. As a wide variety of immunological sensitivities appeared to
blossom in the post-war period and as scientists and clinicians struggled to
expose the mechanisms and meanings of allergic and autoimmune reactions,
allergy became not only a focus of concern for local, national and international health agencies and state organizations but also an increasingly
frequent cause of chronic suffering and disability as well as occasional
personal tragedy.

The rising global incidence and prevalence of allergies immediately generated the spectre of a socio-economic burden of alarming proportions and, as
a result, posed a formidable strategic challenge to the provision of health care
services by modern governments. However, deepening public and professional interest in the personal and political costs incurred by hay fever,
asthma, eczema and food intolerance also created an expansive marketplace
for a rapidly globalizing industrial sector. During the last half of the twentieth
century, the pharmaceutical industry especially began to reap the considerable financial rewards that were made possible by the development and
marketing of anti-allergy products available either over-the-counter or on
prescription. The giant multinational pharmaceutical corporations were not
the only benefactors of a modern plague of allergies. Cleaning, cosmetics and

food industries also responded to, and in some cases fuelled and exploited, escalating public fears of allergic diseases. By the turn of the millennium, colossal amounts of money could be lost or gained through allergy. The aim of this chapter is to trace the emergence of allergy as a global public health problem in the post-war period and to analyse the evolution of commercial and consumer interest in allergies. I shall argue in particular that while mounting evidence of the global spread of allergic diseases undoubtedly generated new economic opportunities, it also fuelled nascent suspicions that certain aspects of modern civilization, including medicine, were making people sick.

Global trends in morbidity and mortality

During the mid-1960s a number of articles in the popular and medical press heralded a new era in the history of allergy. On 27 September 1963 a correspondent for *The Times* reported a wave of asthma morbidity and mortality that had swept through Cuba. Supposedly linked to sudden atmospheric changes, the crisis had resulted in the death of five people and the hospitalization of more than 200 others. In July 1965 the same paper published an account of 'a startling rise in asthma . . . among New York Negroes and Puerto Ricans'. Drawing on prominent contemporary beliefs in the psychosomatic nature of asthma, such outbreaks were initially attributed to 'tensions arising from conditions related directly or indirectly to the civil rights movement'. As Gregg Mitman has cogently argued, however, assumptions about inherent racial predispositions to asthma that permeated attempts to link the epidemic to a vulnerable immigrant psyche were challenged by epidemiological evidence demonstrating that high levels of asthma in certain districts of New York, Chicago and New Orleans were closely correlated with urban poverty. As a result, the wave of American asthma was subsequently reconfigured as a manifestation of urban deprivation and particularly cockroach infestation.[2]

Shortly before revealing putative associations between asthma and race in urban America, *The Times* had also carried brief reports of papers presented at the World Asthma Conference held in Eastbourne in England. Some participants once again concentrated initially on the psychodynamic aspects of asthma, suggesting, for example, that children used their asthma to avoid school or to escape chores at home and that both children and adults could exploit 'asthma to claim attention or to manipulate people or situations'. In considering childhood asthma, however, John Morrison Smith, a consultant physician in Birmingham, injected a sombre note of caution into the debates: 'Death from asthma in any child is really unnecessary', he was reported as

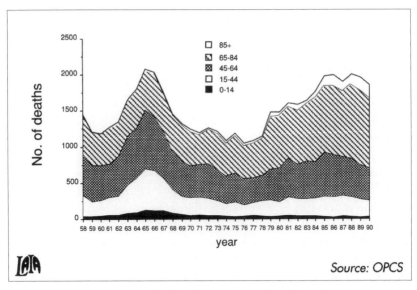

Asthma deaths by age, England and Wales 1958–90 (Office of Population Censuses and Surveys data).

saying. Convinced that better education about the dangers of asthma was essential, he warned that preventable deaths still occurred 'because the physician concerned does not appreciate that a particular child may die and must be treated with that in mind'.[3]

Smith's words proved sadly prophetic. Within a year, Smith was himself contributing to growing medical concerns about what appeared to be an alarming rise in asthma deaths in Britain, particularly in children and young adults. In a letter to the *Lancet* in May 1966, Smith contrasted the general decline in asthma mortality throughout the 1950s with the trend in the early 1960s: in the first five years of that decade, asthma deaths had increased by more than 50 per cent, with the most marked rise in mortality occurring in children over five years old.[4] More detailed epidemiological analysis soon revealed further features of an epidemic of asthma deaths in England and Wales. From 1959 asthma mortality had risen steadily in all age groups, although the trend was especially evident in children between 10 and 14 years old, at which ages the mortality rate had increased eightfold between 1959 and 1966. In addition, studies revealed that the proportion of all deaths between the ages of 5 and 34 that were attributable to asthma had risen from 1 per cent in 1959 to 3.4 per cent in 1966; in children between 10 and 14 years old, the proportional mortality had increased even more dramatically, from 1 per cent in 1959 to 7.2 per cent in 1966.[5] As a result, by 1966, asthma had become 'the fourth most common of the published causes of death', exceeded in children only by road traffic accidents, cancer and respiratory infections.[6]

Given previous understandings of asthma as a relatively mild, non-fatal condition, combined with growing optimism in the post-war period that mortality from infectious diseases was waning and that medicine could cure many life-threatening conditions, it is perhaps not surprising that an epidemic of asthma deaths immediately attracted the attention of the media. A number of articles in *The Times* in the late 1960s pointed to the tragic irony that better management of asthma since the war had not resulted in a fall in mortality and alerted readers to the 'considerable alarm' that the epidemic was causing among patients and doctors. In addition, newspaper coverage noted that rising mortality from asthma was not confined to Britain, but was also evident in certain other industrialized countries; similar waves of asthma deaths were reported, for example, in Australia, New Zealand, Ireland and Norway. Early media reports also raised the possibility that deaths in young asthmatics in these countries might be linked to the over-use of certain inhalers used in the treatment of asthma.[7] Although an iatrogenic cause of the epidemic had already been tentatively broached by contributors to the medical press between 1965 and 1967,[8] towards the end of the decade growing public and professional concerns encouraged epidemiologists to analyse the geographical distribution and possible causes of trends in asthma mortality in greater depth, in the hope of curtailing the outbreak.

As international studies of the epidemic made clear, there were a number of possible explanations for post-war trends in mortality. In the first place, it was possible that the sudden rise in asthma fatalities in the 1960s constituted merely 'an artefact brought about by changes in the diagnostic criteria' used by doctors certifying death.[9] During the late 1950s and early 1960s, pathologists and physicians had certainly attempted to establish a clearer definition of asthma and to distinguish more accurately between asthma, chronic bronchitis and emphysema. Drawing partly on the availability of new treatments, on improvements in spirometry, and on the introduction of the peak flow meter in 1959, many researchers increasingly regarded asthma primarily in functional terms as a form of intermittent airway obstruction that could be reversed by bronchodilators, including corticosteroids. By contrast, chronic bronchitis was defined largely in clinical terms by the presence of a productive cough, while emphysema was characterized principally on a pathological basis as dilatation of the air spaces distal to the terminal bronchioles.[10]

There is anecdotal evidence to suggest that shifting understandings of chronic respiratory diseases in these terms did indeed lead to changes in diagnostic practice in some countries, and especially to the adoption of asthma as a label to describe cases previously diagnosed as bronchitis. In 1979, for example, while reviewing his own experiences as a general practitioner in Devon, England, during the 1960s and '70s (Sir) Denis Pereira Gray, later President of the Royal College of General Practitioners, noted that 'I find now that what I used to call bronchitis is usually asthma'.[11] Similarly, in 1991, Roger Robinson, a former professor of paediatrics in London and associate editor of the *British Medical Journal*, recalled the manner in which a paper published in 1969 had encouraged him to adopt the term asthma in place of the previously popular 'wheezy bronchitis' or 'asthmatic bronchitis' in children.[12] This trend was possibly more noticeable in Britain than in continental Europe or North America where asthma, bronchitis and emphysema were usually regarded as points on a spectrum of chronic lung disease rather than as distinct conditions. However, according to early epidemiological studies, shifting diagnostic practices could not satisfactorily explain mortality trends in the 1960s. As several contemporary commentators argued, since deaths attributable to other chronic respiratory diseases did not decrease while asthma deaths were rising, the increase in asthma mortality could not be construed simply in terms of classificatory changes. Instead, they suggested, the wave of asthma mortality was 'in large part, real and represents a true increase in the annual number of deaths from the disease'.[13]

Having also rejected the possibility that rising mortality could be explained in terms of an increase in the number of patients suffering from asthma or in terms of alterations in the levels of environmental pollutants, epidemiological studies concluded that 'an increase in the case fatality rate' was the most likely explanation for recent trends and tentatively suggested that advances in the management of respiratory diseases might in fact be responsible. Although researchers noted that the increase in asthma mortality did not emerge until nine years after corticosteroids were first made widely available in 1952, they could not entirely discount the contribution of long-term steroid therapy. They pointed out, however, that there was 'a much closer correlation' between mortality rates and 'the use of pressurized aerosols containing sympathomimetics', such as the ß-agonists isoprenaline or orciprenaline, used to relieve the characteristic bronchospasm of an asthma attack. Such bronchodilators had been introduced in Britain in 1960 and consumption had increased more than fourfold by 1966.[14] Subsequent studies tended to confirm growing suspicions that over-use of non-selective ß-agonists might be responsible for the British epidemic of asthma deaths, possibly as a result of cardiotoxicity. Not only did the onset of the epidemic coincide with the introduction of this form of treatment but mortality rates also rapidly subsided once the use of these preparations declined following warnings from the Committee on Safety of Drugs in 1967 and the eventual proscription of direct sales to the British public under Schedule 4B of the Poisons Regulations in 1968.[15]

In spite of early indictments of inhaled sympathomimetic agents, the precise causes of the epidemic of asthma deaths in the 1960s remained (and indeed remain) in dispute. As several commentators noted at the time, the fact that general practitioners (GPS) were not accustomed to recognizing the severity of asthma, the possibility that serious symptoms were masked by palliative treatments, and the failure of doctors adequately to address psychopathological features in some patients might all have contributed to death in individual cases.[16] However, early suspicions of the iatrogenic nature of the British epidemic found indirect support from mortality patterns elsewhere in the world. In 1972 Paul Stolley, from the School of Hygiene and Public Health at The Johns Hopkins University, suggested that many countries, including the United States, were spared an epidemic largely because they did not market or sell large volumes of the highly concentrated form of isoprenaline that was available in Britain.[17] In addition, in the 1970s, New Zealand experienced a second wave of asthma deaths apparently linked to the prescription of a high dose preparation of fenoterol, another relatively non-selective ß-agonist. In a manner analogous to the earlier mortality pattern in the 1960s, this second epidemic began to wane only in 1990 following the withdrawal of fenoterol from the drug tariff.[18]

While debates about the epidemics continued, the wave of asthma deaths during the 1960s had a demonstrable impact on medical and popular understandings of asthma and other allergies. In addition to precipitating new regulations regarding the availability of bronchodilators, the epidemic raised awareness of the dangers of asthma. Deaths from asthma were, of course, not unknown before 1960, but in general most clinicians prior to that time had tended to regard asthma as a relatively mild condition with little impact on life expectancy.[19] From the mid-1960s, however, asthma was reconstructed in both the medical and the public mind as a potentially life-threatening condition requiring expert and urgent medical attention. Although clinicians readily acknowledged that not all asthma was allergic or atopic in origin, the changing clinical features of asthma nevertheless encouraged doctors and patients to reconsider the nature and severity of other allergic diseases. The reconstruction of asthma thus served to divert allergists' attention away from hay fever, which had routinely been regarded as the archetypal allergic disease, towards more severe and more disabling forms of allergy, not only towards asthma but also eventually towards food allergies and allergic forms of eczema.

Significantly, however, the 1960s epidemic of deaths from asthma was only one manifestation of the shifting epidemiology and rising visibility of allergy in the post-war world. Thus, during the last half of the twentieth century, other epidemiological and geographical trends in asthma, hay fever, eczema and food allergies became apparent. In those Western industrialized countries with relatively high levels of allergy during the inter-war years, for example, the incidence and prevalence of allergic diseases increased further during the late twentieth century and specific health service provisions were implemented in many countries to improve treatment and to reduce the burden of illness and lost productivity. More strikingly perhaps, allergic diseases also began to plague the populations of developing countries, many of which had not recognized allergy as a significant health problem prior to the Second World War.

Modern Western trends in allergies were particularly evident in Britain. Following the decline of deaths in the late 1960s, there was a steady rise in both morbidity and mortality rates from asthma in England and Wales (see graph, p. 105). In 1995 a survey conducted by the Department of Health revealed that, in addition to rising trends in mortality, between the 1970s and the 1990s there were significant increases in the levels of self-reported and GP-reported asthma, in GP consultations and hospital admissions for asthma, and in the number of days of certified incapacity as the result of asthma.[20] According to figures obtained from national morbidity surveys, the proportion of the population consulting GPs for asthma increased from 8.5 per 1,000 in 1955–6 to 10.2 in 1970–71, and to 17.8 in 1981–2. This trend was supported by a survey conducted in the west of Scotland, according to which the prevalence of asthma rose from 3 per cent in 1972 to 8.2 per cent in 1996.[21]

The epidemiological pattern of asthma morbidity in Britain during the second half of the twentieth century was mirrored by trends in other allergic diseases. Figures from a survey of the entire population of a single town in the 1970s suggested that during the course of that decade the overall incidence of allergic diseases rose from approximately 23 per cent to 30 per cent.[22] More specifically, between 1972 and 1996 the percentage of a Scottish population suffering from hay fever apparently increased from 5.8 per cent to 19.9 per cent, while the proportion of the English and Welsh population seeking GP consultations for hay fever rose from 5.1 per 1,000 in 1955–6 to 10.6 in 1971–2, and to 19.7 in 1981–2.[23] Similarly, a survey of 1984 revealed a substantial rise in rates of reported eczema in three national cohorts of children born since the Second World War: 'Overall rates rose from 5.1 per cent in children born in 1946, to 7.3 per cent in those born in 1958, to 12.2 per cent in the 1970 cohort.'[24] Figures compiled in 2003 suggested that this trajectory continued, with the prevalence of eczema in Britain increasing roughly threefold between the 1970s and the 1990s.[25]

Notwithstanding the difficulties created by different national criteria for diagnosing allergic diseases and the striking international and regional variations in prevalence, these British patterns of morbidity and mortality were closely reproduced elsewhere in the developed world. In Western Europe a number of studies suggested that the prevalence of asthma, hay fever, allergic dermatitis and drug allergies doubled between the 1960s and the early 1980s. In Switzerland, for example, the prevalence of hay fever rose from an estimated 0.82 per cent in 1926 to 5 per cent in 1958, and to approximately 10 per cent by the 1980s.[26] Beyond Europe, epidemiological studies provided ample evidence of rising trends in most allergic diseases during the second half of the twentieth century, especially in New Zealand, North America and Australia.[27] In 1983 it was estimated that allergies afflicted more than 35 million people in the United States alone, while in 1996 approximately 150 million people were thought to suffer from asthma worldwide.[28] In addition, figures from Japan, which experienced rapid industrialization and an accelerated epidemiological transition during the middle decades of the twentieth century, suggest that rates there also increased significantly. In 1934, when hay fever was identified in 3.5 per cent of a Japanese population resident in California, the condition was reportedly unknown in Japan itself. By contrast, by the early 1980s its prevalence had increased to approximately 5 per cent. Surveys also revealed not only that the prevalence of asthma in Japan appeared to double between 1955 and 1971, but also that the life expectancy of asthmatics was substantially lower than that of the general population.[29]

While allergies were clearly becoming more visible in the developed world during the late twentieth century, the geographical and ethnographical distribution of allergic diseases was also shifting. Perhaps the first concrete evidence for the global spread of allergies came from a survey conducted by Alain de Weck, director of the Institute for Clinical Immunology in Bern, Switzerland. In 1976 de Weck had distributed a questionnaire to members of allergy and immunology societies in South America, Africa, Asia and Eastern Europe. The replies led de Weck to suggest that, although clinical allergy services were often limited in those locations, the health problems posed by allergic diseases in developing countries were not insignificant and that, given the 'emergence of industrialization and better living conditions', they were likely to increase.[30]

Two years later, a meeting of allergists and immunologists convened by the World Health Organization (WHO) reported that, historically, most studies on hypersensitivity had 'taken place in the laboratories and medical clinics of the United States of America and Europe', that is in countries in which rising standards of living and improved health care services had brought infectious diseases and malnutrition under control and in which there had been evident increases in allergy. The report also divided countries into distinct groups with high, medium or low prevalence rates of asthma.[31] Although many developing countries appeared to have low rates, contributors to the meeting presented preliminary evidence that allergy was rapidly becoming a concern in several developing countries undergoing later industrialization and delayed epidemiological transitions. Participants from Indonesia, Kuwait, Nigeria and South America all highlighted both the growing importance of allergic diseases in tropical and sub-tropical environments and the urgent need for improved facilities for training allergists, gathering clearer epidemiological data, diagnosing and treating allergies, and educating the public about the benefits of expert medical advice as opposed to the consumption of unprescribed drugs.[32] Acknowledging these arguments, the meeting concluded that in 'view of the world-wide distribution of allergic diseases and their growing socio-economic importance, the WHO should encourage awareness of allergic diseases as a public health problem in member states'.[33]

Over the next few years, further surveys (some initiated and funded by the WHO) revealed rising trends in asthma, hay fever and other allergic disorders in many developing countries. The most dramatic example of these trends came from studies in Papua New Guinea, which demonstrated that while asthma had been extremely rare prior to 1972 its prevalence in adults had risen to 7.3 per cent by the 1980s.[34] The following decade, further studies suggested that asthma was also emerging in various African countries.[35] Although the WHO recognized the problems created by different national approaches to the definition of allergy and different methods of study, a further WHO workshop in 1984 stressed the impending global impact of allergies:

> Allergic diseases, although seldom life-threatening, affect a large part of the population in industrialized countries and are also becoming an increasing source of morbidity in populations of the developing world. In terms of discomfort in everyday life and of economic losses, allergic diseases certainly deserve to be considered more seriously by public health authorities than may sometimes have been the case in the past. . . . We hope that the considerations and proposals discussed will benefit present and future generations of potentially allergic patients throughout the world.[36]

Deeper investigations into the epidemiology of allergy, such as the world-wide survey coordinated by the Steering Committee of the International Study of Asthma and Allergies in Childhood during the mid-1990s, revealed persistent regional gradients in the prevalence of symptoms of hay fever, asthma and eczema. At the same time, however, they also reinforced concerns about the extent to which allergies constituted a global, rather than merely Western, health problem.[37] Such evidence contributed to the gradual erosion of the familiar social and cultural boundaries of these diseases. Allergy was clearly no longer confined to the Western civilized world, as it apparently had been in the early twentieth century, but was spilling out from the affluent West across borders that had been constructed and maintained on the basis of race, class, gender and geography. Towards the end of the twentieth century, while hay fever continued to be more prevalent in British children from affluent families, asthma was arguably more common and more commonly fatal among lower social classes, thereby mirroring the pattern of morbidity and mortality displayed by most chronic degenerative diseases.[38] In addition, earlier accounts of the male predominance of allergies were also challenged by surveys conducted during the 1970s and '80s, which suggested that while boys did indeed tend to demonstrate greater sensitivity to common allergens and to suffer more allergies than girls the pattern was generally reversed in adult life.[39] As I shall argue in the next chapter, the epidemiological profile of allergic diseases was increasingly regarded not primarily as a product of innate intellectual and educational superiority (although that notion undoubtedly persisted), but as the result of shifting patterns of industrial production and consumption in the modern world.

While debates about the extent and causes of rising trends in asthma, hay fever, eczema, and food and drug allergies continued, the socio-economic burden generated by allergic diseases was immediately clear to modern national and international health organizations. In the early twentieth century, commentators on both sides of the Atlantic had complained that hay fever often necessitated time off work and that asthma constituted a drain on the national economy. According to a brief report on the work of the Asthma Research Council in *The Times* in 1929, for example:

> Asthma cripples from year to year some 200,000 otherwise healthy people. Asthma and its allied disorders rob the world of industry of the work of more than half a million men and women during the winter months of each year. On economic grounds alone some remedy against losses of this magnitude is overdue.[40]

As mortality and morbidity rates rose after the Second World War, both the direct and indirect cost of allergic diseases increased significantly. In Britain, for example, the direct cost of allergies to the National Health Service (NHS), including the cost of prescriptions, medical time and hospital admissions, rose steadily, threatening to 'wreck Norman Fowler's plans for the NHS' according to one observer in 1985.[41] Concern about the potential impact of escalating costs was not misplaced. By the early 1990s the net ingredient cost of prescriptions for asthma alone was £347 million, a figure that constituted 11 per cent of the total NHS prescription cost.[42] At the turn of the millennium, the estimated annual cost to the NHS of treating asthma was about £850 million; by 2004 it had topped £1 billion.[43] However, the indirect costs of allergy from lost productivity and social security payments were often estimated to be even greater. Industrial injury benefit payments for dermatitis (both toxic and allergic) accounted for approximately two-thirds of all benefits paid out for occupational diseases in the 1970s.[44] In 1977 a report from the Asthma Research Council suggested that more than two million days were lost each year through asthma, 'costing more than £2 million in sickness benefits'.[45] By the 1990s the level of certified incapacity from asthma had risen to more than 10 million days per year, and by 2000 the combination of lost productivity and benefits apparently accounted for more than 60 per cent of the total cost of asthma to the nation.[46]

As several international surveys coordinated by the WHO during the 1970s and '80s revealed, the escalating socio-economic burden of allergic diseases evident in Britain was emulated elsewhere. According to the report from a

WHO meeting held in Geneva in 1978, allergic asthma and hay fever were responsible for '85 million days of restricted activity, 33 million days in bed, 5 million days lost from work and 7 million days lost from school' in North America each year.[47] Some estimates of the impact were even more dramatic. In a guide for parents of children with allergies, published in 1973, Claude Frazier, a physician from North Carolina, suggested that more 'Americans suffer from allergy than from any other disease', and that 'annually they lose some thirty-six million school days because of allergic diseases'.[48] In 1968 the cost of hospitalizing patients with asthma in the United States was in the region of $62 million per year.[49] By 1984 the total direct cost of hospitalization, medication and physician time in the treatment of asthma had risen to $1.5 billion. Equally strikingly, the loss of five million days work per year 'equated with $589 million in lost wages'.[50] By 1992 the total cost of asthma alone in the United States was more than $6 billion.[51]

Although comparison between countries often proved difficult because of the operation of different health care systems and different modes of calculation,[52] similarly spiralling patterns of both direct and indirect costs were reported in many continental European countries during the last quarter of the twentieth century. In Italy during the 1970s, for example, asthma was the most frequently reported disease in workers.[53] According to Dr Apostolou, a participant at the XIth International Congress of Allergology and Clinical Immunology in London in 1982, approximately 40 per cent of all visits to the doctor in Greece were due to allergic diseases.[54] In 1984 the WHO estimated that the direct and indirect costs of allergic diseases in Western Europe were roughly US $4 billion per year.[55] More recently, extrapolation of figures from detailed studies in Sweden and France suggested that the total annual cost of the major allergic diseases (asthma, hay fever, and atopic and contact dermatitis) in Western Europe was in the region of 29 billion ECU (approximately US $35 billion). Such findings led the UCB Institute of Allergy to stress the extent to which the emergence of allergic diseases constituted a major socio-economic burden in modern Europe.[56]

The mounting cost of allergies in the modern world can be traced not only to rising levels of allergy but also to greater awareness and shifting approaches to the management of allergic diseases. Early indications of epidemiological trends in asthma in the 1960s and '70s spawned media and public interest in allergies and generated new regional, national and international health policies aimed at reducing morbidity and mortality rates and, ultimately, at curbing the socio-economic impact of allergic diseases. In

Britain, for example, the wave of asthma deaths and rising morbidity in the 1960s precipitated calls for greater education and support for patients with asthma as well as occasional requests for more specific measures, such as non-smoking compartments in aircraft.[57] Widespread public and professional concern also led to the establishment of dedicated asthma clinics and intensive care services, promoted the development and adoption of facilities for self-monitoring and treating asthma at home, and encouraged the creation of an Asthma Charter (published by the National Asthma Campaign), which set out the level of care to be expected under the NHS. Although their value was sometimes challenged, open-door policies, which allowed self-admission to hospital without the need for intervention from a GP, were also introduced in many areas of England and Wales.[58] As the National Asthma Campaign pointed out, by the turn of the millennium, allergies (and particularly asthma) had become a 'hot topic' among members of the British Parliament; in addition to stimulating the establishment of an all-party group on asthma, the subject apparently 'occupied more parliamentary time than any other health condition other than cancer'.[59]

National surveys of rising trends and shifting patient needs were often followed by the elaboration of new guidelines for the management of allergic diseases. These guidelines in turn generated new audits of available services and led to the reformulation of both trends in allergies and the demand for services. In Britain, national guidelines for the treatment of asthma were first established by the British Thoracic Society in 1990 and were regularly updated over subsequent years. The guidelines set out protocols for diagnosing and assessing both children and adults with asthma, advocated a stepwise approach to treatment, established the criteria for emergency admission, and suggested standards for the organization and delivery of care and for patient education.[60] In 1991 the American National Heart, Lung, and Blood Institute (NHLBI) published similar guidelines for the diagnosis and management of asthma as part of a National Asthma Education Program.[61] More broadly, these national initiatives were reinforced by the elaboration of global programmes, such as the Global Initiative for Asthma, coordinated jointly by the NHLBI and the WHO, and the Global Asthma and Allergy European Network, launched in 2003 by a European consortium of research and support organizations. As the WHO had predicted in the 1970s in the wake of the epidemic of asthma deaths and in the face of steadily rising levels of allergic diseases across the world, by the dawn of the new millennium allergy had become a public health and socio-economic problem of global proportions.

In the process, allergic diseases had generated large-scale collaborative international research initiatives and facilitated rapid global expansion of the pharmaceutical industry.

Global networks in allergy

The rising visibility of allergic diseases in the last half of the twentieth century and growing awareness of their socio-economic impact in both developed and developing countries owed much to the emergence of international perspectives on disease in the post-war period and, more particularly, to the global research, surveillance and educational initiatives of the WHO. After operating for two years as an Interim Commission, the WHO was formally founded in 1948 as an attempt to rationalize various international health activities. Its roots were located in the nineteenth-century international sanitary conferences and in the cooperative work of early twentieth-century international health organizations such as the Pan American Sanitary Bureau, the Office International d'Hygiène Publique and the League of Nations Health Organization, all of which were concerned predominantly with the control of infectious diseases or with setting international standards.[62] In its early years, the WHO, like its precursors, adopted a vertical approach to disease control that focused on the identification and eradication of specific endemic and epidemic communicable diseases, such as malaria, tuberculosis, smallpox, typhus and influenza. From the early 1960s, however, the WHO introduced a more expansive and strategic approach to disease prevention and treatment, which included the establishment of an intensified research programme pursued not only at WHO headquarters in Geneva but also in satellite units throughout the world. Significantly, the first central research unit, created in 1963, was dedicated to immunology.[63]

The founding of the WHO immunology unit, under the initial directorship of Howard Goodman, followed a report of five scientific groups invited by the Director-General of the WHO in 1962 'to summarize the present state of knowledge in the field and to make recommendations for future research'. Recognizing that immunology was 'one of the fastest growing fields of medicine' with important implications for many areas of biomedical research and clinical practice, the report established a blueprint for the development of research programmes in immunoprophylaxis, immunopathology, transplantation immunology and immunochemistry.[64] From the unit's conception, manifestations of allergy and hypersensitivity constituted an important strand of the WHO's immunological research agenda, not only in the context of the

WHO's commitment to elucidating immunopathological mechanisms but also in terms of the perceived connections between allergy and immunization.[65] During subsequent decades, the WHO's interest in allergy intensified and the immunology unit made a series of critical contributions to scientific, clinical and epidemiological understandings of allergic diseases, to the training of allergists, to international collaboration among scientists and clinicians, and to the classification of allergy.

In addition to providing an initial protocol for diverse research initiatives in immunology, the WHO also convened scientific groups to consider emergent needs for training immunologists and to evaluate the status and potential contribution of immunology to clinical practice. In both cases, allergy figured strongly in the reports and recommendations made by the expert committees. At a meeting on the teaching of immunology in the medical curriculum held in Geneva in 1966, Dr. A. D. Ado, based in the Department of Pathological Physiology at the Second Moscow Medical Institute, highlighted the variable status of teaching in 'allergology' across the world and stressed the importance of allergy to many areas of clinical practice, including rheumatology, paediatrics, transplantation immunology, respiratory medicine, dermatology, and ear, nose and throat medicine.[66] The committee echoed Ado's concerns about training by noting the general lack of educational opportunities in immunology and allergy even in countries such as Britain and the United States which were 'relatively well-provided by immunologists', and by setting out the minimal requirements for courses in immunology, including coverage of hypersensitivity reactions mediated both by antibodies and by cells.[67] In addition, the committee's report incorporated a memorandum from the British Society for Immunology, which emphasized the manner in which immunological reactions underlay 'a variety of disorders such as autoimmune diseases, allergy and other hypersensitivities'.[68] Critically, the potential contribution of studies of allergy to clinical practice was taken up by a WHO scientific group on clinical immunology in 1971, where, once again, the importance of allergy emerged in a number of clinical domains, including hypersensitivity to infectious organisms, atopic allergy, delayed hypersensitivity and drug allergies.[69]

The WHO responded to these reports on training and research in immunology and allergy in a variety of ways. In the first place, immunology research and training centres were set up in Ibadan (1964–5), São Paolo (1966), Lausanne (1967), Singapore (1969) and Mexico (1969).[70] The purpose of these centres, which were part-funded by the WHO, was to provide training in immunology in developing countries and to generate research initiatives specifically addressing local health problems. At the same time, the WHO offered financial support for specific research and training programmes elsewhere. In the 1960s and '70s, for example, the WHO provided small grants for projects, training courses and research fellowships in immunology and allergy in London, Athens, Egypt and Madrid,[71] as well as funding Alain de Weck's surveys of both the epidemiology of allergic diseases and the availability of clinical allergy services in developing countries. In a memorandum on de Weck's contributions in 1976, Giorgio Torrigiani (who had replaced Howard Goodman as Chief of Immunology at the WHO) stressed that, although the immunology unit had always been closely interested in allergic diseases, the field had not previously been sufficiently mature for effective WHO involvement. By the mid-1970s, however, Torrigiani argued, the situation had changed and 'new findings in basic immunology can now be applied to this field which represents a great public health problem in many countries'.[72]

In addition to funding research and training in allergy, the WHO also contributed to the creation and maintenance of an active international network of allergists and immunologists, thereby furthering the development of scientific internationalism that had emerged initially in the form of trans-national treaties and conventions during the early twentieth century. In 1966 the WHO established a Joint Liaison Committee for Immunology with the Conseil des Organisations Internationales des Sciences Médicales (CIOMS). In order to facilitate international collaboration in immunology, the Committee published a regular newsletter advertising conferences and training courses, relaying information about past and current events, and disseminating the work of the WHO immunology unit and its satellite centres.[73] Three years later, the WHO also assisted in the formation of an International Union of Immunological Societies (IUIS) aimed at promoting interaction between existing national bodies and at facilitating the foundation of new national societies. By organizing international congresses as well as establishing and maintaining channels of communication across the world, the IUIS, WHO and CIOMS together provided a crucial framework for the development of what Bernard Cinader referred to many years later as a 'global family' of immunologists and allergists.[74] It is perhaps no coincidence that the creation of a global network of immunologists in this way occurred at precisely the moment when scientists such as Niels Jerne and Frank Macfarlane Burnet were formulating a network theory of the immune system.[75]

Throughout the 1960s and '70s, the IUIS and WHO also attempted to address a variety of sensitive professional anxieties that had troubled allergists since the creation and expansion of allergy clinics during the 1910s and '20s. As Alain de Weck pointed out in his report on the establishment of allergy research and training programmes, one of the main obstacles to professional development in many countries was 'the lack of recognition by national authorities', a problem that was compounded by the absence of the equipment and techniques necessary for the 'appropriate standardization of allergen extracts'.[76] Such concerns were not confined to developing countries and, as I suggested in the previous chapter, had already hindered the emergence of a recognized speciality of allergy in both Britain and the United States. In 1964 a subcommittee of the International Association of Allergology (founded in 1951) was established specifically to consider requirements for specialization. Three years later, the subcommittee proposed some basic principles for specialist training, most notably the introduction of a certification procedure based on completion of a two-year programme in 'the scientific basis of the speciality as well as the clinical practice of allergy'.[77] Leading allergists discussed these issues further at the International Congress of Allergology held in Florence in 1970. Although the immediate professional difficulties were not resolved, it appeared that many allergists were already embracing a particular strategy to facilitate general acceptance of allergy as a speciality, namely adoption of the title 'clinical immunology and allergy' for departments and societies. While this ploy carried the threat of invasion of the field of allergy by other clinical immunologists, it also provided allergists with an opportunity to expand their clinical remit and boost their professional status.[78]

In December 1969, after nearly seven years of constructive international activity, the WHO published an extensive review of its immunology programme. While the review focused predominantly on developments in the diagnosis and treatment of communicable diseases, it was apparent that the WHO had also stimulated international meetings and collaborative research ventures in immunopathology and immunodiagnosis, including allergy.[79] During subsequent decades, the WHO began to place even greater emphasis on the importance of recognizing the public health impact of allergic diseases and on the need for 'a cooperative international programme'.[80] Accordingly, members of the WHO convened meetings on the epidemiology, socioeconomic burden and prevention of allergic diseases in 1978 and 1984, distributed questionnaires to allergists across the world in order to gauge levels of allergy and the availability of allergists, and attempted to promote the adoption of standard epidemiological tools and definitions.[81] By 1980 allergy was included in the WHO's global medium-term programme in immunology, which stressed the need to evaluate more accurately the impact of allergic diseases in developing countries and to draw up more detailed plans for managing the spread of allergies after consultation with regional centres.[82] In 1983 a further global programme established a clear target: by 1989 the WHO aimed to have assessed the global prevalence of allergic diseases and to have made recommendations for 'preventative and curative measures applicable at primary health care level'.[83]

While the WHO was establishing a framework for extending clinical knowledge and public awareness of the prevalence of allergy in the post-war years, it was also contributing to the elaboration of new classifications of allergic diseases and to the expansion of scientific understandings of the immunological mechanisms involved. In 1946 the Interim Commission of the WHO had taken over responsibility for preparing and publishing the International Classification of Diseases (ICD), which had first found international acceptance as the International List of Causes of Death in 1900. In 1948 the WHO published the sixth revision of the ICD. In addition to providing a standard classification for the purposes of monitoring morbidity and mortality rates, the sixth revision also advocated greater international cooperation and the formation of national committees for gathering data, thereby marking 'the beginning of a new era in international vital and health statistics'.[84]

Reflecting the persistence of theories emphasizing the hormonal basis of asthma and other allergies, such as those propounded by Erwin Pulay and Hans Selye and indeed recognized by the WHO,[85] in both the sixth (1948) and seventh (1955) revisions of the ICD allergic disorders were incorporated in a section that also contained endocrine, metabolic and nutritional disorders, including thyroid disturbances, diabetes mellitus and vitamin deficiency diseases. Separate classification numbers were assigned to hay fever (240), asthma (241), angioneurotic oedema (242), urticaria (243), allergic eczema (244) and a range of other conditions such as allergic conjunctivitis and diverse manifestations of allergy to cosmetics, animal danders, drugs, feathers, dust, food and physical agents (245).[86] In discussions leading up to the eighth revision of the ICD (1965), however, the Australian Medical Statistics Committee questioned the validity of a separate sub-section for allergic diseases (240–45), arguing that attempts to differentiate between allergic eczema and dermatitis or between allergic bronchitis and bronchitis with asthma were unrealistic.

The Australian Committee therefore recommended abolishing the sub-section and transferring individual allergic diseases to appropriate categories according to the organ system concerned.[87] After discussion, the WHO supported the Australian amendments, and when the eighth revision came into effect in 1968 the various allergic diseases were 're-allocated according to the body system affected': asthma (493) and hay fever (507) to diseases of the respiratory system; eczema (691–2) and urticaria (708) to conditions of the skin and subcutaneous tissues; allergic colitis (561) to disorders of the digestive system; and allergic conjunctivitis (360) to inflammatory diseases of the eye.[88] By fragmenting the field of allergy in this way, the eighth revision of the ICD may have served inadvertently to hinder the efforts of allergists to establish a speciality independent of respiratory medicine, paediatrics, ear, nose and throat medicine, and dermatology.

In tandem with its remit to categorize diseases for statistical purposes, the WHO was also committed to clarifying the chemical and cellular mechanisms involved in immunological diseases with the specific aims of promoting solutions to the global spread of allergies, elucidating the role of allergy in infectious diseases, and refining the classification of hypersensitivity states. Attempts to classify hypersensitivity according to the underlying mechanisms and clinical features were not new. In 1923 Robert Cooke and Arthur Coca had suggested distinguishing in the first instance between 'normal' forms of hypersensitivity (such as serum sickness), which occurred in a large proportion of the population, and 'abnormal' forms of hypersensitivity, which were less common and mediated by a 'special mechanism', such as specific antibodies. According to Cooke and Coca, the abnormal forms, which most interested clinical allergists, comprised anaphylaxis, hypersensitiveness of infection, and atopy, each of which demonstrated distinctive clinical and pathological features.[89] In the 1940s and '50s, Arnold Rice Rich extended this approach and divided hypersensitivity into four types: anaphylaxis to foreign proteins, mediated by specific antibodies in the serum; the Arthus phenomenon, a form of intensified and prolonged local reaction to foreign protein; 'pollen type hypersensitivity', or atopic sensitivity, implicated in the pathogenesis of asthma, eczema and hay fever; and, finally, the 'tuberculin type of hypersensitivity', mediated primarily by cells rather than antibodies.[90] More particularly, Rich suggested that while the first three types shared much in common, the mechanisms by which they produced tissue damage differed significantly from those involved in tuberculin-type hypersensitivity.[91]

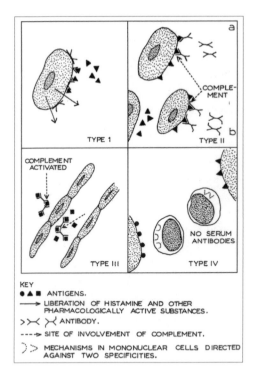

KEY
●▲■ ANTIGENS.
⟶ LIBERATION OF HISTAMINE AND OTHER PHARMACOLOGICALLY ACTIVE SUBSTANCES.
>✕< >✕ ANTIBODY.
--→ SITE OF INVOLVEMENT OF COMPLEMENT.
⟩ ⟩ MECHANISMS IN MONONUCLEAR CELLS DIRECTED AGAINST TWO SPECIFICITIES.

Diagrammatic illustration of four types of hypersensitivity reaction, from Gell and Coombs, *Clinical Aspects of Immunology*.

In the post-war period, renewed interest in the biological, as well as biochemical, features of immunological reactions and in the clinical applications of immunological knowledge facilitated the generation of more refined schemes for classifying hypersensitivity. The most influential scheme, and the one most commonly adopted by scientists, clinicians and international organizations such as the WHO, was developed by two British pathologists, P.G.H. Gell (b. 1914) and R.R.A. Coombs (b. 1921). In the first edition of *Clinical Aspects of Immunology*, published in 1963, Gell and Coombs criticized imprecise usage of the term allergy and advocated a return to the 'sound semantic foundation' established originally by Clemens von Pirquet, in which allergy incorporated both immunity and hypersensitivity. In this context, they went on to suggest that, in order to benefit from new immunological knowledge, allergic reactions should not be classified simply 'in terms of a clinical syndrome, of an anatomical or biochemical lesion' as they often had been, but in terms of the immunological processes involved. Accordingly, Gell and Coombs proposed four basic types of 'allergic reactions underlying disease'.[92]

Gell's and Coombs's Type I reactions (conventionally referred to as anaphylactic or immediate hypersensitivity) were mediated by the release of pharmacologically active substances, such as histamine, from cells passively sensitized by a specific class of antibody, referred to as reagin or atopic antibody. Although the precise nature of atopic antibody remained elusive, this form of hypersensitivity was implicated in hay fever, asthma and certain forms of food allergy and skin reactions. Type II reactions (otherwise referred to as cytolytic or cytotoxic) were initiated by antibodies reacting either with cell surface antigens or with antigens which subsequently became attached to cells. Mediated in many cases by the activation of complement, Type II reactions included transfusion reactions, haemolytic disease of the newborn, 'auto-allergic diseases', and possibly acute nephritis following streptococcal infections. The third category of antibody-mediated hypersensitivity comprised Type III reactions, which included the Arthus reaction and serum sickness. In these cases, antigen was thought to react with antibody either in the circulation or in tissue spaces to form complexes that were 'toxic to cells'.[93]

The final form of hypersensitivity, referred to by Gell and Coombs as Type IV, delayed or tuberculin-type sensitivity, was mediated not by antibodies but by sensitized white blood cells.[94] Early twentieth-century commentators had recognized differences between tuberculin sensitivity and other hypersensitivity reactions, in terms of both the speed of the reaction and its transferability with serum, and the distinction had been utilized in most classification schemes. While working with Karl Landsteiner (1868–1943) at the Rockefeller Institute for Medical Research in the 1940s, Merrill W. Chase (1905–2004) had demonstrated that delayed sensitivity could be transferred by white blood cells from sensitized animals rather than by antibodies. Chase's findings clarified a number of questions about the mechanisms involved in reactions to tuberculin and about the development of immunity in certain diseases, and provided the experimental basis for a classification of hypersensitivity that emphasized immunological processes rather than clinical states. Drawing on evidence of common pathological and immunological features, Gell and Coombs suggested that delayed hypersensitivity operated not only in tuberculosis but also in contact dermatitis, transplantation rejection, and some auto-allergic and parasitic diseases.[95]

Although attempts were made to refine the classification of hypersensitivity according to immunological mechanisms, and although there were persistent disputes about the role of antibodies and other humoral factors in delayed hypersensitivity, the scheme devised by Gell and Coombs was widely adopted by immunologists and allergists across the world.[96] However, while the four categories proposed by Gell and Coombs undoubtedly provided a convenient and rational framework for understanding a range of clinical manifestations of immunological reactivity, they also exposed familiar debates about the language and meaning of allergy. In the first place, their impassioned support for von Pirquet's broad notion of altered biological reactivity clearly ran counter to the manner in which the term allergy was generally employed by scientists and clinicians in the post-war period. Although Gell and Coombs insisted that 'transplantation allergy' and 'auto-allergy' constituted more precise designations than 'transplantation immunity' and 'autoimmunity', it is evident that the latter terms achieved widespread endorsement.[97] Many years later, Coombs continued to lament this linguistic fashion, pointing out that the word autoimmunity was 'misconstrued, absurd, and extremely confusing'.[98] Gell's and Coombs's arguments, however, were routinely ignored and over subsequent decades the meaning of the term allergy was narrowed even further. By the closing decades of the twentieth century, scientists and clinicians preoccupied by rising trends in hay fever, asthma and eczema in particular, used the term allergy to refer almost exclusively to Type I, or atopic, hypersensitivity reactions.[99]

Secondly, Gell's and Coombs's classification revealed recurrent uncertainties about the relationship between immunity and hypersensitivity that had initially been raised by Clemens von Pirquet. In the second edition of their book, published in 1968, Gell and Coombs included diagrammatic representations of the 'allergic mechanisms' (referred to as Modes A, B, C and D) involved in establishing immunity as well as those implicated in disease. Significantly, the putative mechanisms responsible for host resistance closely mirrored the four types of hypersensitivity (or vice versa), since they comprised three forms of antibody-mediated defence in which serum factors and sensitized cells participated in the destruction of the invading organism, and a fourth type of reaction in which 'actively allergized cells' operated in defence of the bodily realm.[100] By drawing explicit parallels between reactions causing tissue damage and those leading to immunity, Gell and Coombs were effectively normalizing the processes of hypersensitivity in much the same way that von Pirquet had attempted to do 60 years earlier. Although many commentators continued to regard hypersensitivity, or allergy, as antithetical to immunity and mediated by qualitatively different mechanisms, the notion that the basis of allergic damage was parallel to immunity found support elsewhere and served to reinforce epidemiological evidence that suggested that, in statistical terms, allergic diseases were increasingly the norm rather than the exception. In a short handbook on allergy published in 1961, for example, Kenneth C. Hutchin (1908–1993) noted that 'allergy is akin to immunity to diseases', and stressed the 'strong resemblance between inherited resistance to disease and the hereditary type of allergy'.[101] As I shall suggest in chapter Six, towards the end of the twentieth century perceived parallels between hypersensitivity and immunity encouraged occasional, albeit contested, reformulations of allergy in teleological terms, that is in terms of its potential contribution to the survival of an individual or species.

Closer integration of allergy into the immunological fold, encouraged by the work of Gell and Coombs, was facilitated by concurrent insights into the nature of the antibody involved in Type I hypersensitivity reactions. For some years, researchers had suspected that the sensitizing antibody responsible for mast cell degranulation and the release of histamine in allergies was IgA, the class of immunoglobulin that, from the early 1960s, had been associated primarily with the defence of mucosal surfaces.[102] In 1967, however, Kimishige and Teruko Ishizaka, working at the Children's Asthma Research Institute and Hospital in Colorado, demonstrated that the antibody responsible for many allergic reactions was not IgA but a newly isolated gamma globulin. The identification of this new class of immunoglobulin, its designation as immunoglobulin E (IgE) and its central role in immediate-type hypersensitivity reactions were confirmed by the WHO in 1968.[103] Significantly, evidence that IgE possessed the characteristic stereo-chemical and antigenic properties of other antibodies, together with the recognition that it constituted a crucial component of human defences against parasitic worms, reinforced beliefs in the biological parallels between hypersensitivity reactions and the mechanisms of host immunity.

According to some allergists, the discovery of IgE constituted a seminal moment in the transformation of clinical allergy from a 'cinderella subject' into a legitimate science, since it helped to constitute aspects of allergy 'which could be identified and measured and which could help to define the disease'.[104] However, while 'the IgE-related immunological explosion' of knowledge, as one reviewer referred to it in 1973,[105] helped to elucidate the precise mechanisms of Type I hypersensitivity reactions, it also led to disputes about the relationship between laboratory tests and clinical assessments of allergic diseases, thereby opening up traditional frictions between experimental and clinical models of allergy. Since the early twentieth century, allergists had adopted skin tests as the most reliable marker of allergic sensitivity and had often played down the relevance of laboratory investigations of anaphylaxis to the study of human allergies. The identification of IgE and the introduction of novel laboratory tests for measuring levels of IgE in 1967 created the possibility that the allergic basis of many diseases might be revealed with more accuracy by specific scientific investigations.[106] However, early hopes that laboratory analysis might 'rapidly replace the more primitive skin test in clinical practice', as one commentator put it in 1989, proved premature.[107] In spite of the WHO's attempts to establish international standards, researchers were troubled not only by technical differences between laboratories but also by the difficulties involved in correlating levels of IgE with the presence or absence of allergic symptoms and in establishing basal IgE levels, which appeared to vary according to age and sex and which were understood to be influenced by both genetic and environmental factors.[108]

In spite of evident difficulties in matching laboratory results to clinical findings, the naming (and blaming) of IgE as the immunoglobulin responsible for many forms of allergic damage helped to shape the broad field of immunopathology and the narrower field of allergy in the late twentieth century. In the first place, recognition that tissue damage was mediated by an immunoglobulin normally present in the serum and responsible for protection against parasitic diseases, together with demonstrations of the role of auto-antibodies in chronic inflammatory diseases such as thyroiditis and rheumatoid arthritis, reinvigorated debates about the the role of host reactivity in pathology, or about seeing disease in terms of 'trouble from within' rather than as the unmediated expression of an external insult. As Ohad Parnes has suggested, this led in turn to the resurgence of more holistic and ecological accounts of disease that emphasized the 'balance between the reparative and destructive reactivity potentials of the body'.[109] Second, IgE offered new opportunities for the pharmaceutical sector to exploit growing consumer interest in allergies. By providing an ostensibly scientific foundation for diagnosing allergies, laboratory measurements of IgE provided the basis for a range of commercial allergy tests available to both doctors and patients.[110] In addition, demonstrations of the pivotal role of IgE in diseases such as hay fever and asthma encouraged closer attention to the cellular and biochemical pathways and mediators of allergic reactions in the hope of identifying new pharmaceutical strategies not only for treating and preventing the rising tide of allergic disease but also for tapping an expanding global market.

Allergy, medicine and money

In 1983 John Morrison Smith, one of the physicians responsible for bringing the post-war epidemic of asthma deaths to medical and public attention, published his personal reflections on the changing treatment of asthma during his professional life. In particular, he reviewed the range of therapeutic options available to respiratory physicians and allergists during the 1950s and '60s. Although some earlier methods of treatment (such as x-radiation for asthma and nasal cautery for hay fever) had largely been abandoned, it is clear that many of the strategies for preventing or relieving asthma, hay fever and other allergic conditions in the post-war period carried a striking resemblance to those routinely prescribed during the late nineteenth and early twentieth centuries. Thus, physicians continued to recommend allergen avoidance, desensitization, breathing exercises and fresh air in open-air schools or mountain resorts as principal therapeutic and prophylactic measures.[111] While the use of some traditional pharmaceutical preparations (such as opiates or asthma cigarettes containing stramonium or belladonna) persisted,[112] it is also evident that doctors and patients had access to an expanding arsenal of pharmacological agents aimed primarily at relieving allergic symptoms.

The pharmacological treatments available for allergic conditions were diverse. A number of remedies, such as Germolene for eczema or Dristan for hay fever, were available over the counter and were widely advertised in popular magazines and newspapers published in Europe and North America and also, in some instances, throughout the developing world.[113] Other preparations were more carefully controlled and available only on prescription. One of the earliest of a new range of treatments introduced in the twentieth century was ephedrine, which as a component of Ma Huang had been included in a number of traditional Chinese remedies for many centuries. First isolated in the late nineteenth century, ephedrine began to attract clinical attention as a treatment for asthma during the 1920s.[114] In addition, various compounds similar to ephedrine were manufactured and marketed for the treatment of hay fever in Britain and the United States. In the 1930s, for example, benzedrine (a proprietary form of amphetamine sulphate) became popular and served to reshape social stereotypes of patients with allergies: according to a commentary in *The Times* in 1938, at the height of the hay fever season, sufferers were inclined 'to put away their notebooks and fumble for the benzedrine'.[115] Although it was soon displaced by adrenaline (epinephrine) in the treatment of asthma, ephedrine continued to be incorporated into commercial

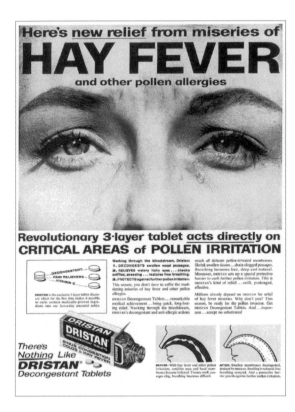

A US magazine advertisement of the 1950s, for decongestant tablets.

preparations well into the post-war period. In the 1960s, for example, the Bayer Products Company was proclaiming the efficacy of Franol (containing ephedrine, theophylline and a barbiturate) or Franol-Plus (with an antihistamine added) for the relief of asthma, bronchitis and hay fever.[116]

Adrenaline had also been isolated and introduced into clinical practice in the early twentieth century, following demonstrations of the pharmacological activity of adrenal extracts in the 1890s and subsequent recognition of the direct bronchodilator effect of adrenaline in the 1900s. During the 1920s injected adrenaline became an important tool in the management of severe asthma and inhaled forms of the drug were also introduced. Awareness of the cardiotoxicity associated with adrenaline and its analogues (linked to their action on both alpha and beta adrenergic receptors), however, led to the introduction of isoprenaline, and the declining use of adrenaline, during the 1940s.[117] Although isoprenaline also demonstrated cardiovascular side-effects, it was not until the late 1960s, shortly after the wave of asthma deaths and the closer regulation of sales of isoprenaline, that the bronchodilator effects of adrenergic agents could be effectively separated from their cardiac effects, and the use of safer, more selective bronchodilators was made possible.

From the late 1930s the place of adrenergic drugs in the treatment of allergies was challenged by the methylxanthines: caffeine, theophylline and aminophylline. Caffeine had been recommended as a treatment for asthma by Henry Hyde Salter and other authors in the mid-nineteenth century, and during the early decades of the twentieth century was included in a number of proprietary asthma preparations. In the 1920s, for example, the British Felsol Company, based in London, asserted that Felsol powder, which combined caffeine with phenazone, anilipyrine and other substances (including the traditional anti-asthmatic lobelia), was 'an ethical non-narcotic preparation indicated in the treatment of bronchial and cardiac asthma, [and] chronic bronchitis'. Citing letters from satisfied doctors, the company's advertising booklet claimed that while 'Adrenaline and other so-called asthma remedies' were temporarily successful in only 50 per cent of cases, Felsol by contrast relieved 80 per cent of patients with asthma.[118] In the 1930s theophylline and aminophylline also became popular, particularly in the United States, and by the 1930s aminophylline had replaced adrenaline in the treatment of acute asthma attacks.[119]

The proliferation of new therapies for allergies during the middle decades of the twentieth century was dependent on dramatic expansion of the pharmaceutical industry. Although a number of manufacturers and retailers had produced various pills and potions from the late eighteenth and early nineteenth centuries, the modern pharmaceutical industry emerged especially in Germany and North America (and to a lesser extent in Britain) during the late nineteenth century, as developments in organic chemistry and physiology made possible the formulation of new pharmacologically active compounds. Driven partly by the increased demand for medicines created by rising population levels and standards of living in the Western world, small businesses expanded. British companies such as Allen & Hanburys, Boots and May & Baker, American firms such as Parke, Davis & Company, and German companies such as Bayer and Hoechst, not only invested in new factories in order to increase production but also established connections with other companies for overseas manufacturing, marketing and distribution of their products. Thus, the American firms Parke, Davis & Company, Abbott, and Burroughs Wellcome all established subsidiary or independent companies and manufacturing bases in Britain during the late nineteenth and early twentieth centuries.[120]

The First World War provided a major impetus to the pharmaceutical industry, stimulating research and development, encouraging partnerships and mergers, and promoting both greater independence and competition within the sector. In particular, many firms continued to expand their overseas activities, laying the foundations for international collaboration (as well as competition) and for the establishment of global pharmaceutical corporations. Drawing on substantial developments in the biomedical sciences, including the isolation of hormones and the development of antimicrobials, during the inter-war years many pharmaceutical companies founded or consolidated dedicated research laboratories and established stronger links with university-based scientists. Intended to increase creativity and productivity, such strategies carried the additional benefits of boosting sales and improving the public image of the industry.[121]

Allergic diseases rapidly became a focus for an expanding pharmaceutical sector. Chemists, druggists and small pharmaceutical firms had been interested in producing medicines for the relief of asthma in the nineteenth century, in particular developing various devices (such as Nelson's inhaler or the bronchitis kettle) for the inhalation of substances that reduced bronchial muscle spasm.[122] In the early twentieth century British and American companies in particular also began to support the production and distribution of pollen preparations used for the diagnosis and treatment of hay fever. In Britain the American firm Parke, Davis & Company was contracted by the Inoculation Department at St Mary's Hospital to market and distribute 'Pollaccine' as well as a wide range of bacterial vaccines. This relationship continued until the 1960s when production was taken over by Beecham Research Laboratories. In the United States, Lederle and Abbott Laboratories and H. K. Mulford Company similarly marketed commercial pollen extracts for use in skin tests and desensitizing treatment.[123] Significantly, the geographical focus of these companies appeared to reflect critical market factors. In 1976, in his survey of the state of allergy for the WHO, Alain de Weck pointed out that up until that time commercial firms had been 'exclusively concerned with problems of industrial countries since the other, for the time being, do not represent a "market"'.[124]

In the middle decades of the twentieth century, and particularly after the Second World War, new understandings of the intercellular mechanisms and inflammatory processes involved in allergy, together with evidence of rising trends in diseases such as asthma, hay fever and eczema, served to stimulate both commercial pharmaceutical and state interest in developing and testing novel medicines. In Britain in the 1950s, for example, the Medical Research Council carried out controlled trials of cortisone acetate in both chronic asthma and status asthmaticus (a form of severe and intractable asthma attack).[125] The importance of such studies lay not only in scientific results of efficacy but also in the financial implications for a National Health Service already strained by rising expenditure on prescriptions and facing a growing epidemic of asthma morbidity. Most therapeutic initiatives, however, came from researchers within the pharmaceutical industry and focused on several discrete strategies: the production of antihistamines, the development of anti-inflammatory corticosteroids, the elaboration of more selective sympath-omimetic bronchodilators and the synthesis of smooth muscle relaxants such as sodium cromoglycate.

As Ulrich Meyer has pointed out, the discovery of the role of histamine in anaphylaxis and allergy encouraged attempts to develop substances that blocked its action, leading for example to the introduction of Torantil in the 1920s and '30s.[126] In 1937 further research was encouraged when Daniel Bovet (1907–1992) and Anne-Marie Staub, working at the Pasteur Institute, reported the antihistamine actions and potential clinical applications of certain pheno-lic ethers.[127] From the early 1940s a number of antihistamines were produced and marketed by European pharmaceutical firms such as Rhône-Poulenc, Hoechst and Bayer, and antihistamines were incorporated in preparations, such as Franol-Plus, which aimed to treat a range of respiratory conditions. The introduction of antihistamines was greeted with considerable enthusiasm on the part of both allergists and pharmaceutical companies. While early medical optimism that antihistamines might alleviate asthma were soon dashed by the results of clinical trials, the new drugs did prove effective in the treatment of hay fever.[128] As pharmaceutical companies were quick to realize, the financial opportunities were as promising as the clinical benefits. In 1955 the British-based firm Allen & Hanburys introduced a new antihistamine, Piriton, based on chlorpheniramine, which had originally been developed by the Schering Corporation in America. As the chairman of Allen & Hanburys made clear, the firm carried high hopes for the new preparation:

> We believe, however, that in Piriton we have made available an antihistamine which comes nearer to the ideal than any other. Being extremely active, its dosage is small, its toxicity low, and the absence of undesirable side effects is a marked characteristic. We believe that this product has a great future.[129]

Although Piriton did indeed become widely prescribed (and subsequently available over the counter) and a central strand of Allen & Hanburys' commercial success in the allergy market, it was soon challenged both by companies producing competing antihistamine preparations and by advocates of familiar techniques such as desensitization. In advertising their diagnostic and therapeutic allergen preparations in 1956, for example, a manual produced by the allergy division of C. L. Bencard Ltd insisted that the involvement of non-histamine mediators limited the impact of antihistamines in 'many cases of hay fever and nearly all cases of asthma, allergic eczema and allergic rhinitis'. In addition, the company's booklet warned that the effects of antihistamines were often transient and that unpleasant side effects were not uncommon. By contrast, it was argued, specific desensitization gave 'prolonged remission of symptoms in a high proportion of cases without continuous medication, and with a minimum of undesirable side effects'.[130] Over subsequent decades, concerns about adverse reactions to early antihistamines, particularly in school children taking examinations, led to the development of non-sedative antihistamines such as terfenadine (Triludan), introduced in the 1980s by Merrell Dow Pharmaceuticals and initially available only on prescription.[131] Awareness of the role of other mediators of inflammation in allergies also encouraged the introduction of drugs that were designed to block the action of leukotrienes or the slow-reacting substance of anaphylaxis (SRSA), which had first been implicated in allergic reactions in the 1940s.[132] Thus, in 1998, Merck launched a leukotriene antagonist, montelukast sodium (Singulair), which received extensive media coverage and which the following year was awarded the Prix Galien for the most innovative and useful pharmaceutical product.[133] In spite of these initiatives, however, Piriton and other early antihistamines remained popular with doctors, patients and health services for the treatment of skin allergies and hay fever. As Pamela Ewan pointed out in a report on hay fever for the Royal College of Physicians in 1989, these supposedly obsolete, primitive antihistamines were known to cause 'sedation in only a proportion of patients, are more effective in some, and are much cheaper'.[134]

During the inter-war years, patients with allergies also benefited from innovative approaches to the treatment of inflammatory conditions such as rheumatoid arthritis, since allergic reactions were known to incorporate a strong inflammatory component. Adrenal extracts were first used in the treatment of asthma in the 1930s, with equivocal results. In 1948, however, American reports of the efficacy of both synthetic cortisone and adrenocorticotrophic hormone (ACTH) in moderating inflammation in patients with rheumatoid arthritis encouraged researchers and pharmaceutical companies in North America and Europe to synthesize the same substances and test them in patients with arthritis and asthma. During the 1950s clinical trials coordinated by the Medical Research Council in Britain indicated the efficacy of both intramuscular and oral cortisone in asthma. However, the adverse effects associated with the long-term use of systemic steroids led to a reluctance on the part of doctors to prescribe them and stimulated attempts to develop locally active compounds for the treatment of both asthma and eczema. In the mid-1950s, for example, hydrocortisone appeared to offer more effective treatment than cortisone for severe inflammatory skin conditions and, in powder form, for asthma.[135]

Subsequent developments in this field were shaped by the takeover of Allen & Hanburys in 1958 by the British pharmaceutical firm Glaxo, which had responded to government challenges by initiating a large project to manufacture corticosteroids. Although Allen & Hanburys continued to trade under its own name, the impact of this shift in pharmaceutical power was evident not just in Britain but eventually throughout the world. In 1963 Glaxo launched Betnovate, which had been developed jointly with the American firm Schering, with whom Glaxo were already collaborating in an attempt to improve overseas sales of the anti-fungal agent griseofulvin. Through skilful advertising, Betnovate rapidly became a market leader in the treatment of inflammatory skin conditions such as eczema and a major source of revenue for Glaxo. Although paediatricians were concerned about side effects and relapses, topical cortisone was recognized to be 'the most valuable preparation in the doctor's armamentorium', capable of transforming 'an itching red oozing skin in a matter of hours'.[136]

During subsequent years, under the research leadership of the Scottish pharmacologist David Jack (b. 1924), Allen & Hanburys in particular strove to develop more potent topically active steroids for the treatment of respiratory diseases and to design pressurized inhalers to improve delivery to the lungs. In the 1960s beclamethasone dipropionate, which had been made available to Jack by Glaxo and incorporated into Propaderm for the treatment of skin conditions, was identified as a suitable candidate for an inhaled steroid. Although early results were not convincing, a British study confirmed the value of inhaled beclomethasone as an alternative to oral steroid therapy.[137] In 1972 beclamethasone was marketed as Becotide for the treatment (or more accurately the prevention) of asthma, and two years later was introduced for the treatment of hay fever as Beconase.[138]

Although, or perhaps because, they revolutionized the management of allergic diseases and contributed substantially to the profits of pharmaceutical companies, corticosteroids were not universally welcomed by allergists on either side of the Atlantic. In particular, clinicians disputed the relative merits of corticosteroids and allergen immunotherapy. While proponents of steroids played down harmful side effects and questioned the ability of allergen immunotherapy to generate clinical improvements, allergists responded by pointing out that the treatment of symptoms was not necessarily the most appropriate approach to allergies and that desensitization had been practised safely and effectively for many years. In a letter to the *Lancet* in 1975, for example, Jonathan Brostoff, a clinical immunologist at Middlesex Hospital in London, emphasized the dangers of certain forms of systemic steroids and complained that an editorial in the same journal had been 'excessively critical of immunotherapy for summer hayfever'.[139] Such disputes should be seen in the context of a rapidly expanding, and increasingly competitive, commercial market for anti-allergy drugs. Although there were clearly international variations in prescribing patterns and trends, and although in the 1970s many novel preparations were yet to be made available worldwide,[140] the potential profits associated with the global distribution of corticosteroids and other anti-allergy remedies were already evident.

In the late 1960s Allen & Hanburys' share of the British (and eventually global) allergy market was increased further with the successful development of a selective bronchodilator. Once again the impetus came from David Jack and his research team. Efforts to synthesize new adrenergic receptor stimulants with selective action on the lungs rather than the heart were brought into sharp relief by the epidemic of asthma deaths in the mid-1960s, in which isoprenaline was thought to be involved. The development of more selective agonists was facilitated by the differentiation between alpha and beta receptors in 1948 and by the further distinction between β_1 and β_2 receptors by Larry Lunts, a chemist working at Allen & Hanburys, in 1967.[141] The following year, the research division at Allen & Hanburys published two articles in which they set out the chemical and clinical features of a novel compound, AH 3365, which was launched in 1969 as a more selective and longer acting beta-agonist than isoprenaline or orciprenaline.[142] Marketed as Ventolin Inhaler, AH 3365 or salbutamol immediately enhanced Allen & Hanburys' commercial standing. According to the company's own account of the development of Ventolin, written to celebrate the thirtieth anniversary of its launch, by 1985 'annual sterling sales had reached £171m; ten years later they exceeded £500m'.[143]

By the early 1970s, salbutamol was also available in tablet and other forms. For example, nebulized salbutamol became increasingly popular in the hospital treatment of acute asthma attacks. Following the practice established in some European countries where domestic nebulizers were common, salbutamol was also administered in Britain via domestic nebulizers at home when NHS funding or private means permitted.[144] However, it was the original, easily recognizable blue Ventolin Inhaler that came to dominate clinical approaches to, and popular images of, asthma. Although regular use of salbutamol was occasionally challenged by concerns about its impact on the long-term management of asthma and although alternative bronchodilators (which were either more selective or combined with steroids) were introduced, inhaled salbutamol became the most widely prescribed inhaler for the immediate control of asthma during the closing decades of the twentieth century. In addition, short-acting β_2-agonists, of which Ventolin was the archetype, were recommended as the first step in asthma management by national and international therapeutic guidelines.[145]

The growing popularity of inhaled bronchodilators such as salbutamol emerged as a graphic reminder of epidemiological trends in asthma and as a potent symbol of wider public concerns about rapid rises in asthma morbidity and mortality. In *Lord of the Flies*, first published in 1954, William Golding had sketched the character of the isolated and delicate asthmatic child familiar to early twentieth-century allergists and psychiatrists studying the allergic constitution: bespectacled, pale, overweight and often ignored by his fellow castaways, Piggy was 'the only boy in our school what had asthma'. In subsequent decades, the public image of asthma began to shift as a number of international athletes acknowledged that they suffered from asthma and as the prevalence of the condition began to increase. By the 1990s overseeing the use of inhalers by rising numbers of asthmatic children had become a major feature of the pastoral duties of school nurses or administrators; no longer a mark of physiological inferiority or singularity, the asthmatic's need for medication apparently conferred both credibility and status.[146] Rather more bizarrely, in 1995 salbutamol's notoriety was also commemorated in the experimental electronic music of Aphex Twin: in a track entitled 'Ventolin', the band incorporated the sound of inhalers.

In the late 1960s the range of drugs available to treat allergies was further boosted by the introduction of sodium cromoglycate. This novel compound was synthesized from a naturally occurring substance, khellin, which was known to act as a smooth muscle relaxant. The development of sodium cromoglycate owed much to the inspiration and persistence of Roger Altounyan (1922–1987), who had worked at Bengers Research Laboratories (part of the Fisons group) since 1956 and who, as a child, had been the model for the character Roger in Arthur Ransome's *Swallows and Amazons* series of children's books. Recognizing the limitations of animal models in asthma research, Altounyan opted to test a range of new compounds on himself, since he had suffered from both asthma and eczema since childhood. After testing nearly 100 compounds using bronchial allergen challenges, Altounyan and his colleagues identified a particular biscromone, FPL 670, with the ability to relax bronchial muscle. The results were published in the *Lancet* and *Acta Allergologica* in 1967.[147] The following year, disodium cromoglycate, applied by a modified Spinhaler, was licensed as Intal, a name derived from the phrase 'interfere with allergy'.[148]

Although its precise mode of action was unknown, disodium cromoglycate attracted immediate interest from allergists and respiratory physicians.[149] In addition, it had a dramatic impact on the financial fortunes of Fisons, rapidly becoming the company's leading product, generating a lucrative global market and stimulating extensive research into the development of analogues that would be active when taken orally. Although early trials at the company's new research facilities in Loughborough proved promising, hopes for an oral alternative to Intal were frustrated. Early compounds, such as FPL 52757, were shown to affect liver enzymes. Proxicromil, or FPL 52787, developed in the late 1970s, looked more promising but animal studies revealed possible carcinogenic properties. Fisons' withdrawal of the drug in 1981 shortly before it was due to be marketed cut over £10m from the company's market value.[150] However, the firm's interest in anti-allergy drugs persisted. In addition to Intal, in the 1970s the company produced Opticrom eye drops, Rynacrom nasal spray, and Nalcrom capsules, which were particularly popular in Italy and Spain for the treatment of food allergies. According to reports of the company's financial fortunes in the wake of the withdrawal of Proxicromil in 1981 and shortly before the patent on Intal was due to expire, Fisons' range of anti-allergy drugs was thought to have 'largely contributed to the huge growth of the group's earnings from pharmaceuticals'.[151]

As the examples of Allen & Hanburys and Fisons demonstrate, the financial benefits to be gained from acquiring a share of the global market for anti-allergy drugs were immense. As private and state expenditure on the treatment and prevention of allergic diseases rose (including the availability and popularity of over-the-counter remedies), the opportunities for pharmaceutical companies to increase their profits soared accordingly. Thus, in the 1990s the market for pharmaceutical products for asthma alone was estimated to be worth in the region of £5.5 billion per annum. In 1995 the best-selling asthma drug worldwide was salbutamol, which GlaxoWellcome had licensed to Schering-Plough for distribution as Proventil in the United States. Glaxo-Wellcome's sales of Ventolin, Becotide and Serevent (and their overseas variants) together amounted to £1.6 billion, making the company the market leader in this field. By the turn of the millennium, every major pharmaceutical company had an anti-allergy product in its top ten commercial sellers. More critically, however, figures suggested that annual sales were also growing significantly. In 1994 the overall sales growth in the asthma market was approximately 14 per cent, markedly higher than the growth rate in either the cardiovascular or the gastrointestinal markets.[152] In 2002 market analysts predicted that GlaxoSmithKline's sales momentum would continue following the introduction of a new asthma treatment, Advair.[153]

Perhaps inevitably, the profits attainable by pharmaceutical companies through the sales of drugs for allergies attracted adverse comments from a number of quarters. Of course, criticism of the industry was not new. In 1933 Charles Forward had bemoaned the fact that 'in this age of commercialism and bureaucracy', manufacturing chemists and research institutes were able to 'make huge profits from the sale of vaccines and similar products', a complaint echoed in A. J. Cronin's comments on hay fever vaccines in *The Citadel*.[154] During the 1930s and '40s the American allergy societies had regularly reviewed their links with the pharmaceutical industry and, in addition to distancing themselves from scientists and clinicians employed by commercial laboratories, had carefully screened advertisements for inclusion in the *Journal of Allergy*.[155] As profits rose after the Second World War, so too did suspicions that pharmaceutical companies were exploiting vulnerable patients for commercial gain. In 1978 a British reporter for *The Times* suggested, in what was presumably an oblique reference to Fisons, that 'the drug company that makes many of the remedies also manufactures a wide range of agricultural chemicals, a common cause of rural hay fever'.[156] At the dawn of the twenty-first century, a number of journalists suggested that the consumption of antihistamines owed more to clever marketing than to demonstrable clinical efficacy, and that people with asthma were 'a vulnerable consumer group' prepared to 'try almost anything to help alleviate the condition'.[157] In addition, they highlighted the manner in which pharmaceutical companies were supposedly promoting multiple allergy syndrome and encouraging the use of antihistamines throughout the year, rather than just during the hay fever season, in order to promote sales.[158] At the same time, a number of alternative practitioners (often operating in direct financial competition with drug companies and orthodox medicine) added their voices to popular concerns by declaring themselves victims of a pharmaceutical conspiracy. In 1997, for example, in a book on the drug-free treatment of asthma that had been developed in the 1950s by the Russian clinician Konstantin Buteyko (1923–2003), Alexander Stalmatski claimed that the Buteyko method was often rejected by asthma experts because it posed 'a serious threat to the profits of drug companies and pharmacists around the world, as well as to the reputations of doctors, hospitals and academics everywhere'.[159]

During the course of its global expansion during the twentieth century, the pharmaceutical industry developed a number of effective strategies for deflecting public criticism and suspicion. Like other companies, those involved in developing and marketing anti-allergy drugs provided financial backing for scientific and clinical studies in universities and research institutes, sponsored research chairs, negotiated deals with laboratories for the production and distribution of allergen preparations, and supported international seminars, symposia and conferences, sometimes in collaboration with the WHO.[160] In addition, pharmaceutical companies funded educational initiatives that included practical manuals and films for doctors (such as those produced by Bencard and Parke, Davis & Company) and leaflets and books for patients, often produced in conjunction with charities devoted to improving both public awareness and professional management of allergic diseases.[161] Finally, the pharmaceutical sector also exploited the power of the media, not only through advertisements in magazines and on television, but also through sponsorship; in 2000, for example, Piriton sponsored weather reports on a British television channel during the hay fever season. Of course, these initiatives often benefited both researchers and patients. At the same time, however, they protected the pharmaceutical industry's investment in developing new treatments for allergic diseases and the rising profits that could be reaped from a global market in allergy.

Exploiting allergy

The financial impact of rising trends in allergic diseases was felt in other industrial and retail sectors during the second half of the twentieth century, both in terms of economic opportunities and in terms of public and political challenges to profit-making and advertising policies. In particular, focusing on allergies became a source of both conflict and revenue for companies in the cleaning, cosmetic and food industries across the world. At the same time, mounting evidence of allergic reactions to an expanding array of pharmaceutical preparations implicated the modern medical profession in the global dissemination of allergic diseases and heightened public anxieties about the impact of the modern domestic and industrial environment on health.

In the first place, growing suspicions of the links between domestic allergens (such as house dust mites and animal danders) and trends in asthma and eczema during the post-war years created opportunities for companies to design and market products (such as vacuum cleaners and bedcovers) aimed at facilitating allergen avoidance. This was not the first time that allergic diseases had stimulated engineering innovations in the cleaning industry. The commercial manufacture of the electric vacuum cleaner by William H. Hoover (1849–1932) in the early twentieth century had initially been driven by a desire to find a solution to dust-induced asthma. In 1907, irritated by the manner in which brushing rugs at work aggravated his asthma, James Murray Spangler (1848–1915), a janitor in a department store in Ohio, had devised and patented a suction machine (his 'carpet sweeper and cleaner') that he hoped would extract dust away from where he was working. Spangler interested first Hoover's wife and then Hoover himself, who bought the patent, established his Electric Suction Sweeper Company, and began manufacturing and selling his first electric vacuum cleaner, Model O, initially in America in 1908 and subsequently across the world.[162] A similar attempt to reduce allergies to straw dust also apparently motivated the production of vacuum cleaners by Bissell.[163]

In the 1980s and '90s, in response to growing public and professional interest in the role of dust in allergy, a number of small companies, such as Medivac Healthcare Limited, HEALTHe Limited, and The Healthy House, began to specialize in designing and distributing vacuum cleaners with high-efficiency particulate air filters, dehumidifiers, mite-proof covers for mattresses, pillows and duvets, and a variety of acaricidal sprays.[164] Attempts to reduce exposure to allergens in this way, or to 'escape the allergen jungle' as one advertising brochure put it,[165] not only drew on early initiatives within the field of clinical allergy, such as the pollen-free chamber or protective masks, but also tapped into traditional Western ideological commitments to creating hygienic homes and into contemporary fears of rising trends in allergies.[166] While such approaches to allergy control were approved in some European countries, where barrier covers were made available through health care providers, in Britain both their efficacy and their legitimacy as medical products

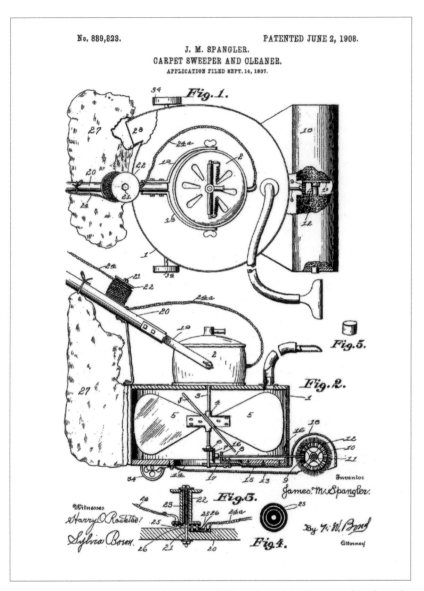

J. M. Spangler's patented 'Carpet Sweeper and Cleaner', 1908 (US Patent and Trademark Office, no. 889,823).

(which would exempt them from VAT) were challenged. However, as critics of the claims made in advertisements for these products implied and as modern fictional accounts of parental anxieties about childhood asthma suggested, consumers continued to purchase expensive vacuum cleaners and other cleaning commodities privately, thereby sustaining a profitable market in anti-allergy devices.[167]

Significantly, the pursuit of profit through the gospel of cleanliness itself created problems. At one level, as I shall argue in the next chapter, increasingly hygienic lifestyles were themselves implicated in rising trends in allergy. In addition, however, dramatic developments in the soap and detergent industry in the post-war years precipitated strident debates about the impact of new occupational and environmental hazards on the prevalence of asthma and eczema. The ability of certain substances (such as soap, silk and wheat flour) to provoke allergic reactions in workers either following inhalation or contact with the skin was well recognized during the early twentieth century.[168] After the Second World War, the incorporation of enzymes in detergents improved the ability of a new wave of 'biological' washing powders to remove stains from clothing and boosted the profits of an expanding soap industry. By 1971 approximately 80 per cent of detergents sold in the United States contained enzymes, resulting in 'retail sales of half a billion dollars'.[169]

A number of researchers, however, began to question the safety of modern detergents, which had already been tentatively indicted as potential causes of cancer by Rachel Carson in her influential exposé of environmental hazards published in 1962.[170] During the late 1960s and 1970s, Michael Flindt, from the Department of Occupational Health in Manchester in the UK, voiced further concerns about the safety of detergents. In several articles, he suggested that proteolytic enzymes derived from Bacillus subtilis could provoke respiratory illness and skin irritation among workers involved in the production of biological washing powders and other detergent products. In 1969, for example, he concluded that 'enzymatic preparations of B. subtilis ('Alcalase' and 'Maxatase') as used in unmodified form in factory conditions had caused sensitisation and allergic chest illness which could be mediated by both type-I and type-III responses'.[171] Significantly, further studies revealed not only the occupational hazard of commercial enzymes but also the potential for chronic low-level exposure to cause asthma and eczema amongst housewives. Flindt's findings provoked bitter disputes between various scientists, government agencies and journalists who supported Flindt's position and leading American detergent manufacturers (such as Proctor & Gamble and Lever Brothers) who, in protecting a lucrative market, 'vigorously defended the safety and efficacy of their enzyme products'.[172]

The political contours of the arguments that ensued were brought out in a lengthy commentary published in the *New Yorker* in 1971. The reporter, Paul Brodeur, supported his fears about an imminent 'public-health hazard of monumental and perhaps irreversible proportions' by quoting the opinions of René Dubos, director of the Department of Environmental Medicine at the Rockefeller University, who suggested that the introduction of any technical innovation should be prohibited until the environmental and human health consequences had been clearly established. At the same time, Brodeur not only exposed the economic interests of the soap and detergent manufacturers but also revealed their startling ignorance of the clinical significance of the problem: at a conference designed to bring the issues out into the open in 1969, the medical director of one of the largest detergent manufacturers was reported to have rejected concerns about enzymes and allergy by insisting that 'in any case, nobody ever dies of asthma'.[173] Manufacturers' attempts to dismiss the problems failed to halt spreading public and professional anxieties. During the 1980s rising levels of occupational asthma and eczema in many developed countries contributed substantially to the economic burden of allergic disease, not only in terms of treatment costs but also in terms of the indirect costs of time off work and sickness benefits.[174] Indeed, in 1982 the British government introduced regulations 'to prescribe occupational asthma as an industrial disease for the purposes of industrial injuries benefit'; according to the regulations, the possible causes included proteolytic enzymes as well as isocyanates, platinum salts, animals and insects, and a variety of fumes and dusts.[175] By the turn of the century, a number of workers had successfully claimed sizeable compensation for work-induced asthma provoked, for example, by contact with flour or chemical disinfectants.[176]

Similar concerns about the allergenic nature of its products also troubled the cosmetics industry in the last quarter of the twentieth century, forcing the industry in new directions and generating high-profile legal cases. Once again, the potential for cosmetics to cause allergic reactions had been recognized much earlier. During the 1950s and '60s, cosmetics were identified as a cause of allergic dermatitis in both ICD 7 (703.6 and 245) and ICD 8 (692.8), textbooks of clinical immunology cited lipstick and other cosmetic products as allergenic, and hair dyes and shampoos were recognized as causes of allergy in various law suits against hairdressers.[177] Critically, in the immediate post-war period, reactions to cosmetics (especially to fragrances) were explained not only in terms of the irritant nature of the chemical constituents but also in terms of idiosyncratic variations in sensitivity. The process of apportioning responsibility in this manner carried significant legal and financial implications. In the case of *Ingham v. Emes* in 1955, for example, the British Appeal Court reversed an award of damages to a client on the grounds that she had failed to notify her hairdresser that she was allergic to the dye; in passing judgement, Lord Justice Birkett concluded that 'the plaintiff was not an ordinary person in that sense at all and, knowing of her peculiarity and failing to disclose it, she disabled herself from relying on the implied warranty'.[178] Equally, in 1956 a domestic guide to 'all medical, marriage and motherhood problems' blamed reactions to cosmetics on the type of 'sensitive skin' that reacted 'unfavourably to intrinsically pure cosmetics, to the eosin (red dye) in lipstick, perhaps, or to the perfume of a soap or powder'.[179] The framing of cosmetic allergies in this way provided the industry with opportunities both to play down the immediate material determinants of cosmetic allergies and to develop new ranges of products that claimed to be designed for 'sensitive skins' or to be 'hypoallergenic'.[180] The financial incentive to advance and protect industrial interests in this way was immense; according to the Women's Environmental Network, by the turn of the millennium British consumers alone were spending £5 billion per year on cosmetics.[181]

In the 1960s and '70s, as the range of synthetic fragrances increased, members of the cosmetics industry established the Research Institute for Fragrance Materials and the International Fragrance Association (founded in 1973), partly in response to an outbreak of a severe form of pigmented contact dermatitis in Japan. The Association in particular attempted to ensure the safe use of fragrances by issuing regulations and guidelines governing the manufacture, handling and testing of fragrances and identifying those ingredients that should not be used.[182] However, the advertising strategies employed by cosmetics companies were increasingly challenged. In the 1980s and '90s, for example, organizations such as the Human Ecology Action League (an American support group for patients with environmental illnesses) began to question the meaning of terms such as 'hypoallergenic' when used in relation to cosmetics.[183] A number of independent studies subsequently revealed that, while consumers believed that the use of 'natural', 'hypoallergenic' and 'dermatologically tested' in advertisements implied that the product was far less likely to cause skin reactions, there were no accepted legal or scientific definitions guiding the application of such terms to particular cosmetics.[184] In spite of efforts to unmask the practices of the cosmetics industry or to expose

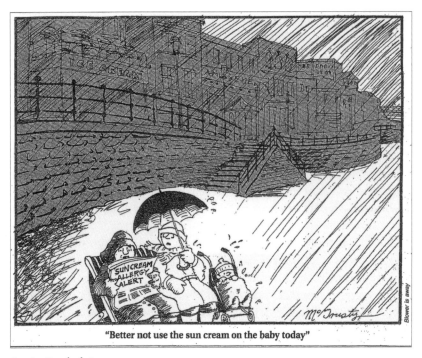

"Better not use the sun cream on the baby today"

Evening Standard, August 2002.

the perils associated with the indiscriminate application of certain lotions and perfumes, and in spite of the attempts of national regulatory bodies, such as the Department of Trade and Industry in Britain and the Food and Drug Administration in the United States, to set clearer standards for the use of terms such as 'hypoallergenic' in marketing material, the industry generally evaded closer regulation of its manufacturing and advertising procedures. As a result, claims on product labels remained 'confusing and potentially misleading' according to some studies.[185] On occasions, the consequences of allergy to cosmetics could be fatal; in August 2000 a woman died following an anaphylactic reaction to hair dyes.[186]

In contrast to the cosmetics industry, the food retail industry was effectively forced to reconsider its manufacturing and food-labelling policies in response to public concerns about allergies. In the post-war period, reports of possible links between childhood allergies and cow's milk led to suggestions that breast-feeding or the use of soy milk might prevent the rise in allergic diseases.[187] Although the nature, and indeed the existence, of a link between cow's milk and allergies was often contested, food manufacturers began to consider ways of developing less allergenic formula milk. Most notably, in the early 1980s, the Swiss food giant Nestlé successfully manufactured a partially hydrolysed formula milk that was intended to reduce mast cell degranulation. According to the company's medical director at that time, Dr Pierre Guesry, Nestlé's interest in allergy was motivated by evidence of rising global trends in allergic diseases and by a belief that allergies constituted one of the major unsolved problems in nutrition. Early clinical trials suggested that the new formula diminished the incidence of wheezing and eczema in children when compared with intact formula milk, and that it was as effective as breast-feeding in preventing the appearance of allergies measured at six months, one year and seven years. Marketed as HA (HypoAllergenic) in Europe and as Goodstart in the United States, Nestlé's new formula milk contributed to the company's emergence as the market leader in nutritional research and as the world's largest food group.[188]

While Nestlé's involvement in allergy research was promoted by awareness of both the health benefits and the financial profits to be gained from developing hypoallergenic products for sale in a global market, contemporary policy changes in the food retail industry were also prompted by broader anxieties about food and allergy. Until the 1990s the primary focus for discussions between manufacturers, doctors, policy makers and the public was the possibility that food additives, such as synthetic preservatives and colourings, might be linked to asthma as well as a range of behavioural disorders in children. During the 1970s and '80s concerns about the role of food additives in hyperactivity in particular generated widespread support for additive-free diets such as that proposed by the American paediatrician and allergist Benjamin F. Feingold (1900–1982).[189] In the mid-1990s, however, anxieties in many Western countries shifted dramatically following a number of tragic deaths linked to anaphylactic reactions to peanuts. Deaths from peanut and nut allergy were regularly reported in the popular press in Britain and extensively discussed in North American and European medical journals. As a result, clinicians across the world advocated immediate action to raise awareness of anaphylaxis, encouraged patients to wear Medic-Alert bracelets, and called for the food industry to label products more clearly 'so that even the smallest amount of potentially lethal foodstuffs may be clearly identified'.[190]

Public and professional pressure for reform was reinforced by guidelines and advice published by state regulatory authorities. In the mid-1990s, for example, several Canadian school boards introduced policies designed not only to reduce the risk of severe allergic reactions to peanuts and other food products in school children but also 'to minimize the legal liability of school boards'.[191] Similarly, in the late 1990s the British Department of Health's Committee on Toxicity of Chemicals in Food, Consumer Products and the Environment established a working group on peanut allergy. In 1998 the group's report suggested that the rise in morbidity and mortality from peanut allergy may have been triggered either by a general increase in atopic diseases or by the increased consumption of peanuts by pregnant and breast-feeding mothers, leading to early sensitization. The trends, however, were also fuelled by substantial changes in the British diet. Following the introduction of peanuts around the Second World War, the regular inclusion of peanuts in pre-packed meals and the growing consumption of Indian, Chinese and Mexican cuisine greatly increased the risk of exposure and allergic reactivity. In addition to highlighting the need for further research, the working group also advised atopic women, and those with atopic partners or children, to avoid peanuts during pregnancy and lactation, and advocated clearer labelling of foodstuffs to indicate the presence of peanuts.[192]

In response to demands from consumers, from national governments and international organizations such as the WHO, and from societies such as the Anaphylaxis Campaign (founded in 1994 by David Reading, whose daughter had died from peanut allergy the previous year),[193] food manufacturers and retailers were forced to provide more detailed information about ingredients and clearer notices about the possible presence of nuts (and indeed other allergens) in products for sale in restaurants and shops. Accordingly, British companies such as J. Sainsbury PLC, Tesco, Marks & Spencer and Thorntons, as well as American firms such as McDonald's, produced their own advice booklets, made available on request full lists of products that might contain nuts and other problematic ingredients, and displayed signs in their stores.[194] While such strategies undoubtedly helped allergy sufferers, they also carried distinct benefits for the food industry. At the start of the twenty-first century, the market for anti-allergy foods, that is foods supposedly free from potential allergens, was expanding considerably. Driven by consumer belief in the prevalence of food allergies as well as by contemporary preoccupations with dieting, body image and nutritional health, in 2002 the British market alone for anti-allergy foods was worth approximately £55 million, with the expectation that it would reach nearly £140 million by 2007.[195]

As these examples from diverse commercial contexts suggest, during the last decades of the twentieth century manufacturing and retail policies and practices were driven not only by concerns about changing patterns of health and sickness but also by economic considerations; the money to be made, or indeed lost, from allergy was often considerable. At the same time, they testify to the manner in which novel constituents of the modern domestic and industrial environment were increasingly implicated in rising trends in allergies. Indeed, for many commentators, the spread of allergies was a potent manifestation of the pathology of progress, a marker of the inevitable downside of Western industrialized lifestyles. Significantly, medicine was not exempt from this critique. As the range of novel pharmaceutical agents proliferated and the consumption of drugs rose after the Second World War, drug allergies appeared to mirror the general epidemiological trends set by hay fever, asthma and eczema. In 1962 the Nobel Prize-winning Australian immunologist Frank Macfarlane Burnet (1899–1985) warned that drug sensitivity was becoming 'the bugbear of modern medicine'.[196] Over the next two decades surveys by the WHO revealed the manner in which drug allergy was 'growing in importance' in both developed and developing countries and outlined the multiple immunological mechanisms and diverse clinical symptoms that could be provoked by adverse reactions to drugs such as penicillin, gentamycin, analgesics and tranquillizers.[197] By the 1980s penicillin was the largest cause of anaphylaxis in the United States, where penicillin allergy was estimated to result in between 400 and 800 deaths per year.[198] Of course, the role of medicine in inducing allergy was not unfamiliar. Clemens von Pirquet's original conception of the term had been inspired by observations of idiosyncratic reactions to serum therapy, and the reformulation of asthma and allergy in the post-war period had arguably been precipitated by the introduction of isoprenaline forte. Like the emergence of allergies to cosmetics, peanuts and cleaning products, however, the gradual eruption of drug allergies as a major form of iatrogenic illness at the end of the twentieth century confirmed beliefs in the manifold hazards of modern civilization.

5

CIVILIZATION AND DISEASE

It is seldom recognized that each type of society has diseases peculiar
to itself – indeed, that each civilization creates its own diseases.

René Dubos, 1961[1]

As the global network of allergists expanded under the aegis of national
immunological societies and the World Health Organization and as public
interest in allergies deepened during the 1960s and '70s, speculative estimates
of the prevalence of allergic diseases in the modern world were replaced by
more substantial empirical evidence of precise geographical and temporal
trends in allergy. Detailed surveys of the global pattern of allergies immediately challenged longstanding beliefs that allergic diseases were largely
confined to the Western world. Indeed, studies of asthma in remote locations
such as Tristan da Cunha, the Maldive Islands and Tanzania revealed prevalence rates often exceeding those found in many developed Western countries. In spite of such evidence from isolated populations, epidemiological
surveys of the prevalence of allergies in migrants who had moved from developing countries to the West, careful analysis of changing patterns of disease
following greater contact between indigenous non-Western populations and
European or North American visitors, and confirmation of a persistent
urban–rural gradient in many forms of allergy, collectively suggested that
some particular feature of Western civilization and urbanization might be
responsible for rising levels of allergic diseases throughout the world. Increasingly regarding the proliferation of harmful allergic reactions as a direct product of the processes of globalization and modernization, epidemiologists and
allergists thus sought to identify the specific 'Westernization factor' that
might explain modern trends in allergy.[2]

Epidemiological attempts to establish the aetiology of allergic diseases
more accurately were, however, beset by methodological and conceptual
problems. Widely differing approaches to diagnosis, conflicting interpretations of statistical evidence, the absence of adequate surveys and sufficient
information from many geographical regions, and the possibility that the
environmental and genetic determinants of allergic sensitivity might vary
according both to location and to the precise clinical manifestation of allergy,
served to render generalizations about aetiology meaningless. Under these

conditions, the communal quest for a rational explanation of global trends in allergies paradoxically became increasingly fragmented as allergists struggled to isolate the discrete factor or factors that might explain local, as well as global, incidence and prevalence rates. In particular, clinicians and scientists around the world focused, often rather narrowly, on the possible impact of distinct health hazards supposedly intrinsic to modern Western lifestyles: shifting patterns of outdoor allergens and air pollution; the proliferation of allergens in the domestic environment; dietary changes; decreasing family size; and the adoption of more hygienic lifestyles. The aim of this chapter is to explore the manner in which the explosion of competing explanations for temporal and geographical trends in allergic diseases during the late twentieth century was framed by growing concerns about the health risks associated with modern civilization.

The risk society

In a short introductory handbook on allergy published in 1961, the physician Kenneth Hutchin considered a range of explanations for rising trends in allergic diseases during the twentieth century. According to Hutchin, whose publications included popular advice books on diet, sex, the health of businessmen and the perils of domestic life, it was possible that allergies appeared to be increasing simply because they were correctly diagnosed more often or because the potential for Western populations to develop allergies had been unmasked by dramatic reductions in mortality rates from infectious diseases and by associated increases in life expectancy. In addition, Hutchin suggested that as the result of greater immunological knowledge allergic reactions were now more commonly implicated in the pathogenesis of conditions previously understood in terms of other causes. As he pointed out, 'the trend of modern medicine tends to point to more and more conditions being due to allergy'. Significantly, however, Hutchin also related contemporary trends in allergies to conspicuous changes in the modern environment and modern lifestyles: 'Last and certainly not least is the increased risk of contact with irritative material in modern life.'[3]

Hutchin was not alone in connecting patterns of allergic diseases to modern living. In the 1950s George Payling Wright (1898–1964), Professor of Pathology at Guy's Hospital in London, had also highlighted the impact of the material environment on trends in health and hypersensitivity:

> The introduction into medicine, industry and domestic life of many new and highly reactive chemicals capable of combining

with proteins in the skin and other tissues has resulted in both men and women being exposed to much greater risks of acquiring allergic diseases now than formerly.[4]

Similarly, in a series of lectures on the interplay between the 'factual and verifiable components' of science and its 'imaginative and emotional determinants', delivered at the Brookhaven National Laboratory in 1960, the microbiologist René Dubos wondered at the dramatic transitions in patterns of disease that had been wrought by fundamental shifts in the fabric of modern lives since the Second World War.

> Coming now to our own times, who could have dreamed a generation ago that hypervitaminosis would become a common form of nutritional disease in the Western World; that the cigarette industry, air pollutants, and the use of radiations would be held responsible for the increase in certain types of cancer; that the introduction of detergents and various synthetics would increase the incidence of allergies; that advances in chemotherapy and other therapeutic procedures would create a new staphylococcus pathology; that alcoholics and patients with various forms of iatrogenic diseases would occupy such a large number of beds in the modern hospital?[5]

Of course, evaluations of the impact of modern lifestyles on health were not new. In the eighteenth century, writers such as George Cheyne, William Cadogan and Thomas Trotter had bemoaned the manner in which intemperance, lack of exercise and over-indulgence in exotic and spicy imported foods were collectively leading to epidemics of nervous diseases, gout and alcoholism among the British upper classes.[6] In the nineteenth century, a similar refrain was taken up by George Beard in America and Charles Blackley in England. According to both Beard and Blackley, the proliferation of a range of nervous disorders, including hay fever, could be traced to substantive changes in the pace and pressure of Western civilization. Indeed, Blackley expressly warned that the prevalence of hay fever would increase as civilization advanced.[7] As Charles Rosenberg has pointed out, such persistent concerns about the pathology of progress proved persuasive not only because they reflected dramatic shifts in the epidemiology of disease in the face of social and economic growth, but also because they provided a vehicle for the expression of extensive reservations about the direction of social and political reform and about the creation of new market relations in emergent capitalist economies.[8]

Notwithstanding evident continuities in the rhetorical force of concerns about the downside of modernity, the language and focus of comments by Hutchin, Wright and Dubos in the 1960s reveal two distinctive features of late twentieth-century formulations of the relationship between civilization and disease, namely a preoccupation with the environmental determinants of allergy and epidemiological interest in the notion of risk. In the first place, post-war commentators betrayed resurgent beliefs that technological and industrial innovations had introduced new environmental sources of disease. As civilization had progressed, so too had exposure to a widening range of substances capable of provoking allergies; by the end of the twentieth century, the human (and indeed other animal) populations of most developed countries were thought to be floating in an expansive ocean of allergens, spawned particularly by the processes of industrialization and urbanization. Thus, allergens were ever-present in the outdoor air, in the home and in the workplace; they lingered in food and drink, emanated from cars and buses, and were released into the atmosphere from toys, electrical appliances and animals; and they constituted potent irritants for skin exposed to jewellery, cosmetics and medicines.

The environmental distribution of allergens generated by modern civilization and the different levels of exposure to those allergens were used to account not only for rising global trends in allergy but also for regional and geographical variations in allergic diseases. Thus the presumed association between allergens and the industrial processes that characterized modern Western society was mobilized to explain the apparent predominance of allergies in urban environments, the increased expression of allergic diseases in migrants moving from rural into urban areas, and the gradient in prevalence between the developed and developing worlds.[9] Significantly, even ethnic differences were often explained in terms of lifestyle and environment, rather than in terms of inherent racial predispositions. Thus in 1986 a report from the WHO cited evidence from the United States, New Zealand, Nigeria and Tristan de Cunha, as well as studies of immigrants, in supporting its conclusion that geographic and racial differences in prevalence were 'more likely to be due to environmental factors such as feeding and the presence of common allergens than to racial, genetic factors'.[10] British studies of trends in hay fever and asthma in the 1980s similarly dismissed genetic factors in favour of modifications in diet or increased 'contamination of the environment by potential irritants'.[11]

Preoccupations with the environmental determinants of allergy did not entirely discourage scientific attempts to clarify the possible role of genetic factors in asthma and hay fever. A familial predisposition to certain allergic diseases (or atopy) had been recognized in the early twentieth century, and various studies during the inter-war years had identified the impact of heredity both on the expression of hypersensitivity and on the age of onset of clinical symptoms.[12] In the post-Second World War period, scientists and clinicians across the world continued to search for the gene or genes that might be responsible for determining immunological reactivity to allergens. In particular, evidence of varying prevalence rates in racial groups sharing a common environment, as well as studies of twins and inbred populations, supported suspicions that genetic factors remained important.[13] The range of scientific investigations of putative hereditary mechanisms was extremely broad. While some investigators exploited novel genotyping techniques in order to identify genes on specific chromosomes (coding for IgE receptors, for example) or to demonstrate linkages with immune response genes, such as those in the Major Histocompatibility Complex,[14] others either employed detailed epidemiological studies in attempts to establish the precise mode of inheritance or explored the putative association between atopic disease and selective immunodeficiency states, most notably IgA deficiency.[15] Thus, although many allergists certainly focused increasingly on the environmental causes of modern trends in allergy, race, ethnicity and family history continued to be regarded as critical predisposing factors and, not unexpectedly, to attract considerable media interest.[16]

Formulations of inheritance as a predisposing factor for the expression of allergy illustrate the second striking feature of the comments by Hutchin, Wright and Dubos, namely their emphasis on risk. During the 1960s and '70s it became increasingly common for clinicians on either side of the Atlantic to evaluate both environmental and genetic causes of allergy in terms of risk; thus, while Hutchin and Wright tentatively referred to the risks generated by exposure to chemical irritants, over subsequent years researchers exploited complex demographic and statistical analyses in order to identify the diverse 'risk factors' operating in allergic diseases.[17] The emergence of risk factor analysis in studies of allergy reflected general trends in epidemiology in the post-war period. The practice of evaluating risk had been developed by the insurance industry during the late nineteenth and early twentieth centuries. Merging probability theory with new statistical tools, insurance companies attempted to predict mortality rates initially according to age and sex, but subsequently 'extended this principle to other characteristics, including occupations, build, and blood pressure, which they termed risk factors'.[18] By the 1960s the results of major studies aimed at identifying risk factors in coronary artery disease and lung cancer, combined with growing interest in devising preventative measures for chronic non-infectious diseases, had served to consolidate the utility of epidemiological assessments of risk. There were, of course, challenges to risk-factor analysis. In the post-war period contemporaries criticized the manner in which it led to victim-blaming, tended to displace laboratory research and clinical experience, and carried problematic legal implications. More recently, historians and social scientists have also exposed the manner in which the 'culture of risk management' provided state agencies with a powerful means of moralizing and regulating certain forms of supposedly dangerous individual and group behaviour.[19] Nevertheless, in the decades after the Second World War the identification and reduction of risk increasingly dominated clinical, epidemiological and public health conceptions of disease.

In the field of allergy, as in studies of cancer and heart disease, the range of potential risk factors was understood to be broad, encompassing genetic determinants of disease, bodily and mental characteristics, environmental and occupational factors, and various lifestyle triggers such as diet, smoking, levels of exercise, alcohol consumption and hygiene.[20] Indeed, one of the striking features of new epidemiological preoccupations with risk was the manner in which the causation of disease was now conceived in complex, multifactorial terms rather than in terms of a single aetiological agent, an approach that had previously been popularized by germ theories of disease during the late nineteenth century. As a number of sociological studies have suggested, the multifactorial assessments of risk espoused by epidemiologists were routinely shared by patients and their families, who also understood the cause of their allergies in terms of interactions between environmental, lifestyle and genetic factors.[21] It is important, however, to recognize that there were distinct socio-economic, political and cultural features of late twentieth-century discourses on risk. In the 1980s the influential German social scientist Ulrich Beck explicitly linked the emergence of risks, and the intellectual and political meanings of risk, to the processes of modernity. 'Risk may be defined', he argued, 'as a systematic way of dealing with hazards and insecurities induced and introduced by modernization itself. Risks, as opposed to older dangers, are consequences which relate to the threatening force of modernization and to its globalization of doubt.'[22] From this perspective, modern risks (conceived by Beck largely in terms of environmental pollutants) were the inevitable product of capitalist strivings for wealth: 'In advanced modernity the social production of wealth is systematically accompanied by the social production of risks.'[23] Thus, historically, formulations of risk emerged in those parts of the world where 'genuine material need' had been reduced 'through the development of human and technological productivity' and where new hazards had been 'unleashed to an extent previously unknown'.[24] Under those circumstances of environmental uncertainty, people were living precariously on what Beck termed 'the volcano of civilization'.[25]

Both the emergence of risk-factor analysis and environmentalist exposés of the historical determinants and the political and moral contours of risk discourse encouraged scientists and clinicians to focus more energetically on unmasking the external environmental, rather than internal genetic, causes of allergy. In many ways, this process ran counter to clinical preoccupations with individual patterns of sensitivity, which allergists routinely attempted to reveal with skin tests and to modify with desensitization. In addition, environmental approaches to allergy challenged the legitimacy of the pharmaceutical industry's commitment to deeper laboratory research into the biochemical mechanisms of allergy and the subsequent development of drugs that modified immunological reactivity. However, in line with emergent ecological sensibilities that highlighted the dangers posed by Western civilization to the global environment as well as to health, the risk factor approach to the prevention of disease facilitated new models of clinical intervention and health policy that prioritized the identification of those threatening aspects of modern lifestyles that might explain both global trends in allergic diseases and periodic exacerbations of symptoms in individual patients. Thus, just as cancer specialists strove to detect the presence and potency of new carcinogens in the late twentieth century, so too allergists toiled to characterize new allergens that might be floating in the atmosphere, lurking in the material constituents of the indoor environment, or concealed in food, drink and drugs.

Pollen and pollution

From the first stirrings of allergy in the mind of Clemens von Pirquet in the early twentieth century, pollen released into the atmosphere from grasses, trees, shrubs and flowers constituted the archetypal allergen. Feared by hay fever sufferers, revered by allergists for its biological potency, captured and measured by aerobiologists, dissected by botanists, manipulated and

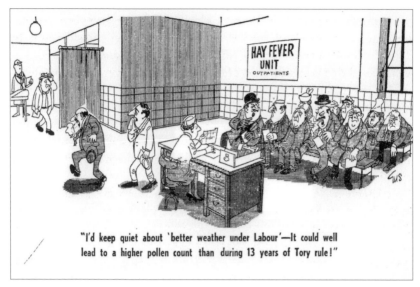

"I'd keep quiet about 'better weather under Labour'—It could well lead to a higher pollen count than during 13 years of Tory rule!"

Evening News, June 1970.

commercially exploited by drug companies, employed by forensic scientists and palaeologists as a tool for dating suspicious deaths,[26] and celebrated by historians as a form of dust that defied historically constructed boundaries between pure nature and impure civilization (or between purity and pollution),[27] pollen also generated research institutes dedicated to its study, such as the National Pollen Research Unit in Worcester, England, and was exploited by cartoonists as a potent vehicle for political parody. Perhaps more strikingly, at the turn of the millennium the liberal dissemination of pollen in the global atmosphere was identified in popular culture as the quintessential symbol of ecological disharmony, as a metaphor for drug abuse and sexual licence, and as an evocative marker of the crisis of modernity. References to pollen thus appeared in creative outbursts as diverse as Marilyn Manson's lyrical 'Diamonds and pollen', 'The pop singer's fear of the pollen count' by The Divine Comedy, and Jeff Noon's stark metaphorical cyberfantasy, aptly entitled simply *Pollen*, which imagined the devastation wrought by nature's revenge against the cancerous spread of the urban landscape.[28]

Soon after pollen had been identified as the elemental cause of hay fever and subsequently framed as an exemplary allergen, longitudinal regional studies and sweeping national and international surveys rapidly exposed temporal trends and geographic variations in pollen concentrations in the atmosphere. The seasonal distribution of different pollens released from trees, grasses and flowers was immediately evident to botanists and allergists and specific cycles of exposure were used to account for contrasting national patterns and individual manifestations of hay fever. While most British sufferers experienced the symptoms of hay fever in the summer months as the result of the grass pollen season, American hay-feverites were more fearful of the autumnal release of ragweed pollen. In other countries, sufferers were plagued predominantly by tree pollen released into the atmosphere according to botanical rhythms and climatic conditions: when hay fever was first described in Japan, it appeared to be triggered most commonly by pollen from the Japanese cedar tree, while in southern France, China and Italy, plane and cypress trees provoked the greatest allergic responses. Similarly, asthma was apparently uncommon in Kuwait until the importation of *Prosopis* trees in the 1950s.[29] Pollen thus constituted not only a global allergen, responsible for hay fever and asthma across the world, but also an allergen with peculiarly local or regional distribution and significance.

As allergists and botanists, often working either for or in conjunction with pharmaceutical companies, began to compile detailed pollen maps and to distribute daily pollen counts during the middle decades of the twentieth century, they also revealed the close association between levels of atmospheric pollen and climatic conditions.[30] Thus, studies in the 1960s, '70s and '80s demonstrated the influence of wind speed and direction and heavy rainfall on the pollen content of the air.[31] Features of the built environment, as well as climatic variations, were also thought to determine patterns of pollen in urban spaces. The relative absence of trees and grasses in heavily built-up areas, in addition to the dispersal of pollen by turbulent winds around tall buildings, generally served to lower the pollen count in cities and towns.[32] As Gregg Mitman has shown, however, in some locations the successful colonization of inner city wastelands and parks by ragweed proved especially problematic in early twentieth-century North America, prompting local and national public health and agricultural services to establish policies designed to eradicate this urban dissident.[33] In New Orleans during the 1910s, for example, the commissioner of public works made available 20 convicts 'who cleared the streets and side-walks of the outer sections of the city of the weeds, in accordance with a map prepared by the topographic committee' of the American Hay-Fever Prevention Association.[34] Similar efforts to exterminate or control what British aerobiologists referred to as the 'super allergenic urban weed' were made in Montreal during the 1930s and subsequently in Japan and several European countries infected by ragweed seeds imported accidentally from North America.[35] Such concerns about pollen pollution in towns and cities continued to shape debates about urban planning and agricultural policies deep into the twentieth century; at the European Allergy Workshop in 1998, for example, one contributor exposed the absurdity of continuing to plant birch and *Fraxinus*, two intensely allergenic trees, in towns and the grounds of infant schools.[36]

Carefully established temporal and geographic variations in atmospheric pollen counts were used to explain national and seasonal patterns of hay fever and asthma. In the post-Second World War period, seasonal fluctuations in pollen concentrations were also mobilized by clinicians seeking to account for observations that the prevalence of allergies in children varied according to the month of birth. In the 1970s a number of British studies suggested that children, especially girls, born between December and February (that is, just before the major release of grass pollen into the atmosphere) exhibited a greater prevalence of hay fever than children born at other times of the year; by contrast, asthma was more common in children born between May and October, shortly before the autumnal rise in house-dust mite concentrations.[37] While research in other countries revealed slightly different monthly associations, dictated by seasonal patterns of pollen release from major allergenic plants in those locations, and while some authors contested the consistency of the findings, the results of subsequent studies tended to confirm the general principle that exposure to allergens in early life increased the expression of atopic diseases.[38] Allergists generally explained the association in terms of immunological immaturity: transient deficiency in IgA in young babies was thought to leave the immune system vulnerable to allergenic challenge.[39]

However, while aerobiological studies of pollen helped to clarify certain epidemiological features of hay fever in the modern world, other trends remained enigmatic. In particular, it became clear that pollen levels could not explain the rising trends in hay fever that were evident in most developed countries in the last half of the twentieth century. Indeed, as a number of authors suggested, while the prevalence of hay fever was increasing on both sides of the Atlantic from the 1960s, both the length of the pollen season and levels of pollen in the atmosphere were steadily declining as the result of urban expansion, the cultivation of less prolific pollen-producing plants, the deleterious effect of car pollution on plant life, and shifting agricultural practices, such as early harvesting to make grass silage.[40] Faced with this apparent paradox, as well as with reports of the greater prevalence of hay fever in cities than in rural areas and with evidence that farmers' children were less likely than their peers to suffer from hay fever, allergists and respiratory physicians turned to alternative explanations for modern trends in allergies. In particular, they sought both to identify additional allergenic components of the outdoor atmosphere and to determine the possible impact of changing patterns of environmental pollution on the manifestations of allergy.

Biological constituents of the outdoor environment other than pollen were known to provoke not only local manifestations of allergy, such as hay fever and asthma, but also systemic, sometimes life-threatening, anaphylactic reactions. Perhaps the most well-known threat came from stinging insects. Severe idiosyncratic reactions to bee and wasp stings had been described in ancient medical texts and over subsequent centuries doctors had reported occasional fatalities.[41] In the late nineteenth and early twentieth centuries, as interest in both toxins and hypersensitivity blossomed, reports of complications, including sudden death, appeared regularly in medical journals.[42] At that time, adverse reactions to stings were generally explained in terms of the direct action of a toxin or as the result of the injection of 'an urticaria-producing bacillus' along with the venom.[43] However, shortly after Charles Richet and Clemens von Pirquet had set out the major experimental and clinical features of anaphylaxis and allergy, clinicians began to suspect the involvement of immunological mechanisms in the pathogenesis of reactions to bee and wasp stings. Thus, in 1914 a British physician, A. T. Waterhouse, proposed that the sudden onset of symptoms, the cardio-respiratory effects and the history of previous exposure were all 'strongly suggestive of anaphylaxis'.[44] Allergists consequently attempted to desensitize patients against stinging insects, initially with whole body extracts until, in the 1950s, Mary Hewitt Loveless (1899–1991) introduced the use of pure venom, carefully extracted from the venom sacs, for both diagnostic and therapeutic purposes.[45]

In spite of the development of more effective prophylaxis and indeed better therapeutic measures (such as convenient preparations of adrenergic agents), anxiety about insect stings and the perils of outdoor life at certain times of the year persisted. In the 1950s insect stings were estimated to account for nearly one death each week in the United States, leading clinicians on both sides of the Atlantic to call for greater education of patients and doctors about the benefits of desensitization and about the importance of carrying emergency supplies of oral isoprenaline or injectable adrenaline.[46] Although this advice was subsequently echoed in newspaper articles which referred to 'the annual nightmare' of the wasp season for allergy sufferers and which advised patients to keep emergency kits close at hand,[47] some clinicians suggested that the risk of severe or fatal reactions had been overestimated and that allergists were alarming the public unnecessarily. In the 1980s, for example, Howard S. Rubenstein argued that the risk of suffering from a fatal bee or wasp sting in the United Kingdom was one in five million; similarly, he pointed out that annual deaths from stings in the United States (approximately 40) were dwarfed by deaths from motor accidents (50,000), drowning (6,000) and lightning (115). In a summary that neatly reflected contemporary preoccupations with the epidemiology of risk, Rubenstein concluded not only that patients should be liberated from 'unrealistic fears of highly improbable events' but also that, given the inability of doctors to identify children 'at risk', the use of immunotherapy (which was expensive and also potentially dangerous) could not be justified.[48] As I shall argue in chapter Six, while some commentators acknowledged the validity of Rubenstein's 'warning against an exaggerated fear of bee stings', debates about the value of immunotherapy in such cases continued to haunt modern allergists.[49]

Bees and wasps were not the only outdoor insects and arachnids thought to be responsible for allergic reactions. During the second half of the twentieth century, allergists in various geographical locations also described hypersensitivity reactions (including skin irritation, asthma and rhinitis) to midges, mites, fire ants and locusts: in 2003, for example, a swarm of locusts in central Sudan apparently triggered an asthma epidemic in which eleven people died and more than 1,500 were admitted to hospital.[50] In addition, allergists began to recognize more clearly the role of mould or fungal spores in the atmosphere. The possibility that inhaled spores might operate as potent aeroallergens in asthmatic patients had been suggested by Willem Storm van Leeuwen in the 1920s, and his ideas had initiated collaboration between allergists and mycologists in British hospitals and allergy departments.[51] During the post-Second World War period, allergists and respiratory physicians around the world became increasingly interested in determining the allergenicity of fungal spores in domestic, occupational and outdoor environments. In particular, spores from *Aspergillus fumigatus* were implicated in a specific form of allergic alveolitis occurring most commonly in farmers exposed to mouldy hay (when it was referred to as farmer's lung) and in people who kept birds (pigeon-, bird- or budgerigar-fancier's lung). Studies revealed not only that allergic bronchopulmonary aspergillosis was mediated by a mixture of Type I and Type III (and possibly Type IV) hypersensitivity reactions to spores in the atmosphere but also that genetic factors might be important.[52] Although the role of *Aspergillus* in other cases of asthma remained unclear, fears that mould allergies (and other conditions) were being spread by flocks of feral pigeons led to attempts in some countries to devise strategies (much like earlier ragweed elimination policies) aimed at culling the wild bird population and reducing the burden of zoonotic diseases. In 2003, for example, concerns about the health risks posed by birds in Trafalgar Square in London encouraged Ken Livingstone, the Mayor of London, to introduce fines for anyone caught feeding the pigeons.[53]

While exposure to fungal spores was well recognized as an immediate trigger of allergic reactions in certain individuals, it was not implicated in rising global, or specific national, trends in allergy. Indeed, it would appear that the number of people keeping pigeons in Britain, for example, fell during the period in which asthma was increasing in both frequency and severity.[54] Thus, in addition to exploring changing concentrations of allergens in the outdoor environment, allergists were forced to consider the possibility that other atmospheric factors, most notably air pollution, might be responsible for aggravating allergies. Historically, doctors had recognized a link between levels of atmospheric smoke and fumes, on the one hand, and respiratory conditions, on the other, at least since the seventeenth century, and indeed sporadically for much longer.[55] It was during the Industrial Revolution of the late eighteenth and early nineteenth centuries, however, that urban smoke was identified as a major and spreading health hazard in Britain and subsequently in other modernizing countries. As industrial expansion and urbanization led to the increased, but often inefficient, combustion of coal in domestic as well as manufacturing settings, smoke pollution became a problem not only in London and large British provincial industrial centres such as Manchester, but also in Europe (Essen and Cologne, for example), North America (Chicago, Pittsburgh, Ohio and Pennsylvania), Canada (Toronto), Japan (Osaka), Australia (Melbourne), and indeed elsewhere.[56]

During the middle decades of the nineteenth century, doctors and politicians expressed growing concerns about the impact of atmospheric smoke on health. As Bill Luckin has shown in a number of articles on air pollution in Britain in the late nineteenth and early twentieth centuries, the weekly returns of the Registrar-General regularly attributed the excess deaths in the capital from bronchitis, pneumonia and whooping cough to a combination of London fog and pollution.[57] These concerns persisted into the early decades of the twentieth century, underwriting contemporary interest in open-air colonies for consumptives and open-air schools for children with tuberculosis, bronchitis and asthma, and fuelling the fashion for taking holidays in mountainous or coastal 'respiratory resorts', where the air was supposedly cleaner and more invigorating than the polluted urban atmosphere. Of course, rural or coastal open-air colonies and schools offered patients with respiratory disorders much more than merely cleaner air; improvements in health were also attributed to better diets, physical exercise and removal from the pressures and stresses of home. Nevertheless, the promotion of clean air as both a preventative and therapeutic measure testifies to contemporary Western concerns about the impact of urban air pollution on public health.

In the late nineteenth and early twentieth centuries, anxieties about the economic and medical repercussions of rising levels of air pollution stimulated a number of initiatives on both sides of the Atlantic. In Britain, public health legislation incorporated tentative smoke abatement clauses, the government initiated official inquiries and, in 1912, established the Advisory Committee on Atmospheric Pollution, and pressure groups such as the National Smoke Abatement Society (later the National Society for Clean Air), which was formed in 1929 by the merger of societies in London and Manchester, campaigned for greater state regulation of pollution.[58] In a similar vein, Chicago City Council introduced the first American air pollution law in 1881 and during the first half of the twentieth century many other North American industrial cities, such as St Louis and Pittsburgh, introduced more effective regulation.[59] However, legislation, government inquiries and local activism made little overall difference to levels of smoke production in the late nineteenth and early twentieth centuries in either Europe or America. Political reluctance to interfere with industrial interests, debates about the precise impact of pollution on health (including occasional suggestions that the urban atmosphere might be of benefit to asthmatics)[60] and continuing ideological commitments to the domestic hearth as a symbol of individual and national prosperity, collectively served to undermine arguments for reform.[61]

During the inter-war and immediate post-war years, opposition to government intervention began to crumble, primarily as the result of highly visible international air pollution episodes in which large numbers of people died, most notably in the Meuse Valley in Belgium in 1930, in Donora, Pennsylvania, in 1948 and, perhaps most significantly, in London in 1952. During the 1930s and '40s a combination of climatic conditions and pollution had periodically generated dense 'smogs' (a term first coined in 1905 to describe the combination of smoke and fog) in London and other cities, leading to rises in morbidity and mortality from respiratory and cardiac diseases.[62] In December 1952, however, a thermal inversion trapped a particularly deep and impenetrable layer of smog over London. As visibility decreased dramatically, transport in the capital became virtually impossible and accidents multiplied.[63] In addition, both hospital admissions and mortality rates rose sharply, with most patients being admitted for, and dying from, heart and respiratory problems. Prompted by extensive public alarm, evident in newspaper editorials and correspondence, speakers in Parliament argued vehemently for an immediate government inquiry and more effective legislation before another severe winter smog plunged the country into further turmoil.[64] Although the government attempted to delay intervention, claiming that there were more pressing priorities (such as the growing housing crisis), a Committee on Air Pollution, chaired by the South African engineer and industrialist Sir Hugh Beaver (1890–1967), was appointed in July 1953.[65]

In addition to evaluating the economic burden of pollution, the Beaver Committee drew a number of conclusions about the impact of atmospheric pollution on health. First, it acknowledged that the smog of 1952 had been 'accompanied by an immediate and sudden rise in both illness and mortality' and that approximately 4,000 people had died as a direct result of the smog during the first three weeks of December 1952. Second, the Committee presented evidence that at the height of the smog deaths from bronchitis had increased nine-fold, deaths from pneumonia four-fold, and deaths from other respiratory diseases in the region of five- to six-fold, figures that suggested that the smog in 1952 was far more severe than previous air pollution episodes.[66] More strikingly, in its Final Report the Committee also noted with some concern that the death rate from bronchitis in Britain was 50 times higher than the death rate in Denmark and that mortality rates from pneumonia and bronchitis were far higher in urban than in rural areas. Although the urban–rural gradient was less marked for other respiratory diseases, and although it was recognized that factors other than air pollution (such as climate or housing, for example) contributed to these comparative figures, the Committee deduced that there was 'a clear association between pollution [especially by smoke and sulphur dioxide] and the incidence of bronchitis and other respiratory diseases'.[67] The apparent correlation between visible smoke pollution and lung diseases led the Beaver Committee to demand remedial action for what was identified as 'one of the most urgent problems to-day in the field of environmental hygiene'.[68]

The London smog of 1952, like the Donora incident in America, eventually proved a catalyst for the introduction of a national clean air policy in Britain, embodied in the first Clean Air Act of 1956.[69] According to some historians, the smog can also be regarded as a conspicuous historical example of the impact of pollution on asthma.[70] However, retrospective interpretations that suggest that mortality during winter air pollution episodes was linked to exacerbations of asthma are not supported by contemporary evidence. Although the Beaver Committee acknowledged the influence of air pollution on bronchitis and pneumonia, morbidity and mortality from asthma did not figure overtly in its calculations. Subsequent surveys of the impact of pollution on respiratory health tended to reinforce this perspective. Neither a report from the Ministry of Health in 1954 nor one published in 1970 by the Royal College of Physicians identified a causative link between urban air pollution, on the one hand, and asthma morbidity and mortality, on the other.[71] While there were occasional reports of asthmatic symptoms induced by pollution, such as 'Tokyo-Yokohama asthma' or 'asthmatic bronchitis' occurring in American military personnel stationed in Japan during the 1940s and '50s, it appeared that in most instances these were examples of bronchitis provoked by irritants rather than cases of asthma.[72]

Although contemporary American studies focusing expressly on the possible connection between sulphur dioxide concentrations in the atmosphere and asthma attacks also failed to identify a clear relationship,[73] scientific concerns about the hazards of sulphur dioxide in asthmatics persisted. In the early 1980s, for example, research in California suggested that asthmatics might be more sensitive to lower levels of sulphur dioxide than the rest of the population. The evidence was immediately mobilized by scientists and environmental pressure groups in their efforts to encourage the Environmental Protection Agency (EPA) to set lower limits on acceptable levels of air pollutants. Such calls for reform were stridently resisted by industrial manufacturers. Concerned about the impact of new regulations on productivity and profits, the utility, petroleum and chemical industries not only responded by suggesting that the EPA should 'abandon its concern for such subgroups and set standards that protect only against significant risk of adverse effects in the general population', but also were reported to have offered financial inducements to members of the Senate Committee on Environment and Public Works.[74] Although the EPA did gradually introduce revised standards during the 1980s, efforts to regulate specific industrial pollutants more closely were undermined by new concepts of exposure, in which total exposure to a range of indoor and outdoor pollutants was deemed a more accurate measure of risk.[75] At the same time, as clinical and epidemiological attention was switching to the effects of smoking as a risk factor for respiratory disease, interest in the impact of outdoor air pollution on asthma (and indeed chronic bronchitis) tended to fade.[76]

Waning concerns about the role of air pollution in asthma and other allergic conditions may also have been driven by observations that, during the period when asthma was known to be increasing, atmospheric pollution by smoke and sulphur dioxide (and possibly other pollutants) was declining in most developed countries. In Britain, for example, emissions of sulphur dioxide and black smoke clearly fell in the wake of the Clean Air Acts of 1956 and 1968.[77] However, as the Beaver Committee had intimated in the 1950s, and subsequent international studies also suggested, measures of the effects of pollution on health needed to include assessments of the impact of pollutants from traffic rather than merely industrial processes. From the middle decades of the twentieth century, increased emissions from cars and buses encouraged researchers to consider the role of pollutants discharged during petrol and diesel combustion either as causes or initiators of asthma or as factors that could provoke asthma attacks in certain patients. The evidence proved ambiguous. In spite of occasional epidemiological reports suggesting that vehicle pollution might explain patterns of asthma and hay fever and the exacerbation of symptoms in individual patients, and in spite of laboratory evidence demonstrating the role of pollutants on lung function in animals,[78] the link between levels of traffic and trends in allergy remained speculative and contested. Thus, comparative studies charting the prevalence of asthma in Germany following the opening and removal of the Berlin Wall in 1989 and subsequent political reunification in 1990 showed paradoxically that allergies were less common in heavily polluted East German cities than in their West German counterparts. Likewise, several other cities or regions with high levels of atmospheric pollution, such as Athens in Greece and parts of China, generally experienced low levels of asthma. By contrast, some countries with relatively clean air, such as Scotland and New Zealand, demonstrated high rates of allergic diseases during the second half of the twentieth century.[79]

In the 1990s scientific scepticism about the role of air pollution in shaping modern global patterns of allergic diseases was substantiated by inquiries conducted by the British Committee on the Medical Effects of Air Pollution and by a working party of the British Society for Allergy and Clinical Immunology.[80] In 1995, for example, the British Society confidently concluded that:

There is limited evidence at the moment to support the idea that air pollutants are responsible for the increased prevalence of asthma and allergic disease in countries with a 'western' lifestyle. Worldwide, where increased incidence of allergic disease has been convincingly documented over time, allergen exposure has more obviously been responsible than exposure to air pollutants.[81]

Significantly, however, the reluctance of experts to indict pollution as a cause of epidemiological trends failed to dispel public suspicions and concerns. Towards the turn of the millennium, television programmes and articles in the popular press continued to convey widespread anxieties not only that outdoor pollution was aggravating asthma in particular patients but also that traffic-related pollution was fuelling modern trends in allergy. Thus, in 1993, a television documentary reproached the British government for failing to pay attention to the serious nature of asthma and for continuing to allow main roads to be built through residential areas.[82] Similarly, columns in national and local newspapers, as well as the educational material released by environmental pressure groups, exposed the manner in which 'dirty cities and polluting factories' in America and Britain were putting 'lives at risk' by inducing lung cancer, heart disease, and asthma.[83] As Ulrich Beck pointed out in the 1980s, dissonance between lay perceptions and the findings of expert committees was to be expected in societies transfixed by risk: one of the defining characteristics of the modern risk society, Beck suggested, was the existence of demonstrable fissures between scientific and social rationality in evaluating and dealing with the hazards of civilization. According to him, such disjunctions were determined partly by the tendency of modern science simply to chart the regional distribution of pollutants rather than attempting to assess their particular impact on individual people, and partly by the failure of scientists to acknowledge that 'the same pollutants can have quite different meanings for different people, according to age, gender, eating habits, type of work, information, education, and so on'.[84]

Persistent public beliefs in the impact of pollution on asthma were shaped primarily by personal experiences of the manner in which symptoms were provoked by air pollution episodes. Anecdotal accounts to this effect were reinforced by clinical reports that pollution could, in certain circumstances, exacerbate breathing difficulties in individual patients with established disease. It is possible that public concern was also intensified by broader anxieties about the effects of environmental pollution on general health and about the impact of traffic exhaust fumes and urban smog on the modern environment.[85] Significantly, however, while the public continued to focus on outdoor air pollution as a major cause of ill-health (including allergies) and to indict national governments and international health organizations for failing to address global patterns of pollution, clinicians, epidemiologists and laboratory scientists were turning increasingly to factors in the indoor environment and westernized lifestyles that might explain modern geographical and temporal trends in allergic diseases.

Allergy and the modern home

In the late nineteenth and early twentieth centuries, clinicians had sometimes advised patients with hay fever and asthma to spend more time indoors during the pollen season. In the last half of the twentieth century, by contrast, the indoor environment itself was implicated in shaping the modern distribution of allergic diseases. Driven partly by evidence that global patterns of outdoor air pollution could not adequately explain trends in allergy and partly by observations that people were spending an increasing proportion (up to 90 per cent) of their time indoors, allergists began to conceive modern domestic and occupational environments as potentially pathogenic. Of course, interest in the home and workplace as possible breeding grounds for disease was not new. As Nancy Tomes has suggested, around the turn of the nineteenth into the twentieth century growing awareness of the role of germs in human diseases provoked widespread anxieties about domestic hygiene. The ensuing 'battle with bacteria' not only provided substantial commercial opportunities for the manufacturers of innovations such as white porcelain toilets, vacuum cleaners, refrigerators, disinfectants and new forms of packaging, but also promoted novel fashions and social customs intended to reduce the spread of germs.[86] Significantly, the advent of antibiotics in the mid-twentieth century did not quell anxieties about household germs; in addition to effectively exploiting both the post-war explosion of consumerism and contemporary emphases on the role of women in maintaining domestic harmony and health, the manufacturers of cleaning products, such as soaps, detergents and disinfectants, also took advantage of continuing fears about the diverse microscopic dangers lurking in the modern home.[87]

In the mid-twentieth century, allergists also recognized the importance of the home environment as they documented substantial improvements in the symptoms of asthmatic children when they were removed to open-air schools or mountain retreats. In such cases, the dangers of the home were thought to be both material and emotional. While interest in the psychogenic aspects of allergy certainly persisted, dramatic changes in the domestic environment in developed countries during the 1960s and '70s encouraged allergists and epidemiologists to focus more exclusively on identifying possible allergens in the modern home that might account for emergent trends in allergies and that might, at the same time, suggest new means of avoidance. According to some commentators, indoor air pollution subsequently became 'the single most important emerging air quality issue of the 1980s',[88] prompting national surveys in many countries and inspiring global inquiries into the health risks (including allergies and cancer) posed by a range of new contaminants contained within, and emanating from, building materials, furnishings and other consumables.[89]

Although allergists were increasingly aware that gas, smoke, paint fumes and various volatile organic compounds in the indoor environment could exacerbate the symptoms of allergy, in the post-war period they tended to concentrate, along traditional lines, on the allergenic qualities of house dust. For many centuries, clinicians and patients had recognized that dust in the home and workplace aggravated the symptoms of asthma. In the early twentieth century, as asthma, hay fever and eczema were brought together under the rubric of allergy, clinicians graphically demonstrated the ability of dust extracts to provoke positive skin reactions and to induce allergic symptoms.[90] As a result, although its role in allergy remained contested and although the precise constituent of dust responsible for provoking allergies remained mysterious for many years (leading John Freeman to denounce it as an 'allergic bogy'),[91] dust became, like pollen in the outdoor environment, the archetypal indoor allergen.

Enduring interest in the relationship between house dust and allergies was tempered by the knowledge that dust comprised a mixture of many different components, including human and animal danders, feathers, bacteria, moulds, algae, and the remains of food, insects and plants.[92] As a number of studies revealed, many of these substances could induce allergic reactions. Cats and dogs, for example, had been known to provoke asthma and rhinitis in the nineteenth century, and in the early twentieth century animal danders from pets were identified by both American and European allergists as potent domestic allergens.[93] Although some allergists initially rejected the notion that hypersensitivity to animal dander was a frequent cause of asthma or rhinitis, subsequent studies led researchers to conclude that pets constituted an important cause of domestic allergies in the modern world, particularly in certain geographical locations such as Northern Scandinavia.[94] Indeed, at the turn of the millennium, the growing importance of allergies to domestic animals motivated an American company to attempt to produce 'transgenic' designer pets with the allergen genes deleted.[95]

In the 1960s, however, Reindert Voorhorst (b. 1915) and his colleagues in the Department of Allergology at Leiden transformed understandings of the role of dust in allergy by demonstrating that, in most circumstances, the major allergenic component of dust was not animal dander but the ubiquitous mite, *Dermatophagoides pteronyssinus*.[96] The possibility that microscopic mites might be involved in asthma had first been suggested by a German physician, Hermann Dekker, in 1928. Significantly, in implicating mites in asthma, Dekker had highlighted the manner in which modern modes of living were creating the conditions necessary for the proliferation of mites and other harmful biological products:

> It is, nevertheless – one can apply oneself to the question of an asthma mite as one likes – a hygienic anachronism that the modern cultivated person sleeps in beds which are a mockery of all the rules of hygiene, in beds of which the contents are mainly soiled in the year long, daily use through dust, fungal spores, bacteria, and from the effect of the damp bed warmth, an opulent breeding ground of fungi, yeasts, and harmful vermin, in beds which often for years and tens of years are not cleaned, for one cannot seriously call the beating, leaving out in the sun, of voluminous bedding, a cleaning! A completely neglectful chapter of hygiene! All the worse, that for sure asthma is not the only illness to arise from mites.[97]

Dekker's suspicions were eventually confirmed by Voorhorst and his associates, who not only demonstrated a close correlation between dust allergy and skin reactivity to *D. pteronyssinus*, but also established the role of temperature and humidity in determining the concentration of mites in house dust. Voorhorst's conclusions, and the subsequent identification of a potent allergen in mite excretion products, were readily accepted by allergists around the world and effectively initiated global research into the biology and ecology of the house-dust mite. In particular, a number of studies (which were often reported in the media) revealed the prevalence of mites in bedding, carpets, soft furnishings and toys, clarified the impact of humidity on mite populations and the role of regular cleaning in reducing levels of mite infestation, and demonstrated the capacity for mites to provoke not only asthma but also eczema and rhinitis.[98]

Significantly, greater knowledge of the ecology of mites generated new understandings of seasonal, climatic, geographical and occupational variations in the prevalence of asthma and other allergic diseases. As a variety of studies in the 1960s and '70s suggested, fluctuations in mite populations could account for higher levels of allergy in children born during the late summer months, as mite levels were rising, and for the exacerbation of symptoms during the autumn.[99] The regional distribution of allergies was also traced to the effect of specific climatic conditions on mites. For example, both the prevalence of 'climate asthma' in certain coastal regions of South Africa and the increased incidence of asthma in damp houses situated near rivers were explained in terms of the regional variations in humidity that encouraged the proliferation of mites in those locations.[100] Conversely, improvements in asthmatic symptoms at high altitude were related to lower levels of house dust mite in conditions of low temperature and low humidity.[101] In addition, while regular bed cleaning was promoted as a means of reducing mite populations, it was also recognized that bed making constituted an occupational hazard for cleaners and housewives, thereby helping to explain the higher incidence of mite sensitization in women.[102]

One of the principal attractions of the house-dust mite theory, however, lay in its ability to account not only for the distinctive seasonal, climatic and geographic distribution of allergies but also for global temporal trends in asthma, rhinitis and eczema. As evidence for the role of mites in allergies deepened, allergists began to explore the possibility that, as Dekker had intimated in 1928, domestic fashions and cleaning practices might be causing the modern epidemic of allergies. During the late twentieth century, the use of fitted carpets increased dramatically, particularly in those countries that experienced a surge in asthma morbidity and mortality, such as New Zealand and Britain; for example, by 2000 approximately 98 per cent of British homes had fitted carpets compared with 16 per cent in France.[103] At the same time, the composition of carpets and other home textiles was transformed by the introduction of artificial fibres, by the use of tufted instead of woven carpets, and by manufacturers' attempts to design carpets in which the dirt and dust sank to the lower layers, thereby maintaining the floor's clean surface appearance.[104] The consequences of these technical developments were to render modern carpets more resistant to effective vacuum cleaning, to facilitate the retention of water at the base of the pile or in the underlay, and to increase the survival and proliferation of house-dust mites. By the turn of the millennium, researchers estimated that as many as 100,000 mites might live in one square metre of carpet and that mite allergen levels in carpets could be between six and fourteen times higher than those on smooth floors.[105]

Other major changes in domestic fashions, which appeared to facilitate the proliferation of house-dust mites, were often driven by broader political and economic considerations. In the mid-1970s the Organization of Petroleum Exporting Countries (OPEC) dramatically increased the price of oil in an attempt to exert pressure on the West following the outbreak of war in the Middle East. Faced by rising fuel costs and rampant inflation, householders in many developed, temperate countries immediately became more conscious of the need to conserve energy and to reduce heating bills. As a result, home owners installed insulation, replaced older windows with double glazing, and endeavoured to prevent draughts around doors. Such energy-saving measures tended to reverse a traditional emphasis on the beneficial effects of domestic ventilation and were encouraged in some countries by specific tax credits. The net effect of these alterations was to decrease ventilation, increase humidity and provide a convenient environment for mites to thrive in carpets, bedding and other soft furnishings.[106] While these trends might have been offset to some extent by the manner in which central heating dried the indoor atmosphere, thereby reducing mite concentrations, the overall impact of major changes in home design and fabrics was to increase exposure to domestic allergens such as mites and animal dander, particularly among modern Western populations.

Evidence that sensitivity to house-dust mites was possibly responsible for many cases of asthma, rhinitis and eczema led to the formulation of specific therapeutic and preventative strategies. In the first place, allergists conducted trials that evaluated the efficacy and safety of hyposensitization with partially purified, commercially prepared mite extracts. While some writers were sceptical about the supposed benefits of hyposensitization and anxious about side effects, others reported substantial improvements in asthmatic symptoms, as well as a reduction in the need for other therapies following a course of injections.[107] Drawing on knowledge about the ecology of mites and on studies suggesting that mite levels were low in hospitals as the result of the frequent changing and laundering of bed linen and the regular washing of mattresses, clinicians also devised meticulous cleaning regimes aimed at reducing domestic mite concentrations.[108] While a number of surveys identified significant improvements in self-reported symptoms and measurable reductions in bronchial hyper-reactivity, physicians recognized that many of the allergen-avoidance protocols tested in controlled trials were too demanding for patients and their carers to reproduce at home or that some cleaning methods (such as the use of conventional vacuum cleaners) tended to increase, rather than decrease, mite concentrations in the indoor atmosphere. As a result, allergists often warned that the most effective means of minimizing exposure to mites was simply to remove carpets.[109]

Professional and public awareness of the link between levels of house-dust mite and trends in allergies also spawned commercial opportunities, not only for pharmaceutical companies to market mite vaccines,[110] but also for the cleaning industry to devise and sell acaricidal sprays, mattress and pillow protectors, air conditioners, and vacuum cleaners fitted with high efficiency particulate air filters.[111] Preoccupations with mites also encouraged allergists to offer advice to patients about simplifying the interior design of their homes in order to reduce exposure to indoor allergens. During the inter-war years, well before the identification of *D. pteronyssinus* as the mite responsible for many allergies, allergists had offered patients and their parents precise instructions on how to prevent the accumulation of dust; these included removing or regularly cleaning rugs, curtains and pictures, dusting floors and furniture with a damp or oiled cloth, vacuuming, and excluding animals from the house. In extreme cases, allergists had suggested adopting Storm van Leeuwen's notion of an allergen-free (or 'miasm-free') chamber that was hermetically sealed and ventilated with filtered air.[112]

In the post-war years, such advice proliferated as allergists attempted to establish the principles on which allergy-free homes should be run.[113] Significantly, the preference for simple domestic furnishings was shaped not only by new understandings of the relationship between the indoor environment and allergy, but also by modern architectural trends that emphasized the importance of clean, spacious, functional and uncluttered interiors and by traditional anxieties about the spread of germs. During the early twentieth century, designers and social reformers on both sides of the Atlantic had denounced both Victorian homes, with their pillows, drapes and other soft furnishings, and Victorian attire as repositories of dust and breeding grounds for germs.[114] As concerns about the control of infection at home persisted into the 1950s and '60s, the identification of the role of dust in allergy and evidence that allergic diseases were increasing in frequency and severity effectively reinforced the efforts of designers, architects, and the authors of domestic advice books, as well as the commercial manufacturers of disinfectants and other cleaning products, to promote the gospel of cleanliness.[115] At the end of the twentieth century, this trend encouraged the construction of eco-friendly houses and 'low-allergen' residential developments, in which 'pile carpets and papered walls' were to be replaced by 'the pared-down Mediterranean look', in order to improve 'energy levels and well-being at the same time'.[116]

While approaches to the modern indoor environment reflected both clinical and public preoccupations with patterns of infectious and allergic diseases, they also revealed broader cultural stereotypes relating particularly to class and gender. As several contemporary commentators made clear, substantial national and regional differences in domestic fashions and house-keeping practices, as well as environmental factors such as dampness and overcrowding, could explain widely divergent levels of allergic diseases in different racial and ethnic groups and in different classes.[117] As some histori-ans have suggested, however, the crusade for domestic cleanliness on both sides of the Atlantic was also framed by the attempts of middle-class reform-ers to improve the habits and homes of the working classes and, in some cases, of immigrant communities.[118] Ironically, like the advice given to hay fever sufferers to travel during the pollen season, many of the strategies recom-mended to householders for the avoidance of germs and allergens in the indoor environment (such as changing furnishings and decor or improving sanitation) may well have been beyond the means of many working-class families.

It is also evident from contemporary medical literature that the burden of maintaining domestic health was thought to lie clearly with mothers. In a popular advice book on allergy published in 1976, for example, Doris J. Rapp (an American paediatric allergist and clinical ecologist) and A. W. Frankland noted that it was 'impossible (and unnecessary) for a busy housewife to keep the entire home allergy-free'.[119] Similarly, in 1982, a study of house-dust mites in homes in Bristol in England warned that any technique for removing dust mites 'should be simple and quick so that it is likely to be carried out efficiently over a long period by unsupervised mothers in their own homes'.[120] While such pronouncements (as well as advertisements for clean-ing products directed specifically at housewives) undoubtedly reflected the domestic reality of many women's lives in the second half of the twentieth century, they also reinforced gendered divisions of labour and reiterated traditional preoccupations with the role of mothers in the pathogenesis of allergies, already apparent for example in formulations of 'smother love' and asthma in the 1940s and '50s.[121]

At the turn of the millennium, debates about the role of house dust in asthma encountered a new twist. In 2000 a report from an American study, published in the *Lancet*, suggested that certain factors (bacterial endotoxins) present in dust protected infants against the risk of developing allergies.[122] Accounts in the daily press immediately rejoiced in the knowledge that people who were 'allergic to housework' (not surprisingly illustrated by a woman dusting a television set while her young daughter played in the foreground) could now be reassured that 'a little bit of dirt can be a good thing'.[123] The central role of house dust in allergies was also challenged by evidence that exposure to alternative allergens both at home and in other indoor environments might be critical. A stream of investigations thus explored the manner in which insects, plastics, flour, chemicals, coffee and castor beans, latex, isocyanates in paints, and a range of other substances present in schools, offices and factories as well as homes might be fuelling trends in allergy.[124] Such studies did not displace clinical interest in the role of house-dust mites. However, by drawing attention to the broader physical conditions in which modern populations lived and worked, they prompted allergists and epidemiologists to attempt to identify novel lifestyle factors that might have increased the risk of exposure, or modified measurable biological responses, to allergens in the contemporary environment.

Lifestyle and disease

During the course of the twentieth century, there were profound changes in the lifestyles of people in both developed and developing countries. In addition to the broader processes of urbanization and industrialization, which transformed the outdoor environment as well as patterns of work and leisure, the volume of traffic on roads, railways and in the air increased as people travelled faster and further. Diets were altered not only by the global exchange of national cuisines but also by the decline of breast-feeding and by the introduction of synthetic preservatives and colourings, and a range of new chemicals were incorporated into medicines, detergents, pesticides, paints and perfumes. At the same time, technological innovations, such as the television and computer, combined with shifting domestic fashions to alter radically the indoor environment and to encourage more sedentary lifestyles. As the number of electronic gadgets rose during the course of the century, average family size fell in most Westernized societies, leading some market researchers to suggest that the television was 'today's new family member'.[125]

It is not surprising that dramatic modifications in modern lives were implicated in rising trends in allergies and indeed many other 'diseases of affluence', such as cancer, heart disease, diabetes and obesity. Towards the end of the twentieth century, a considerable volume of international research was aimed at determining whether substantial changes in the Western diet were responsible for the increasing prevalence of asthma, hay fever and eczema. In particular, studies focused not only on the role of well-established allergens (such as eggs, milk and wheat) but also on the introduction of a richer, more varied diet that exposed people to relatively new or exotic allergens, such as peanuts and kiwi fruit, and on the preponderance of pre-packed meals and 'junk food' containing high levels of salt and artificial additives.[126] An investigation in Saudi Arabia, for example, concluded that a traditional rural diet of local fresh vegetables, milk, rice, chicken and fruit (as opposed to the urban preference for imported and processed foods) reduced the risk of asthma in children.[127] As I shall argue in the next chapter, although the reality of food allergies was contested in the late twentieth century, persistent professional and public concerns about the role of food additives in allergic diseases not only encouraged greater regulation of the food industry and boosted the popularity of 'allergen-free' foods, but also helped to foster the emergence of clinical ecology as a prominent, but controversial, branch of medicine concerned primarily with the identification and elimination of hidden health hazards in the environment.

Interest in the relationship between food and allergy also generated research into the relative impact of breast-feeding and formula milk. Studies published in the inter-war period had already suggested that feeding cow's milk to infants increased the incidence of infantile eczema.[128] According to susbsequent research conducted during the 1970s and '80s, breast-feeding, especially during the early months of life when IgA levels were low, resulted in either a reduced incidence or the later expression of allergies. In 1978, for example, Heinz Wittig and his colleagues in Florida provided evidence that the age of onset of allergies was significantly later in breast-fed (average of 7.1 years) than in bottle-fed children (average of 4.5 years).[129] However, advocates of breast-feeding as a means of reducing or deferring the expression of allergy were challenged by studies demonstrating that a number of potent allergens and industrial contaminants could pass to a child through the mother's milk. Thus, in 1988 Italian researchers demonstrated a greater incidence of positive skin-prick tests to common allergens in breast-fed children.[130] Several years later, independent studies published in the *Lancet* similarly concluded that allergens in breast milk (derived, for example, from the mother's diet) might serve to sensitize predisposed infants and that breast-feeding could increase the risk of developing atopic diseases.[131]

Contemporary preoccupations with the pivotal role of mothers (and less obviously fathers) in fashioning the pre-natal and early childhood environment that might precipitate allergies was also evident in studies of parental smoking. Of course, as some commentators made clear in the 1970s, a statistical link between allergies and smoking did not necessarily simply indicate that cigarette smoke initiated or exacerbated respiratory symptoms in allergic patients; it could also be interpreted as evidence that atopy constituted a risk factor for smoking-induced bronchial irritability.[132] Nevertheless, subsequent studies served principally to stress a causal relationship between passive smoking and levels of childhood asthma. In the 1990s it was estimated that nearly 400,000 cases of asthma in the United States were caused by parental smoking, either by the mother during pregnancy or by either parent during the child's early life.[133] Such attempts to assess the contribution of passive smoking to the incidence and prevalence of allergy were motivated not only by growing concerns about the health impact of global trends in smoking but also by nascent interest in the prenatal origins of adult disease and in the role of maternal risk factors in asthma.[134]

While preoccupations with the impact of modern lifestyles on health clearly reflected substantial changes in patterns of production and consumption, they also reconfigured traditional anxieties about the dangers of civilization or about the manner in which Western consumer culture was habitually promoting wealth at the expense of health. Thus, many late twentieth-century critiques of Western lifestyles, with their focus on poor diet, smoking and the lack of physical exercise, manifestly echoed eighteenth-century denouncements of the role of intemperance and gluttony in the aetiology of gout and nervous instability, Thomas Beddoes's early nineteenth-century account of consumption in the affluent classes, or late nineteenth- and early twentieth-century fixations with the apparent association between madness and civilization.[135] In spite of evident continuities in the rhetoric, however, post-war debates about allergy also revealed a novel strand to the pessimistic sentiments of civilization's discontents, one that blamed the astonishing advent of allergies on rapid developments in medicine and standards of hygiene as well as on material changes in the indoor and outdoor environments and dramatic transitions in Western lifestyles.

In the late 1980s David Strachan, an epidemiologist at the London School of Hygiene and Tropical Medicine, published his findings from a large study of the epidemiology of hay fever and eczema. The results were remarkable: 'Of the 16 perinatal, social and environmental factors studied the most striking associations with hay fever were those for family size and position in the household in childhood.'[136] Thus, the more children there were in a family, and particularly the greater number of older siblings present, the lower the prevalence of hay fever and eczema. In evaluating his results, Strachan tentatively proposed what became known in subsequent discussions as 'the hygiene hypothesis':

> These observations do not support suggestions that viral infections, particularly of the respiratory tract, are important precipitants of the expression of atopy. They could, however, be explained if allergic diseases were prevented by infection in early childhood, transmitted by unhygienic contact with older siblings, or acquired prenatally from a mother infected by contact with her older children. Later infection or reinfection by younger siblings might confer additional protection against hay fever.[137]

Significantly, the hygiene hypothesis not only offered an explanation for contemporary epidemiological variations according to family size in Western developed countries, but also provided a speculative biological rationale for the social, geographical and historical distribution of hay fever that had been identified by pioneers in the field, such as Bostock, Blackley and Beard.

> Over the past century declining family size, improvements in household amenities, and higher standards of personal cleanliness have reduced the opportunity for cross infection in young families. This may have resulted in more widespread clinical expression of atopic disease, emerging earlier in wealthier people, as seems to have occurred for hay fever.[138]

Strachan's emphasis on family size and hygiene was not entirely new. In the 1950s John Freeman had suggested that allergic diseases were more common in children with few or no siblings.[139] In 1976 a note in the *Lancet* had also warned that 'allergic diseases may be the price man has to pay for increasing hygiene in an environment abounding in highly allergenic materials'.[140] However, while Freeman had explained 'the extraordinary prevalence of the Only Child in the Allergy Clinics' in terms of emotional suffocation,[141] proponents of the modern hygiene hypothesis preferred to couch their explanations in terms of immunological maturity. Low levels of early childhood infections, they argued, resulted in imbalances in the immune system (such as the polarization of T-cell subsets towards T_H2 responses) with the resultant production of primitive or immature immunological reactions to potential antigens and the emergence of autoimmune diseases as well as allergies.[142]

Although Strachan himself later raised doubts about the plausibility of the hygiene hypothesis,[143] the possibility that there was a downside to modern Westernized hygienic lifestyles attracted considerable attention from journalists who not only publicized scientific accounts of the perils of sterility but also exposed growing circumstantial support for the hygiene hypothesis from a range of international investigations. Some studies, for example, noted that children in day-care nurseries tended to experience more infections and to develop fewer allergies than children cared for on their own at home.[144] Similarly, there appeared to be an inverse relationship between population levels of parasitic infections (in which IgE constituted a major protective mechanism) and the expression of allergic diseases, a relationship that not only helped to explain the lower prevalence of allergies in tropical climates but also prompted suggestions that allergies might be treated by artificial injections with parasites.[145] More critically and more contentiously, some commentators pointed to the increasing use of antibiotics and the growth of childhood immunizations in Western societies as possible triggers for rising trends in allergies, since both forms of medical intervention might conceivably reduce the opportunity for supposedly normal immunological maturation. This suggestion found particular support from studies of children who followed an anthroposophic lifestyle and who therefore had limited exposure to antibiotics or vaccinations but a diet rich in fermented vegetables containing live lactobacilli.[146]

Intriguingly, preoccupations with the manner in which the modern hygienic environment might be responsible for the emergence of new patterns of disease reversed older epidemiological and cultural fixations with dirt. In the wake of the Industrial Revolution and the identification of pathogenic germs, dirt was construed by late nineteenth-century doctors and social reformers as one of the greatest threats to public health. As the result of a combination of improved nutrition, medical advances and the adoption of preventative sanitary measures both inside and outside the home, morbidity and mortality from infectious diseases declined dramatically in most developed countries. However, it is possible that the relatively successful battle waged by Western medicine and civilization against bacteria and other microorganisms was responsible for unleashing a new plague of chronic immuno-logically mediated diseases upon the world. Driven partly by the financial interests of the pharmaceutical and cleaning industries, the pursuit of personal cleanliness and domestic hygiene appears to have disturbed individual immunological balance as well as the global ecological equilibrium. If the hygiene hypothesis is to be believed, modern industrial society has generated novel risks to health that can be contained only by artificial exposure to older forms of dirt and disease. At the dawn of the new millennium, Western scientists in particular were paradoxically advocating treating allergies with bacteria-laden tablets or probiotics designed to restore a supposedly natural ecological harmony and to promote protective, rather than destructive, forms of immunological reactivity.[147]

The volcano of civilization

According to allergists, by the close of the twentieth century many modern populations were living in an allergenic world, one that had been created and fashioned by dramatic transformations in indoor and outdoor environments, in lifestyles, and in culture and commerce. The industrial society had thus spawned new risks to health and longevity, including the perils of greater exposure to dust, pollen, pollutants, insects, animals, chemicals, medicines and food capable of triggering severe, and sometimes fatal, allergic reactions. At one level, the threat of an avalanche of allergies submerging modern society appeared to be real. During the course of the late twentieth century, allergies to a widening range of novel substances were described in the medical and popular press: patients were shown to be allergic to peanuts, fruits, various constituents of soaps, detergents and shampoos, anaesthetics and antibiotics, and even to body fluids such as semen. According to some newspaper accounts, people also demonstrated bizarre allergies to electricity and sunlight, and allergic diseases began to affect different organs in new ways, evidenced by the appearance of certain forms of immunologically mediated conjunctivitis caused by the use of contact lenses.[148]

As the range of potential allergens increased, so too did the apparent frequency, severity and complexity of allergic reactions. In 1979 only two cases of latex allergy had been reported in medical journals. By the end of the twentieth century, however, natural rubber latex allergy, causing both dermatitis and asthma, was not only a well-recognized occupational hazard among health care workers using surgical gloves but was also evident in children and adults exposed inadvertently to latex in toys, clothes, balloons, and the handles of squash rackets, stimulating the establishment of latex allergy support groups in some countries.[149] Strikingly, sensitivity to latex also appeared in the form of 'latex fruit syndrome', in which patients exhibited cross-reactions to proteins in latex and those in certain foods, notably bananas, avocado pears and chestnuts. More specifically, latex allergy was linked to allergic reactions to kiwi fruits, which were first introduced to British and American supermarkets as a luxury item in the 1960s and which caused increasing numbers of severe allergic reactions during the last two decades of the twentieth century.[150]

The growing severity and frequency of allergic reactions clearly influenced patients' perceptions of their conditions. According to a survey conducted by Asthma UK in 2004, patients with asthma often felt that they were 'living on a knife edge', fearful that the next attack of breathlessness would be their last. As one contributor to the report commented: 'I feel like I'm living with a time bomb and if I have a bad attack I say to myself: "Is this the one that will kill me?".'[151] Notwithstanding the evident reality of patients' experiences and fears, some commentators questioned whether the global blossoming and worsening of allergies at an epidemiological level in the post-war period was a biological reality or an illusion created by expansive media coverage.[152] The evidence proved equivocal. While late twentieth-century accounts insisted that the range of allergens and the prevalence of allergy did increase spectacularly after the Second World War, articles and textbooks published during the inter-war and immediate post-war years indicate that earlier generations of allergists had not only already recognized a comprehensive range of putative allergens but had also asserted, in a comparable manner, that a substantial proportion of Western populations was already troubled by allergies prior to the rapid expansion of medical reports and media interest.[153] In addition, it is apparent that, notwithstanding the emergence of sporadic reactions to exotic substances, most cases of hay fever, eczema and asthma in the late twentieth century were triggered by a fairly narrow range of familiar allergens, namely pollen, house dust, animals and certain foods.

It is possible, therefore, that the global epidemic of allergies carefully charted by allergists and epidemiologists, sensationally revealed by the media, and deeply dreaded both by patients and by national and international health organizations was, in some senses, imagined. As Ulrich Beck pointed out in the 1980s, health risks could be both 'real and unreal', shaped not only by knowledge of the past but also by fear of the future. The modern risk society was thus 'a catastrophic society', in which the 'exceptional condition threatens to become the norm' and in which the evaluation of risk was largely shaped by 'projected dangers of the future'. According to Beck, widespread and tenacious fears that the volcano of civilization was on the verge of erupting, thereby unleashing a plague of allergic diseases, cancers and other conditions on inhabitants of the modern world, served both to promote public awareness of new threats to health and to encourage the elaboration of national and global strategies aimed at reducing risks. In words that echoed the growing apprehensions of asthmatic patients, as well as political calls for health care reforms, Beck suggested that 'the time bomb is ticking. In this sense risks signify a future which is to be prevented.'[154]

As Beck's words suggest, pandemic concerns about an outbreak of allergies that was thought to be sweeping the world during the closing decades of the twentieth century can be understood not only in terms of the production and dissemination of novel allergens by Western civilization but also in terms of contemporary preoccupations with risk assessment and related anxieties about the manner in which modern civilization had generated unfamiliar, but preventable, environmental and public health hazards. The depth and focus of mounting fears about the proliferation of allergy and the magnitude of public consternation at the broader environmental risks generated by modern consumer culture were both acutely evident in debates about the aetiology and ecological significance of total allergy syndrome, a novel clinical affliction that had first appeared in embryonic form in the post-war years but which began to attract more expansive medical and media coverage in the early 1980s.

In the middle decades of the twentieth century, several authors had suggested that various ill-defined local and systemic clinical symptoms might be caused by previously hidden or unsuspected allergies. Thus, in the 1930s Warren Vaughan had argued that 'minor allergy' might explain a range of non-specific manifestations of ill-health, such as headache and fatigue.[155] In the 1950s and '60s American allergists and paediatricians extended this notion to suggest the possibility of a discrete allergy syndrome that was found more commonly in women but which was distinct from nervous fatigue. According to Claude Frazier in 1963, for example, the 'allergic tension-fatigue syndrome is a systemic manifestation of allergy in much the same way and may, in fact, be a syndrome brought on by gastrointestinal reaction to food mainly, or drugs or an inhalant.'[156] Frazier's formulation of a non-organ-specific allergy syndrome, marked by chronic fatigue and triggered particularly by constituents of modern diets, drew heavily on the work of food allergists and clinical ecologists, who from the mid-twentieth century had been describing the broad range of symptoms that could be precipitated by previously indiscernible food sensitivities.[157]

In the early 1980s, at precisely the same time that public, professional and political anxieties about AIDS were emerging, reports of more malignant systemic reactions to the Western environment began to appear in both the medical and the popular press. Thus, journals, newspapers and magazines began to highlight the plight of certain patients, often middle-class women, who appeared to be hypersensitive or allergic to multiple elements of the modern industrial environment. In sensitive patients, exposure to chemicals and pollutants in the urban, occupational or domestic atmosphere could precipitate symptoms ranging from debilitating headaches, muscular fatigue and mental lassitude to life-threatening cardio-respiratory collapse or severe psychological disturbance. In language that betrayed escalating environmentalist concerns about the perils propagated by the material constituents and cultural preoccupations of late modernity, the condition became known variably as total allergy syndrome, multiple chemical sensitivity, environmental illness or twentieth-century disease.

Although clinical interest was probably most evident among North American clinical ecologists and allergists, the first 'popular victims' of total allergy syndrome were two young British women, Sheila Rossall and Amanda Strang, who came to public attention in 1982. Newspaper coverage revealed that both Rossall and Strang exhibited signs of hypersensitivity to common foods and chemicals (such as chlorine, petrol, nylon, plastics and ink), and that both women had attempted to alleviate their condition by retreating into specially prepared sterile environments.[158] Over subsequent years, clinical ecologists, allergists and journalists described further cases of total allergy syndome, as well as sporadic examples of what were thought to be related manifestations of environmental sensitivity: children who were apparently 'allergic to nearly all food' or workers who suffered from 'sick building syndrome'.[159]

From the earliest incarnation of the new syndrome, clinical ecologists claimed that multiple chemical sensitivity constituted a form of allergic disease in which diverse, and often non-specific, symptoms were mediated by specific immunological reactions to substances ingested or inhaled from the environment. However, even as the immunological parameters of the condition were being constructed, the biological reality of total allergy syndome was being systematically challenged by the orthodox medical profession. In October 1982, while Sheila Rossall was flying home after a two-year period of treatment at an allergy clinic in Dallas, allergists congregating at an international conference in London were denying the possibility that anyone could be allergic to the twentieth century: according to one contributor, it was 'a nonsense, an American nonsense'.[160] Subsequent reviews not only harshly criticized the concept of environmental illness but also implied that cases of multiple chemical sensitivity were more usually caused by psychological disturbances or specific psychiatric conditions than by demonstrable or quantifiable immunological processes.[161]

Uncertainties about the legitimacy of the diagnosis and professional disagreements about the aetiology and pathogenesis of total allergy syndrome were ruthlessly exposed in the media. While television documentaries challenged both conventional and alternative accounts of chemical sensitivities, newspaper cartoons immediately ridiculed the notion of total allergy syndrome when it first appeared in 1982, and mobilized the condition as a convenient medium for social comment and political satire.[162] In his film of 1996, *Safe*, which was billed as a 'chilling environmental horror story' of the physical and psychological traumas experienced by a middle-class American woman suffering from chemical sensitivities, Todd Haynes not only criticized modern society and conventional medicine for failing to address the existential dilemmas faced by sufferers but also indicted alternative health care philosophies for prioritizing the individual pursuit of health and happiness at the expense of collective social action aimed at reducing pollution and limiting or

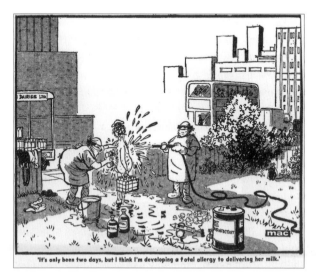

'It's only been two days, but I think I'm developing a total allergy to delivering her milk.'

Daily Mail, October 2002.

The Sun, October 1982.

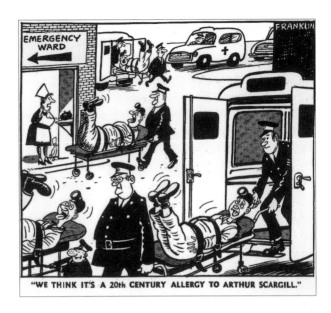

"WE THINK IT'S A 20th CENTURY ALLERGY TO ARTHUR SCARGILL."

reversing environmental degradation. As Matthew Gandy has argued, Haynes's treatment of chemical sensitivity also constituted a disparaging commentary on middle-class preoccupations with order and security, on widespread anxieties about the emergence of new diseases such as AIDS, and on the demise of the political Left in America.[163]

In spite of scepticism, and sometimes open hostility, from conventional physicians, cinematographers and cartoonists, clinical ecologists and environmental activists continued not only to defend the biological and existential reality of total allergy syndrome but also to claim an even deeper ecological significance for the condition. According to the science writer Peter Radetsky, people with environmental illness served as 'advanced scouts, providing a warning of what might happen to the rest of us if we don't watch out'. Employing a series of poignant case histories, Radetsky suggested that against 'their will, simply because of their unwanted susceptibilities, they function as prophets, by their example crying doom for a society in which industry, with its essential chemicals and toxic byproducts, is in the driver's seat'.[164] Radetksy's forewarning of future health risks resonated with other denouncements of the perils of modern civilization. For one correspondent to the *New York Times* in 1997, increases in certain forms of childhood cancer constituted evidence of the 'downside to the pleasures and indulgences of existence at the end of the 20th century'.[165] The following year, in an essay review on obesity published in the *New Yorker*, Malcolm Gladwell similarly highlighted concerns that over the previous 30 years 'the natural relationship between our bodies and our environment – a relation that was developed over thousands of years – has fallen out of balance', leading to the emergence of new epidemics of chronic ill health.[166]

Although some environmentalists controversially suggested that the popular litany of environmental deterioration, ecological imbalance and social disintegration comprised more myth than reality,[167] rising trends in allergies, heart disease, cancer, diabetes and obesity reinforced suspicions that modern Western society was making people sick. Together with the global epidemic of hay fever, asthma and eczema, the appearance of multiple chemical sensitivity in particular fuelled fears that even the apparent triumphs of Western civilization carried catastrophic consequences that would come to haunt those affluent classes and countries that had served as the principal architects of those successes. Thus, while improved standards of domestic hygiene and environmental sanitation, new therapies and the growth of the modern consumer society all contributed to the decline of infectious diseases and increased life expectancy that typified Westernized societies, they also threatened to unleash unpredictable risks to health. As René Dubos pointed out in 1961, modern Western medicine was implicated in this paradoxical process: 'Most unexpected, perhaps is the fact that medicine is creating new disease problems by reason of its very successes.'[168] With barely concealed satisfaction, Ulrich Beck referred to this self-destructive process as the 'boomerang effect': 'The agents of modernization themselves are emphatically caught in the maelstrom of hazards that they unleash and profit from.'[169] At the turn of the millennium, therefore, allergy not only highlighted the manner in which modern industrial society had created new global health risks, but also constituted a conspicuous symbol of what many alternative practitioners, ecologists and environmentalists regarded as an evolving crisis of modernity.

6

RESISTING MODERNITY

> Each historical period elects its own metaphors for talking about
> the body.
>
> Anne Marie Moulin, 1991[1]

In 1948 the Scottish doctor and playwright James Lorimer Halliday (1897–1983) published a polemical monograph on psychosocial medicine in which he outlined the multifarious ways in which civilized Western society was making modern populations sick. Renowned for his studies on the role of emotional factors in rheumatoid arthritis and asthma and a founding member of the Glasgow Psychosomatic Society, Halliday acknowledged that increased access to food, medical care and hygiene in Britain since the late nineteenth century had undoubtedly resulted in 'progressive improvement in the indices of its "physical health"'. However, the parallel disruption of established patterns of employment, family life, religion, commerce and politics had conversely initiated a progressive deterioration in the 'social health' of many communities. Social disintegration and the creation of a 'sick society', Halliday argued, was manifest in declining fertility, increased incidence of psychosomatic disorders, rising rates of sickness and absenteeism from work, deepening unemployment, juvenile delinquency, class war and regional nationalism, mass emigration, the decline of religious faith, and the popularity of escapist pursuits such as gambling.[2]

In seeking to explain the causes of modern trends in health and happiness, Halliday drew two general conclusions: first, that 'purely physical approaches' to understanding patterns of sickness were insufficient and should be supplemented by psychological methods; and second, that since the causes and features of social disintegration were evident throughout the developed world, it was necessary to examine and challenge the 'roots and growth of this Western civilization, including those of its typical economy, the market economy'.[3] Although Halliday was positive about the possibility of engineering social reintegration and encouraging a decline in psychosocial disorders, other commentators in the post-war period were less optimistic. Indeed, during the last half of the twentieth century, rising trends in allergic diseases, cancer, heart disease and stress, as well as declining fertility rates in many developed countries, were collectively employed to expose the manner in which supposedly artificial Western lifestyles and modern capitalist economies were damaging health. In addition to issuing strident warnings about the dangers of uncontrolled industrial expansion and unregulated commercial enterprise, critics of modern civilization also called for greater individual and political resistance to the destructive forces of modernity and for a return to nature. In this chapter, I want to examine the ways in which notions of resistance and nature not only characterized debates about the aetiology, diagnosis and management of allergic diseases but also came to permeate disputes about the professional organization of allergy services in the late twentieth century. At the same time, I want to explore the manner in which allergy was adopted as a convenient metaphor for the diverse physical, psychological and social perils facing modern populations.

Returning to nature

In a brief but provocative article published in a leading daily newspaper in February 2004, Prince Charles, heir to the British throne, indicted a familiar panel of suspects supposedly responsible both for rising trends in allergic diseases and for various other biological disturbances. According to the prince, reduced human fertility, chemically induced cancers, sex changes in fish and the emergence of allergy as a global public health problem could collectively be traced to increased exposure to untested chemicals in the environment and food chain. Pointing to evident links between allergy, on the one hand, and outdoor and indoor air pollution and modern Western lifestyles, on the other hand, Prince Charles's formulation of the medical consequences of an environmental crisis echoed earlier formulations of the downside of modernity. At the same time, the prince also mobilized pervasive contemporary fears about the perils of unrestrained and unbalanced technological and social progress as well as more specific anxieties about the pollution of the environment with pharmacologically active substances. These anxieties had been most clearly expressed in the 1990s by advocates of the 'environmental endocrine hypothesis', according to which the seepage of industrial and agricultural chemicals into the environment was disrupting the endocrine systems of both humans and animals and leading to a range of reproductive, immunological and developmental abnormalities.[4] At the dawn of the new millennium, Prince Charles echoed these environmentalist concerns with his own words of warning:

> Our disregard for the delicate web that sustains our environment
> is leading to its degradation . . . Factors associated with western

society, such as overeating, lack of exercise and an obsession with hygiene, as well as our exposure to a myriad of chemicals from products whose effects we are only just learning about, are conspiring to weaken our defence against the environment. Our children are paying the price.[5]

In setting out his solutions to the explosion of allergic diseases in the modern world, Prince Charles highlighted two critical dimensions of popular and professional debates about allergy. In the first place, he emphasized the lack of available orthodox medical resources to cope with expanding patient demand and suggested that, given the inadequacy of specialist allergy services in Britain, doctors and nurses needed 'greater support in helping to advise and treat patients with serious and increasingly complex allergy problems'. Second, he advocated fighting allergies with 'more traditional, "natural" approaches' to health care. Referring both to growing patient requests for greater access to complementary medicine and to promising results from clinical trials of acupuncture, homoeopathy, herbal medicine and controlled breathing in the treatment of asthma, Prince Charles argued that, by prioritizing prevention, the development of an integrated approach to allergies 'need not mean huge additional expenditure', but, conversely, carried the prospect of alleviating the future social and economic burden of allergies.[6]

Prince Charles's appraisal of the problems posed by allergies was ostensibly motivated and largely moulded by epidemiological patterns of morbidity and mortality from asthma, hay fever and eczema. In addition, however, his comments were shaped by popular critiques of modern consumer and industrial society that were already evident in Halliday's writing but which were subsequently fostered and fashioned by the counter-culture of the 1960s. Thus while Prince Charles's formulation of the hazards of modern civilization reiterated traditional concerns about the pathology of progress, his ardent appeal for a return to nature also echoed the particular 'body-centred, anti-industrial, and global version of an environmental imaginery' that had been effectively forged during the decades immediately following the Second World War.[7] As Roy Porter and others have suggested, the proponents of complementary medicine played a critical part in, and themselves benefited from, post-war romantic appeals to a simpler, less polluted past as a model for future developments: 'it is clear that much of the allure of modern alternative medicine lies in its ability to link philosophies of sickness to a wider disaffection with, and a critique of, industrial society, nostalgically evoking myths of golden ages of health, and seeking a return to Nature, through herbal remedies, natural cures, spiritualism, jogging and ginseng'.[8] From this perspective, Prince Charles's passionate call to resist the iniquitous spread of modern Western lifestyles and to pursue a more balanced and coordinated approach to health care reflected not only broader political endeavours to reverse the processes of environmental degradation and redress ecological disequilibrium, but also contemporary psychological and spiritual aspirations for global harmony and individual salvation.

Of course, the fallacies embodied in post-war naturalistic millennial dreams were evident even as they were being imagined. In the late 1950s and early 1960s, for example, the microbiologist René Dubos cogently cautioned against the proliferation of beliefs in the possibility of an uncritical rejection of modernity and an unrestrained return to a state of nature:

> But the state of equilibrium never lasts long and its characteristics are at best elusive, because the word 'nature' does not designate a definable and constant entity. With reference to life there is not one nature; there are only associations of states and circumstances, varying from place to place and from time to time.[9]

The historicism evident in Dubos's brand of ecological sensitivity also warned against accepting utopian visions of future health and sanity:

> Whether they be medical or political, utopias imply, as pointed out earlier, a static view of the world. In reality, however, societies are never static. Nothing is stable in the world – men change, and so do all their problems. We can indeed expect a 'new chapter in the history of medicine', but the chapter is likely to be as full of diseases as its predecessors; the diseases will only be different from those of the past.[10]

Some years later, Dubos's eloquent pleas for a more dynamic and historically sensitive interpretation of ecological relations found support in Ulrich Beck's critique of the 'naturalistic fallacy of the ecological movement'. Although he recognized the emotional appeal of attempting to return to nature, Beck insisted that modern notions of nature were themselves deeply problematic and socially contingent: 'Thus even nature is not nature, but rather a concept, norm, memory, utopia, counter-image . . . There are manifold reminders of the fact that the meanings of "nature" do not grow on trees but must be reconstructed.'[11] For Dubos and his successors, the solution to this disciplinary crisis was to encourage a more balanced, evolutionary and ecological perspective, according to which health and disease were to be regarded as products of an ever-changing equilibrium between internal and external environments. Drawing on the doctrines of the nineteenth-century French physiologist Claude Bernard (1813–1878) and on Hippocratic notions of universal sympathy, Dubos envisaged health, survival and fitness primarily in terms of the ability 'to resist the impact of the outside world'. Significantly, according to Dubos, historical and emotional factors, as well as the immediate material environment, played a distinct part in determining the individual's ability to resist or adapt:

> In most cases, the effect produced by any stimulus is conditioned by the biological and social history of the group and by the past experience of each individual. In other words the manner of response is predetermined not only by the molding effect of selective evolutionary forces but also by the accidents of personal life – from allergic idiosyncrasies to acquired patterns of behaviour ... The effects of the physical and social environment cannot be understood without knowledge of individual history.[12]

Dubos's explicit reference to allergy as a field where 'manifestations of the past' could be effectively demonstrated in the living organism and his deliberate linkage of biological and psychological phenomena clearly contained echoes of Charles Richet's formulation of the notion of parallel humoral and psychological personalities. It also transported crucial elements of Clemens von Pirquet's expansive conception of allergy as a general form of altered biological reactivity forward into the post-war period. At the same time, Dubos's words concealed intimations of increasingly contentious debates about the meaning of allergy in the modern world. As allergic diseases blossomed and as concerns about environmental devastation deepened during the last half of the twentieth century, allergy became a pivotal pawn in politicized debates about the manner in which, as Halliday and many other commentators had argued, modern society was making people sick. Allergy thus constituted a readily discernible, and scientifically validated, marker for both past and present degradation of the natural environment as well as a potent metaphor for physical and psychological disaffection with, and resistance to, the structures and values of modern industrial and commercial life. In the process, the expanding scale of allergy emerged as a crucial issue in debates about the allocation of finite state resources and as a turbulent battleground in the conflict between conventional Western biomedicine and alternative holistic approaches to health and society.

Unmet needs

During the second half of the twentieth century, public, professional and political concerns about the socio-economic burden of allergic diseases were mirrored by anxieties about the impact of allergies on the quality and longevity of individual lives, particularly in Britain where mortality and morbidity appeared to be the highest in the world. At the start of the new millennium, for example, fears about allergic diseases were convincingly captured in a report published by Asthma UK. This charitable organization, which had first emerged in the 1920s as the Asthma Research Council before becoming the National Asthma Campaign, was 'dedicated to improving the health and well-being of the 5.1 million people in the UK with asthma' through the more proficient coordination of research and the generation and maintenance of mechanisms and facilities for educating patients and their families. Reinforcing the results of previous surveys into patients' experiences of living with asthma conducted during the 1990s, the Asthma UK report, *Living on a Knife Edge*, offered powerful evidence of the reality and depth of the personal traumas endured by people with asthma. Focusing especially on those with severe asthma, the survey revealed that 'as many as one in six report weekly attacks so severe that they cannot speak, one in five say they are seriously concerned that their next asthma attack will kill them, and few feel any optimism that the future holds out hope of a better life'.[13]

Asthma UK's pleas for health care providers and governments to pay greater attention to the problems of asthma and to target resources at those 'whose asthma fails to respond to current treatments' were supported by sporadic evidence that asthma was regularly under-diagnosed, that the public remained ignorant of the seriousness of asthma attacks, and that the provision of educational action plans served to improve self-management and to reduce asthma morbidity.[14] Anxieties about the spreading impact of asthma were reproduced in debates about allergic diseases in general, encouraging widespread public and media demands for improved services for allergy sufferers and their families. In 2003 a survey by the Royal College of Physicians of London pointed out that 'deep anxiety' about allergies was often the product of a 'lack of information' and highlighted the manner in which patient demands for help were usually met not directly by members of the medical profession, who had limited training in allergy, but by the various independent charitable bodies dedicated to the field of allergic diseases.[15]

Throughout the twentieth century, charities had played a crucial role in promoting research into allergies and educating patients and doctors in many countries. In Britain, from the 1920s, the Asthma Research Council had been pivotal in developing the speciality, funding research projects, establishing clinics and drawing attention to the needs of patients. In North America, similar educational and promotional activities were performed by the Asthma and Allergy Foundation of America, which was founded in the 1950s as a voluntary, non-profit organization aimed largely at allergy sufferers and their families but which, like the Asthma Research Council, retained strong links with professional allergists through its Medical-Scientific Council.[16] In the immediate post-war period, comparable societies for the study of asthma and other allergic conditions were also founded in Australia and New Zealand as well as many European countries.

During the closing decades of the twentieth century, the range of activities and the focus of these charities expanded, reflecting not only growing global concerns about rising trends in allergic diseases but also dramatic developments in the delivery of health care services and communication technology. In Britain, the National Asthma Campaign established collateral support societies for patients, families and friends, published a journal, launched a telephone helpline and website, endorsed a variety of educational products particularly for children with asthma, drafted the Asthma Charter which set out 'the basic rights of all people with asthma', and in conjunction with the British Thoracic Society and British Lung Foundation constituted the Lung and Asthma Information Agency which published regular fact-sheets about respiratory disease.[17] Often motivated by patients' experiences of the limitations of state medical provisions for people with allergies, during the 1980s and '90s the National Asthma Campaign was joined by other charitable organizations dedicated to improving allergy services and disseminating information to patients. New organizations included the National Society for Research into Allergy, formed in 1980, the British Allergy Foundation (later Allergy UK), established in 1991, and the Anaphylaxis Campaign, founded in 1994.[18] In some instances, societies concentrated exclusively on particular manifestations of allergy, exemplified by the focus of the American Food Allergy Network or the National Eczema Society, which started operating in Britain in 1975.

By the turn of the millennium, these charities (and a number of web-based organizations) were being inundated with requests for help and information. While Allergy UK received approximately 45,000 enquiries and dispatched 250,000 fact-sheets annually, the National Eczema Society fielded more than 20,000 enquiries each year, and the Anaphylaxis Campaign dealt with 20,000 enquiries annually and sent out 140,000 leaflets to patients, schools, hospitals and doctors' surgeries.[19] In addition, charities often produced or endorsed popular educational books on allergy aimed at supplementing medical advice.[20] However, it is a notable irony that as public demand for information and support expanded in the wake of an apparent epidemic of allergies, clinical and public health facilities for the diagnosis and treatment of allergic diseases declined. This pattern was most evident in Britain. In 2002 a Department of Health definitional survey of specialist services for allergy noted that although organ-based physicians, paediatricians and immunologists supervised approximately 100 clinics for specific forms of allergic disease, there were only six specialist centres in England (three in London, and one each in Cambridge, Leicester and Southampton) that provided full-time clinical services for patients with allergy. In the light of what was regarded as an 'extremely poor' level of national provision for patients with allergies, the Department of Health joined forces with the British Society for Allergy and Clinical Immunology to form a National Allergy Strategy Group and proposed the development of specialist centres aimed at raising the quality of services available to patients and general practitioners.[21]

In 2003 the parlous state of clinical allergy in Britain was further revealed by a report from the Royal College of Physicians, *Allergy: The Unmet Need*. Lamenting the fact that previous reports from the College had had little impact on the evolution of clinical facilities, and emphasizing the gulf that existed between the need for, and the availability of, appropriate professional services, this survey outlined diverse obstacles to the provision of effective treatment and advice:

> There is a major shortage of allergy specialists, with only six fully staffed clinics in the UK, that have developed mainly around research interests. Allergy barely features in the undergraduate medical curriculum, and the lack of specialists means virtually no clinical training is available. Opportunities for postgraduate clinical training are limited. Knowledge of good allergy management in practice is therefore minimal or non-existent.[22]

Recognizing the importance of developing specialist services for children with allergy and adopting 'a "whole system" approach in which allergy is treated as a condition in its own right, and not as a series of diseases depending on the organ system involved', the Royal College recommended a number of strategies for future improvements. In particular, the report advocated the establishment of regional allergy centres, the creation of new consultant posts and specialist training schemes, and the generation of improved educational opportunities for general practitioners and practice nurses. In addition, the College highlighted the need for greater central state recognition of, and financial responsibility for, provincial allergy services and exhorted patient support groups to continue to expose the inadequacy of services.[23]

The issues raised by the Royal College's report were immediately taken up by journalists who not only stressed the inability of the National Health Service to cope with increasing numbers of allergy patients but also emphasized the manner in which inadequate services were putting lives at risk.[24] However, while the situation in Britain at the dawn of the new millennium certainly appeared sensationally stark, it is significant that concerns about both the relatively lowly status and the gradual contraction of allergy services were neither new nor indeed exclusively British. In the late 1970s the Dutch allergist Reindert Voorhorst had complained about the manner in which, throughout the world, 'chairs for allergology are established only with extreme difficulty and the number of lectures on allergology attended by physicians before their graduation can be counted on the fingers of one hand'.[25] Some years later, reflecting on the challenges facing allergists at the start of the twenty-first century, Stephen Wasserman (an American allergist who had been consulted by the Royal College of Physicians when it was preparing its report on allergy services in Britain) reviewed some of the struggles that North American allergists had experienced in their efforts to procure professional recognition for their discipline. In particular, Wasserman pointed out that the failure of early allergists to standardize diagnostic and treatment protocols, the predominantly out-patient focus of clinical allergy, its preoccupation with pathological mechanisms rather than organ-based lesions, and the tendency for national health agencies to support 'the most reductionist research possible', had collectively served 'to isolate allergy from the mainstream of medicine and paediatrics'.[26]

Wasserman's analysis of the factors that inhibited clinical allergy from 'assuming its full place in American medicine' was astute. The decline of allergy services in Britain and in some other countries at the end of the twentieth century was indeed deeply rooted in the history of clinical allergists' struggles to forge an independent medical speciality during the early and middle decades of the century. More particularly, however, the professional problems facing modern allergists can be traced to doubts and debates about their central therapeutic strategy, allergen immunotherapy. As I suggested in chapter Three, since its introduction to the clinics at St Mary's Hospital in London in the early twentieth century, prophylactic vaccination against hay fever, asthma, insect stings and other conditions had constituted 'the corner-stone of allergy practice' around the world.[27] Indeed, in spite of persistent concerns about the standardization of allergen extracts, about its mode of action, and about the safety and efficacy of the procedure, by the post-war period immunotherapy had achieved almost cult status among allergists and their patients, becoming the treatment of choice in venom allergies in partic-ular but also being regularly employed in hay fever, asthma, and certain drug allergies.[28]

During the 1970s and '80s, however, grumbling concerns about immunotherapy intensified. In 1971, in an editorial in the first edition of *Clinical Allergy*, Jack Pepys complained that, in view of the many difficulties associated with it, hyposensitization occupied 'too prominent a place at present'.[29] Pepys's belief that objective evidence for accurately evaluating immunotherapy was not yet available was compounded by sporadic reports in both the medical and popular press of deaths among British patients in particular. In 1980, for example, a British general practitioner reported the death of a patient undergoing desensitization for hay fever and asthma and warned that injections should not be administered 'without the availability of oxygen and a skilled assistant'.[30] Three weeks later, in a letter to the *British Medical Journal*, Pamela Ewan responded to the report by suggesting that impressions of benefit from immunotherapy were 'often based on anecdote' and that the introduction of new drugs had rendered obsolete the need for desensitization, which was 'potentially dangerous and often ineffective'.[31] Ewan's disparaging remarks were immediately rebutted by A. W. Frankland (John Freeman's successor as director of the allergy clinic at St Mary's), who pointed out that the risks were associated only with certain allergen prepara-tions, that there was 'no doubt' that 'specific immunotherapy does give benefit', and that it was inappropriate to 'damn all hyposensitisation injections as dangerous'.[32]

The tensions evident in this British exchange were expressed more overtly elsewhere. In 1986, in the wake of ongoing international debates about the need for more careful trials of desensitization and for improved standardiza-tion of extracts,[33] the editors of *Clinical Allergy* solicited the opinions of physicians with competing views on desensitization in the treatment of asthma. The case against immunotherapy was made by I.W.B. Grant, a consultant chest physician from Scotland. In addition to rehearsing prominent reservations about efficacy and safety and about the failure of allergists to conduct controlled trials of the procedure, Grant also maligned the character of many practitioners by alluding to the traditional stereotype of the clinical allergist originally depicted by A. J. Cronin in The Citadel. 'Senior physicians', he wrote, 'may recall with cynicism the financially profitable cult of hyposensitisation with haphazard mixtures of numerous allergens practised by unscrupulous self-styled allergists in the years before beta$_2$-agonists, sodium cromoglycate and corticosteroid aerosols became available'. Pointing out that it was difficult to understand how desensitization had 'withstood scientific scrutiny for so long', Grant concluded that 'had immunotherapy as currently practised been introduced only recently, it would not have been approved by the Committee on Safety of Medicines', a point often reiterated in subsequent debates.[34]

Immunotherapy was defended by two Danish allergists, H. Mosbech and B. Weeke, from the Allergy Unit at the State University Hospital in Copenhagen. Acknowledging the need for 'more systematic and controlled studies', and carefully distancing themselves from the 'mysticism, scepticism or even wild enthusiasm' often associated with immunotherapy, Mosbech and Weeke diligently surveyed the evidence in support of the procedure before concluding that desensitization did indeed 'have a role in the treatment of selected patients with allergic asthma'.[35] Not surprisingly, in the 'great debate' that subsequently erupted in the journal, the positive approach to immunotherapy adopted by Mosbech and Weeke generated more support from correspondents than Grant's blanket indictment of desensitization. For example, several allergists openly criticized Grant's cynicism and emphasized the disadvantages of modern drug treatments. However, the correspondence clearly illustrates the extent to which allergists acknowledged the potency of Grant's scepticism and were concerned about their professional reputation. Although one contributor generally endorsed the optimism expressed by Mosbech and Weeke, he also insisted that immunotherapy should not 'be undertaken in an uncritical, homoeopathic fashion by unenlightened enthusiasts, but in an ordered supervised way by specialists, based on strict diagnostic criteria and with proper supervision of treatment'.[36]

In October 1986 the debate was interrupted by a decisive intervention from the Committee on Safety of Medicines, which issued a warning in the

British medical press about the dangers of employing immunotherapy as a treatment for allergic disorders. Responding in particular to anxieties about the risk of death associated with the use of desensitizing vaccines, especially in patients with asthma, the Committee recommended that such vaccines 'should be used only where facilities for full cardiorespiratory resuscitation are immediately available' and that 'patients should be kept under medical observation for at least two hours after treatment'.[37] As many commentators around the world noted with dismay, the Committee's recommendations and its subsequent guidelines essentially proscribed the use of allergen immunotherapy by general practitioners in Britain. The impact of this prohibition on the credibility of clinical allergy and on the availability of allergy services was immediately apparent. According to a report prepared by A. J. Frew, secretary of a working party established by the British Society for Allergy and Clinical Immunology, in 'the absence of a system of hospital based allergy clinics, allergen immunotherapy in the United Kingdom was effectively abolished overnight'.[38]

Concerns about the dangers of desensitization were less marked in other countries, where deaths attributed to the application of diagnostic skin tests or to treatment with allergen extracts were apparently rare, possibly as a result of the use of different commercial allergen preparations. In 1990, for example, two clinicians from The Johns Hopkins Asthma and Allergy Center pointed out that allergy clinics at the Roosevelt Hospital in New York had administered more than one million injections without a single fatality between 1935 and 1955, and that subsequent surveys had revealed that only 46 deaths had occurred in total in the United States between 1945 and 1985.[39] Nevertheless, the Committee's intervention in 1986 initiated a series of intense arguments among an international community of allergists eager to challenge the Committee's restrictive proclamation. In a stream of position papers, articles and correspondence, individual allergists and professional societies in Britain, North America, central and southern Europe, and Scandinavia attempted to counter prejudices against immunotherapy and to rehabilitate clinical allergy within the realm of modern scientific medicine by stressing that diagnosis and treatment should be performed only by experienced allergists, by conducting trials aimed at identifying the 'true risk:benefit ratios' of immunotherapy, and by reasserting the previously acknowledged value of immunotherapy in the treatment of allergies to stinging insects.[40] In addition, allergists attempted to distance themselves from a variety of seemingly related, but unconventional, forms of therapy, such as enzyme potentiated desensitization, oral immunotherapy, bioresonance and neutralization therapy. Enzyme potentiated desensitization, in particular, was dismissed by many allergists as 'yet another form of alternative allergy treatment founded on dubious scientific principles'.[41]

Sanctioned by a memorandum from a combined meeting of the World Health Organization and the International Union of Immunological Societies,[42] and by statements from the European Academy of Allergology and Clinical Immunology, the general consensus among a global network of allergists debating the role of immunotherapy was that, while improvements in standardization were certainly desirable, the Committee on Safety of Medicines had overestimated the risk:benefit ratio and had imposed unnecessary restrictions on practitioners. In particular, most allergists argued that the Committee's requirement for patients to be kept under observation for two hours was excessive, and that 30 minutes' surveillance was sufficient. As a result, in many countries (most notably the United States and Scandinavia) allergen immunotherapy continued to comprise 'one of the most frequently administered treatments', and in North America occupied 'one of the first places in the treatment of adolescents'.[43]

In Britain the outcome was remarkably different. Although British allergists continued to stress the value of immunotherapy, the persistent concerns about safety, efficacy and standardization that had been exposed by the Committee's deliberations in 1986 served to undermine the professional status of allergy and contributed to the subsequent contraction of state-financed facilities for the treatment of allergic diseases identified by the Royal College of Physicians in 2003. Crucially, factors other than specific concerns about immunotherapy may have accentuated this process. At one level, clinical allergy (like many other specialities) was a victim of the intrusion of competitive market forces into the organization and distribution of state-governed health-care services and of the financial constraints experienced by, and imposed upon, the National Health Service during the 1980s and '90s. At another level, however, the bargaining position of clinical allergists in this market economy was compromised by their tendency to resist the processes of modernization within medicine. While John Freeman's idiosyncratic approach to diagnosis and treatment may well have suited the holistic ethos of both hospital and private practice during the inter-war period, his professed antagonism to the brave new world of clinical trials, standardized treatment protocols and state regulation contributed to the marginalization of the discipline in the post-war decades. Although allergists occasionally claimed that the discovery of IgE in 1967 had rescued their speciality from its equivocal status as a 'cinderella' subject and enabled it to 'join the ranks of science',[44] for many commentators clinical allergy remained a speciality more closely linked to the individualistic and empirical philosophies of alternative medical practitioners than to the ostensibly objective ideologies and procedures of modern Western medicine. Thus, in an article in *The Times* in 2003, Theodore Dalrymple (a practising doctor) suggested that 'the whole idea of allergy remains slightly disreputable because it is so fertile a field for quacks who prey on hypochondriacs'.[45] In parallel fashion, allergen immunotherapy was routinely dismissed as a 'specialist procedure with few indications'.[46]

It is ironic that while allergists were being forced to defend themselves against accusations of quackery their patients were turning increasingly to alternative practitioners for relief. In April 1992 a report from the Royal College of Physicians' Committee on Clinical Immunology and Allergy acknowledged that the rapid expansion of clinics offering alternative forms of treatment since the 1980s and the growing tendency for patients to consult alternative practitioners reflected 'dissatisfaction with the allergy care available under the National Health Service'.[47] Although the report was sceptical about the efficacy of many alternative treatments, subsequent surveys, both in Britain and North America, suggested that patients were continuing to move away from conventional forms of therapy during the last decade of the twentieth century. Studies conducted by the National Asthma Campaign, for example, revealed that more than 50 per cent of patients with asthma had tried complementary therapies.[48] Similarly, in 2003, the Royal College of Physicians noted, with characteristic cynicism, that the severity of symptoms suffered by many people with allergies had not only 'forced the public to look outside the NHS' but had also facilitated the 'proliferation of dubious allergy practice in the field of complementary and alternative medicine, where unproven techniques for diagnosis and treatment are used'.[49] Of course, the trend towards alternative sources of healing was not confined to allergies; sales of herbal medicines for depression, for example, clearly soared during the 1990s.[50] Nor were professional conflicts between orthodox and heterodox practitioners entirely new; throughout the eighteenth and nineteenth centuries licensed doctors on both sides of the Atlantic had strained to clarify the boundary between 'regular' and 'irregular' practitioners and to exclude a variety of unlicensed quacks and empirics from the confines of what was increasingly regarded as official, government-sponsored medical practice.[51] However, debates about the treatment of allergy in the late twentieth century were peculiarly indicative of a deepening rift in the fabric of modern medicine and society.

The political economy of allergy

Throughout the twentieth century, patients with allergies regularly employed a wide variety of both over-the-counter and prescribed remedies to relieve their conditions. As the reports from the Royal College of Physicians suggest, however, in the closing decades of the century British patients were increasingly prepared to consult alternative practitioners and to experiment with an expanding range of unconventional treatments. At a broader geographical level, international medical journals and the media regularly reported the results of clinical trials and recounted patients' experiences with alternative remedies such as homoeopathy, acupuncture, ayurvedic remedies, iridology, hypnosis, and herbal medicines including butterbur, local honey or bee pollen, and yamoa. In addition, various 'natural' dietary regimes, ranging from the 'nature cure' promoted by the naturopath Harry Benjamin and others at mid-century through dianetics programmes adopted by Scientologists in the post-war period to macrobiotics, became popular in many developed, as well as developing, countries.[52] Patients and clinicians across the world also became interested in the Buteyko Method for treating asthma which, although ostensibly in line with more traditional interests in the role of physiotherapy and exercise in asthma, offered a radically different approach to management. In the 1950s Konstantin Buteyko, a Russian clinician, had suggested that hyperventilation and reduced levels of carbon dioxide were responsible for asthmatic symptoms. As a result, he devised a 'revolutionary treatment' for asthma intended to retrain patients' breathing patterns. This alternative form of drug-free treatment was evaluated by trials in Russia and Australia and attracted considerable media interest and public support in the 1990s.[53]

With very few exceptions, alternative approaches to the diagnosis and treatment of allergic diseases were dismissed by conventional clinicians. Although some orthodox medical practitioners acknowledged that evidence of efficacy was growing in some instances (most notably in the case of herbal remedies used to treat eczema),[54] they also highlighted the unreliability of unconventional diagnostic tests, the absence of adequate clinical trials of complementary remedies, the potential risks of unregulated therapies, the variable quality of commercial preparations and the cost of many alternative treatments.[55] Of course, as some alternative therapists were keen to point out, debates about the relative merits of alternative and conventional approaches to allergic diseases (and many other conditions) were framed by political and professional, as well as evidential, issues. Approaches to allergy that indicted modern industrial and commercial processes and advocated drug-free treatment regimes not only challenged the fees and status of conventional practitioners, who in many countries were still struggling for recognition and reward, but also threatened the profits of the pharmaceutical, cleaning, cosmetics and food industries.[56]

These political and professional tensions were particularly apparent in late twentieth-century debates about clinical ecology or environmental medicine, an approach to allergies that had first been coherently formulated by an American allergist, Theron G. Randolph (1906–1995), in the 1950s and '60s. Randolph had graduated in medicine from Michigan in the 1930s and practised as an allergist in Wisconsin and Michigan before setting up in private practice in Chicago in 1944. Increasingly convinced that food allergy was the prime cause of many illnesses, he began to lobby government agencies and industry for clearer guidelines governing the labelling of processed foods. Randolph's activism on this issue led to his exclusion from the Northwestern University Medical School, the loss of a research grant from a food manufacturer and increasing professional isolation. Nevertheless, he continued to practise as an allergist and to publish papers and monographs on food sensitivities.[57]

In 1951, some years before the publication of Rachel Carson's influential exposé of environmental pollutants, Randolph provoked further debate amongst allergists by suggesting that 'increasing pollution of the environment from chemicals was a major source of chronic illness'.[58] In subsequent years, Randolph dedicated his professional life to exploring the environmental determinants of disease, founding the Society for Clinical Ecology (subsequently the American Academy of Environmental Medicine) in 1965, establishing his own Ecology Unit or Environmental Control Unit for diagnosing and treating food and chemical sensitivities, and inspiring a number of clinicians to continue the battle against pollution of the environment and food chain.[59] In Britain, his work was taken up especially by Richard Mackarness (1916–1996), who had met Randolph in the 1950s and who applied Randolph's ideologies to the treatment of patients with mental illness at Basingstoke Hospital in England. In the 1980s Mackarness's book, Not All in the Mind, which was dedicated to Randolph, was credited with having 'done most in the past decade to bring before the general public the more widespread implications of allergy'.[60]

The central tenets of clinical ecology as it emerged in the post-war period were relatively uncomplicated. Employing an expansive definition of allergy that was reminiscent of the work of Clemens von Pirquet, Randolph believed that a wide range of physical and mental symptoms were the product of biological sensitivities to common foods, natural inhalants and chemical pollutants in both the outdoor environment and the home. Headaches, arthritis, asthma, hay fever, fatigue, abdominal symptoms, depression and anxiety, for example, could all be stimulated by the material constituents of everyday life. Randolph's approach was not unfamiliar to clinical allergists, who regularly regarded hay fever, asthma, eczema and food allergies as idiosyncratic reactions to substances that had been ingested, inhaled or touched. There were, however, significant differences between clinical ecology and allergy. In the first place, Randolph insisted that allergic reactions could be provoked by regular exposure to low levels of many non-toxic, and supposedly non-allergenic, substances. Second, he argued that in addition to causing immediate symptoms (characteristically seen in hay fever and asthma), allergy could also precipitate a variety of ill-defined chronic conditions. In these cases, which he linked explicitly to the physiological and psychological processes involved in addiction, the relationship between the food or chemical responsible and the biological reaction was often masked or hidden by the body's adaptive processes, rendering diagnosis difficult. In order to overcome this problem, Randolph and his peers employed elimination diets followed by challenge tests with suspected foods and chemicals, rather than using the skin tests preferred by mainstream allergists.[61]

Clinical ecologists also differed from allergists in their understanding of the mechanisms involved in allergies and in their approach to treatment. While conventional allergists focused largely on IgE-mediated hypersensitivity reactions and referred to other forms of sensitivity as intolerance rather than allergy, clinical ecologists implicated a much wider range of immunological, neurological and hormonal factors in the pathogenesis of allergy.[62] In an interview published in 1983, Randolph demonstrated his scathing disregard for allergists' narrow preoccupations with IgE.

> The allergists are stuck in a trap of their own making. There are numerous mechanisms in allergy. It's ridiculous to limit the concept of hypersensitivity to the one mechanism of IgE. They're trying to make it an exclusive practice. They won't give up. Why? Because they are blockheads.[63]

Treatment in a clinical ecology unit also diverged from conventional approaches that were aimed primarily at altering individual patterns of immunological reactivity using either desensitization or an array of pharmaceutical agents such as antihistamines, bronchodilators and corticosteroids. By contrast, clinical ecologists emphasized the importance of avoiding noxious substances by devising specific diets (such as the 'rotary diversified diet') tailored to the individual patient's susceptibilities and by creating a safe environment or 'oasis within the polluted world', within which patients could retreat and recover from the hazards of modern civilization.[64]

The intellectual and pragmatic precursors of clinical ecology and the professional, social, political and cultural contexts in which the discipline began to flourish in the post-war years were complex. At one level, it may not have been a coincidence that Randolph practised in Chicago, where animal ecologists such as Warder Clyde Allee (1885–1955) and Alfred Edwards Emerson (1896–1976) had developed a school of ecology that prioritized the role of the environment over heredity and which exercised romantic notions of cooperation, harmony and holism rather than competition.[65] However, although the emergence of ecology as a field of study might have provided a local context for the development of environmental medicine, Randolph himself did not locate his ideas within the broader ecological tradition but preferred to stress the clinical origins of his discipline. In the first instance, the ecological vision cultivated by Randolph and propagated by Mackarness and others clearly drew heavily on the studies of early twentieth-century pioneers in the field of food allergy. Soon after Charles Richet and Clemens von Pirquet had introduced the notions of anaphylaxis and allergy, a number of clinicians and scientists, such as the Irish-born physician Francis Hare (1857–1928),[66] began to interpret idiosyncratic reactions to certain foods in immunological terms and to suggest that food allergy might constitute the underlying mechanism in a miscellany of clinical conditions, including asthma, eczema, migraine, mood disturbances and dyspepsia.[67] More particularly, Randolph borrowed from the ideas and discoveries of several leading American allergists: Albert H. Rowe (1889–1970), who had been inspired by the work of Charles Richet and his French colleagues on 'l'anaphylaxie alimentaire' and who had introduced elimination diets in the treatment of food allergies during the 1920s and '30s;[68] Herbert J. Rinkel (1896–1963), who had formulated the concept of 'masked allergy' following observations on his own reactions to eggs;[69] and Arthur F. Coca (1875–1959), who had explored the notion of 'familial nonreaginic food allergy' in 1943 and who had devised the pulse test to identify problematic foods.[70]

During his early years as a clinician, Randolph had developed close connections with Rowe, Rinkel and Coca, and Mackarness had met Albert Rowe during a visit to the United States in 1963.[71] When Randolph and Mackarness began to disseminate their own work to a clinical and broader public audience, they explicitly acknowledged their debt to their predecessors, two of whom (Rowe and Rinkel) were also honoured at the First International Congress of Food and Digestive Allergy, held at Vichy in France in 1963.[72] However, as clinical ecologists began to distance themselves further from mainstream allergy through the adoption of novel diagnostic and therapeutic protocols, they also exploited contemporary developments in other areas of the physiological and pathological sciences. In particular, both Randolph and Mackarness appropriated the concept of 'adaptation' from the work of the Austrian physician Hans Selye (1907–1982), who spent most of his professional life in Canada and who was regarded by Mackarness as one of the 'immortals of medical research', alongside Louis Pasteur, Frederick Banting and Alexander Fleming.[73] During the 1930s and '40s Selye began to study physiological responses to stress (defined as the 'wear and tear caused by life') and to suggest that many clinical conditions (including allergies, rheumatoid arthritis and hypertension) should be understood not merely as signs of externally inflicted damage, but as 'manifestations of the body's adaptive reactions, its mechanism of defense against stress'.[74]

Coining the phrase 'general adaptation syndrome' to describe the combined neurological, immunological and endocrinological responses to stress, Selye outlined three principal stages of the stress syndrome: the alarm phase, in which the body was thought to react immediately (especially through the production of corticosteroids) to combat stress or shock; the stage of resistance or adaptation, in which physiological defence mechanisms attempted to maintain homoeostasis in the face of persistent exposure to 'stressors'; and the stage of exhaustion, at which point even the body's auxiliary channels for containing stress could no longer maintain equilibrium.[75] Significantly, it was this notion of distinct temporal shifts in response to external stress that clinical ecologists such as Randolph and Mackarness adapted in order to explain allergic reactions to environmental agents. During the alarm phase, initial exposure to certain foods and chemicals precipitated immediate forms of hypersensitivity, such as hay fever, asthma and anaphylactic shock. Subsequent exposure, even at low levels, activated adaptive mechanisms that masked the nature of the causal relationship between the allergen and symptoms, and, paradoxically, led to physiological and psychological dependence on the offending substance. In extreme cases, continued exposure eventually led to extensive collapse of the adaptive processes and the generation of florid disease, such as multiple chemical sensitivity or even death.[76]

The notion of adaptation or resistance to environmental stresses articulated by Selye, Randolph and Mackarness in the post-war period paralleled René Dubos's contemporaneous formulation of health as the ability to adapt to the outside world. The political and biological principles of clinical ecology also resonated with the concerns of the modern environmental movement as it emerged in the 1960s. Of course, environmental sensitivity was not new in that period but had been evident in some form in many countries at least from the middle years of the eighteenth century.[77] Since the late nineteenth century, various smoke abatement societies on both sides of the Atlantic had campaigned for greater protection of the built and natural environments, for limiting the ill-health caused by environmental pollution, and for reducing the incomplete and wasteful combustion of fuel. During the twentieth century, political attention to environmental issues was also prominent in Britain, North America and many other countries well before the emergence of the modern environmental movement. Environmental concerns were evident, for example, in the rise of urban planning (regulated in Britain by the Green Belt Act of 1938 and by the Town and Country Planning Acts of 1932, 1944 and 1947), the creation of national parks in the United States and Australia around the end of the nineteenth century and subsequently in Britain from the 1950s, and the establishment of areas of national beauty in Britain under the Countryside Act of 1949.[78]

According to many environmental historians, however, the modern environmental movement did not emerge with any force until the 1960s, appearing at that time as 'a fusion of public health and preservation concerns' on a global scale.[79] Initiated in particular by Rachel Carson, whose 'frontal assault' on the use of pesticides in Silent Spring attracted considerable public and media interest after its publication in 1962,[80] modern environmentalism had developed rapidly into an international movement by the 1970s, embraced by religious leaders as well as scientists and politicians and attracting as much support in developing countries such as India and China as in the developed world.[81] In 1970 Time magazine declared 'the environment' the issue of the year; the environmental pressure groups Greenpeace and Friends of the Earth were founded in 1971; and the 1970s was labelled the 'environmental decade' by

Life magazine.[82] First formed in 1975, the Green Party was attracting votes in European elections by the 1980s.[83] In Britain, the creation of the Department of the Environment in 1970 perhaps marked the official start of the gradual greening of British politics, a process that accelerated, but was also deeply contested, during the 1980s and '90s.

The evolution of global environmental sensitivities in the post-war period was driven in part by international disputes about the apparent conflict between economic development and environmental protection and more particularly about the limits of sustainability.[84] In addition, modern environmentalism was shaped by greater recognition of the impact of environmental change on health at individual, national and global levels,[85] by the emergence of mass consumerism and rapid technological development in Western countries in the post-war years, and by the political upheavals and challenges to established authority generated by, and expressed in, civil rights movements and campaigns against the nuclear arms race.[86] Significantly, the evolution of grass-roots environmental activism, made possible through television and other forms of mass communication, in turn provided fertile ground for the growth of clinical ecology. In sympathy with environmentalist critiques of modern industrial and commercial society, which many believed to be polluting the environment with toxic chemicals, clinical ecologists began to challenge the ideologies and presumptions of modern Western civilization. For Randolph, the need to identify more healthy forms of energy and basic materials, thereby preventing the efflorescence of allergies, operated 'with, not against, environmentalism'.[87] Suggesting that civilization had altered 'our natural balance with the environment', Randolph claimed a pivotal role for his discipline in the struggle to resist the multiple hazards of modernity: 'Clinical ecology shows us how to restore the balance between man and his environment under the condition of advanced civilization.'[88] For Randolph and others, clinical ecology thus offered robust strategies for survival in a 'poisoned world'.[89]

Few aspects of modern life escaped the ecological critique. Pharmaceutical, cosmetics, food and petrochemical industries were castigated by Randolph and Mackarness for initiating and sustaining rising trends in allergies and addictions, a refrain that was echoed in the popular press: 'The scale of chemical adulteration of foodstuffs is scandalous, and it is, of course, in the interests of commerce and industry to perpetuate the general ignorance among the public of the widespread use of such chemicals as tartrazine, monosodium glutamate, nitrate, butylated hydroxy toluene (BHT), butylated hydroxy anisole and sodium benzoate.'[90] In addition, clinical ecologists came into direct conflict with orthodox medical practitioners by explicitly aligning themselves with the supposedly anarchic convictions expressed by the Austrian-born sociologist and former Roman Catholic priest Ivan Illich (1926–2002), who suggested that modern medicine had become a major threat to health through its reliance on 'incriminated substances'.[91] As Randolph was acutely aware, neither the medical profession nor those with extensive commercial interests in industrial expansion embraced such stridently anti-modern sentiments. In particular, the theories and practices of clinical ecology were scathingly rejected as misguided and dangerous, and patients with multiple sensitivities to common substances (such as tap water) were often ridiculed and dismissed as suffering from 'pseudo-allergy' or 'false food allergy',[92] with the implication that in many cases symptoms were merely psychosomatic. Although the report of 1992 from the Royal College of Physicians accepted the role of environmental factors in allergic diseases, it disputed the manner in which clinical ecologists and other alternative practitioners adopted vague definitions of allergy, employed unsubstantiated diagnostic tests (such as provocation-neutralization tests, hair analysis and kinesiology), and engineered treatments that were unconfirmed by objective scientific evidence and which encouraged patients to adopt severely restricted diets.[93] Similar resistance was expressed elsewhere, particularly in debates about total allergy syndrome. As Michelle Murphy has eloquently pointed out, orthodox American practitioners 'greeted this newly emergent illness with more than skepticism', proclaiming multiple chemical sensitivity 'an illegitimate diagnosis'.[94]

During the closing years of the twentieth century, some scientists and clinicians attempted to forge a compromise between clinical ecologists and their detractors. Echoing earlier formulations of the complex aetiology and pathogenesis of asthma as well as scientific studies by Hans Selye, Erwin Pulay and others, they sought to integrate holistic, ecological interpretations of allergy with modern biomedical understandings of disease by exploring the physiological interactions between neurological, immunological and hormonal processes of adaptation to environmental change.[95] In spite of such efforts to defuse evident professional and political tensions, debates about multiple sensitivities to everyday foods and chemicals in the environment became increasingly polarized. On one side, those paying allegiance to the biological and political tenets of clinical ecology continued in their efforts to expose the perils of the modern industrial and domestic environment. Anecdotal evidence presented in the form of case histories by alternative practitioners was endorsed by sensational media portrayals of the tragedies suffered by patients who were referred to by Richard Mackarness as 'chemical victims', and by quasi-religious denouncements of what had allegedly become a 'chemical-oriented society'.[96] From this perspective, people with the symptoms of food allergy and environmental illness, for whom 'the ordinary spaces of late-capitalist life' had become uninhabitable,[97] not only constituted examples of 'bodies in protest' against both the materiality and materialism of modern society but also served as portents of impending ecological disaster. 'Multiple chemical sensitivity', wrote Steve Kroll-Smith and H. Hugh Floyd in 1997, 'is the latest evolution in a series of environmental warnings and technological accidents to occur in the latter decades of the twentieth century.'[98]

Conversely, most conventional practitioners continued to denounce the theoretical underpinnings of clinical ecology, to contest the biological reality of many food and chemical sensitivities, and to challenge the evolutionary and political significance of environmental illness. 'Food allergy', reported the Royal College of Physicians in 2003, 'is the cause of much controversy.'[99] While the report recognized the existence and clinical importance of demonstrable IgE-mediated, and sometimes life-threatening, allergic and anaphylactic reactions to various foods (such as peanuts, shellfish, eggs and milk), it was hesitant to accept the more extravagant claims of alternative practitioners that allergy was responsible for a wide variety of systemic somatic symptoms. Preferring to use the term food intolerance, rather than allergy, in these cases, the report highlighted the inherent difficulties in establishing a scientific rationale for treatment: 'Food intolerance is a more difficult and poorly defined area, where there is much less evidence on which to base practice'.[100] Other commentators were less diplomatic, not only stressing the 'large discrepancy between the high prevalence of self-perception of allergy in the general population and the very low prevalence of allergy detected by objective methods', but also suggesting that many patients with environmental illness exhibited primarily psychiatric, rather than immunological, disorders.[101]

Clinical scepticism spilled over into, and was perhaps partly incited by, representations of allergy in the popular press. At the turn of the millennium, feature articles in British newspapers regularly derided contemporary obsessions with food allergies as fashion, fantasy or fad, rather than fact. Situating concerns about allergy within broader cultural preoccupations with dieting and body image, journalists suggested that, contrary to the claims of clinical ecologists, many allergies were indeed 'all in the mind'.[102] More critically, they emphasized the manner in which allergy had become 'the medical Zeitgeist', comprising merely a 'pseudo-epidemic' which not only neatly captured modern anxieties about pollution but also, in the case of food allergy, reflected middle- and upper-class obsessions with the impact and implications of modern dietary habits on health and social status: 'In fashionable circles, what you push to the side of the plate is deemed to have a greater bearing on your health than what you eat off it.'[103]

Disputes about the biological authenticity of chemical sensitivity and food allergy and about the scientific legitimacy of clinical ecology were framed by disagreements about the most appropriate means of evaluating modern forms of diagnosis and treatment. While conventional practitioners and state health care organizations generally insisted on large randomized controlled trials as the only means of objectively determining clinical efficacy, alternative healers routinely resisted the statistical method, preferring instead to emphasize the centrality of individual experience and the primacy of personal narratives. 'The emphasis here is on the word *you*', wrote Randolph and Moss in 1980, 'this is an individualized approach. It concerns the interaction between you and your own particular environment, which is different from anyone else's.'[104] In addition, as clinical ecologists pointed out, disputes about chemical sensitivity were fuelled by industrial concerns about the commercial and political implications of ecological principles. Advice to avoid or limit the consumption of drugs and commonly eaten foods did not endear Randolph and his colleagues to the pharmaceutical and food industries, which were profitably 'mining a rich seam' of 'high-anxiety purchasers'.[105] Significantly, at the heart of many of these modern controversies about the physical and existential reality of multiple sensitivities to chemicals and food and about the validity of clinical ecology lurked a range of familiar disputes about the technical definition, evolutionary purpose and metaphorical meanings of allergy.

Meanings and metaphors

During the course of the twentieth century, the definition of allergy had been systematically narrowed by clinicians and scientists. By the 1930s clinical allergists on both sides of the Atlantic had moved away from Clemens von Pirquet's original broad notion of altered biological reactivity and were focusing primarily on human hypersensitivity. Over subsequent decades, the conventional clinical meaning of allergy was compressed even further.

Although orthodox physicians acknowledged the clinical relevance of non-IgE-mediated hypersensitivity reactions as well as the role of non-immunological mechanisms in adverse responses to environmental agents, they tended to concentrate predominantly on what were referred to as the 'classical atopic diseases', such as hay fever, asthma, urticaria, atopic eczema, bee-sting allergies, and some food and drug allergies, in which the symptoms were induced by the exaggerated production of IgE, mast cell degranulation, and the release of mediators such as histamine.[106] In an American textbook of immunology published in 1997, for example, Mark Peakman and Diego Vergani noted that, for the sake of clarity, they would 'confine the use of the term "allergic" to those reactions that are initiated when mast-cell bound IgE interacts with its target antigen, known as an allergen'.[107] Similarly, in a supplement of *Nature* devoted to allergy and asthma in 1999, William Cookson pointed out that, for pragmatic purposes, the terms allergy and atopy were synonymous.[108]

To the consternation of orthodox physicians, including many allergists, clinical ecologists tended to adopt a more nebulous and flexible definition of allergy that carried conspicuous vestiges of the expansive ideas formulated by Clemens von Pirquet. In an exposition of the field of clinical ecology published in 1980, Randolph and Moss defined allergy as 'any individualized reaction to an environmental substance occurring in time'.[109] Similarly, Mackarness refused to be constrained by convention and explicitly applauded early studies of food allergy that were 'empirical and clinical, in line with von Pirquet's original, wide biological view of allergy'.[110] For clinical ecologists, allergy also incorporated not only those reactions that appeared rapidly and were mediated by the immune system but also a miscellany of conditions in which the effects of susceptibility became evident only over periods of several days, weeks or months. These broader, more elastic definitions of the term allergy were sustained in the writing of many alternative (and indeed some conventional) practitioners, particularly in North America.[111]

Disparities between conventional and alternative definitions of allergy were deeply embedded in, and compounded by, disputes about the evolutionary or teleological importance of allergic reactions. From the orthodox Western medical perspective, allergy traditionally comprised a form of immunity gone wrong, an example of the failure of immunological defence mechanisms to operate normally. Thus, although Jules Bordet and other early twentieth-century clinicians and scientists acknowledged that anaphylaxis and allergy were closely related to immunity, they nevertheless believed that anaphylaxis was 'an accident in the course of the defence'.[112] This interpretation of allergy and anaphylaxis was reiterated by subsequent writers. In 1959, for example, in a passage that revealed not only contemporary preoccupations with charting the evolution of immune responses but also broader cultural visions of political tolerance and global harmony (perhaps shaped by his flight from Germany to England in 1933), the physician Carl Prausnitz reflected philosophically on the meaning of allergy.

> Since undoubtedly allergy is a phase of immunity, might one say, from a finite, egocentric point of view that Allergy is Immunity gone astray? . . . Might one assume that most individuals during embryonic existence acquire Immuno-Tolerance to a wide variety of foreign proteins and their breakdown products as they pass through the placental circulation; but that some individuals, perhaps hereditarily predisposed, fail to do so and are then ready under given conditions of exposure to produce antibodies? Might we dream of a future in which mankind has learned to re-establish, together with general human tolerance, some measure of Immuno-Tolerance?[113]

The notion that allergy constituted a deviant immunological reaction appeared in other locations. Most notably, it fuelled the search for new therapeutic strategies aimed at damping down allergic responses and underwrote assumptions and interpretations of the hygiene hypothesis that postulated that, under certain conditions, the immune system was diverted away from its intended function of protecting the body against pathogenic invasion towards the production of destructive responses to seemingly innocuous external and internal substances. Significantly, even the discovery that IgE-mediated mechanisms possibly conferred protection against parasitic worm infections failed to dispel suspicions that hypersensitivity reactions involving IgE essentially constituted immunological aberrations that served no teleological purpose.[114]

The conventional view of allergies and indeed autoimmune diseases as immunological anomalies or paradoxes was largely driven by narrow preoccupations with the protective role of immunity and by a persistent conviction that the immune system was designed primarily to distinguish between self and non-self. However, as several commentators pointed out during the 1990s, there were alternative ways of understanding the immune system that encouraged a re-evaluation of the individual and evolutionary utility of allergy. In 1991, for example, Margie Profet, from the Division of Biochemistry and Molecular Biology at the University of California, suggested that allergic reactions served in many cases to protect the body against toxins and carcinogens. Pointing out that the 'specialized mechanisms that collectively constitute the allergic responses appear to manifest adaptive design', she proposed that allergy comprised a last line of defence against toxins when other mucosal or humoral defence mechanisms had previously proved ineffective; although inconvenient and debilitating, sneezing, coughing and vomiting served to expel harmful substances that would otherwise penetrate and damage the body. In line with clinical ecologists, Profet argued that rising trends in allergy simply reflected physiological responses to the proliferation of unavoidable toxins in industrial societies. Although Profet recognized that allergy often conferred the danger of discomfort and occasionally death, she suggested that in both individual and evolutionary terms the benefits 'conferred by adaptive allergies' often outweighed the risks. From this perspective, IgE was to be reconfigured as an 'immunobiological hero' rather than a villain.[115]

In the mid-1990s Polly Matzinger, from the National Institute of Allergy and Infectious Diseases in Bethesda, similarly challenged conventional interpretations of immunity, autoimmunity and allergy. Highlighting the problems posed by presuming that the immune system functioned exclusively by discriminating between self and non-self, Matzinger suggested instead that all immune responses, including those hypersensitivity reactions leading to tissue damage, were initiated by alarm signals released from injured cells. In the case of autoimmunity and allergy, the immune system was not necessarily malfunctioning but instead responding to danger signals provoked by mutations or environmental pathogens and toxins. Echoing von Pirquet's emphasis on the pivotal role of bodily reactivity in determining the manifestations of disease, as well as Richet's notion of humoral personality, Matzinger's 'danger model' emphasized the role of immune responsiveness in preserving biological identity and integrity.[116]

These novel theories of immunological function offered a critical counterpoint to traditional interpretations of allergy. In both cases, the symptoms of allergy no longer signified an aberrant individual whose immune system was to be modified and manipulated by drugs and desensitization. On the contrary, allergy constituted a crucial form of resistance to both external and internal dangers, a protective reaction of considerable individual and evolutionary consequence. Interestingly, allergy was occasionally thought to carry other protective properties. Thus, in addition to implicating immunological reactivity in the ageing process (in a manner reminiscent of Clemens von

Pirquet's notion of 'Allergie des Lebensalters'),[117] clinicians postulated that allergy might also protect against malignancies. Noting an inverse correlation between cancer and atopy, some studies advocated the induction of atopy as a form of treatment in patients with cancer.[118]

More intriguingly, allergy remained a condition, or set of conditions, with a distinctive social and cultural geography. During the twentieth century, commentators regularly echoed a prevalent opinion, expressed in earlier decades by Morell Mackenzie, E. M. Forster and others, that allergy conferred some form of innate intellectual or creative superiority. In the 1930s, for example, researchers at Guy's Hospital in London supposedly provided some evidential support for popular beliefs that asthmatic children 'tend to be of "superior intelligence".[119] Similar presumptions surfaced in later discussions of the prevalence of asthma and hay fever in leading literary and musical figures. In the 1980s, in their introduction to a series of articles on 'asthma and human excellence', which explored the lives of Arnold Schoenberg, Alban Berg, Seneca, Charles Darwin, Marcel Proust and others, the editors of the *Journal of Asthma* argued that 'superior intelligence, creative genius, extraordinary personality, and/or social prominence have been associated with asthma often enough to raise the question of a nonrandom occurrence'.[120] Although this inference clearly ran counter to epidemiological evidence that asthma and other allergic conditions were associated more with poverty and deprivation than with social prominence, the notion that allergy constituted a mark of cultural distinction persisted. As several commentators on the fashion for food intolerance pointed out towards the end of the century, the possession of an allergy signified sensitivity and refinement: 'Waving away a dish with a feeble cry of "I like it, but it doesn't like me" lifts the sufferer romantically above their less discriminating dining companions'.[121]

As these comments suggest, the notion of allergy increasingly conveyed a miscellany of broad cultural, as well as technical scientific, meanings. Thus, paradoxically, while allergists were intentionally restricting the definition of allergy to IgE-mediated hypersensitivity reactions, popular usage was expanding the boundaries of the term to incorporate a wide variety of physical and psychological conditions. In 1960 Milton Millman pointed out that allergy was 'a word that in recent years has come into everyday language. The magazines, newspapers, and movies have made the public allergy conscious.' In the process, the meaning of allergy had become more elastic and fluid. 'The lay meaning of allergy in its colloquial form', wrote Millman, 'has come to mean anything or anybody that irritates a person, physically or mentally.'[122]

Vernacular usage did not go unchallenged. During the second half of the twentieth century, clinicians persistently reiterated the earlier attempts of John Freeman and Arnold Rice Rich to resist what they regarded as distortion of the language of allergy. In 1961 Kenneth Hutchin complained that the word allergy 'was both over-worked and abused because nine times out of ten it is used in the wrong way'.[123] Ten years later, in the opening issue of *Clinical Allergy*, Jack Pepys similarly bemoaned the manner in which terms such as allergy and atopy had become so 'confused and so prejudicial to the subject that some authorities would prefer them abandoned'.[124] And in 1974, in a straightforward introduction to the concepts of adaptation and stress, Hans Selye pointed out that many modern scientific terms (including stress) had been appropriated and manipulated in this way: 'Such terms as "Darwinian evolution," "allergy," and "psychoanalysis" have all had their peaks of popularity in drawing-room or cocktail-party conversations; but rarely are the opinions about them based on a study of technical works written by the scientists who established these concepts.'[125]

In general, allergists were unable to resist popular appropriation of the term. In the closing decades of the twentieth century, allergy was increasingly employed to signify a bizarre assortment of physical idiosyncrasies, personal antipathies, psychological aversions, marital disagreements, commercial conflicts and international tensions. Stretching the semantic boundaries of allergy made possible a myriad of metaphorical and comical meanings that paralleled, and perhaps even partially eclipsed or mocked, serious references to rising epidemiological trends in allergic diseases. As Theodore Dalrymple sardonically commented, it 'is curious how a real and genuine problem such as allergy should almost always bring in its wake, as a kind of doppelgänger, a shadow-form that exists only in the minds of men'.[126] In the late twentieth century, people proudly described themselves as being allergic to Mondays, work, crowds, mornings, their mothers-in-law or day-time television, a cultural phenomenon that was sometimes ridiculed, but nevertheless implicitly acknowledged, by cartoonists.[127] Although satirical exploitation of the notion of allergy was largely light-hearted, the term sometimes conveyed darker meanings. During bitter debates about European economic and monetary union in 1997, Jacques Delors, former President of the European Commission, accused German politicians 'of having an allergy towards southern European states'.[128] The following year, the friction evident during negotiations surrounding the merger of two leading multinational pharmaceutical companies, Glaxo and SmithKline Beecham, was heralded as an 'allergic

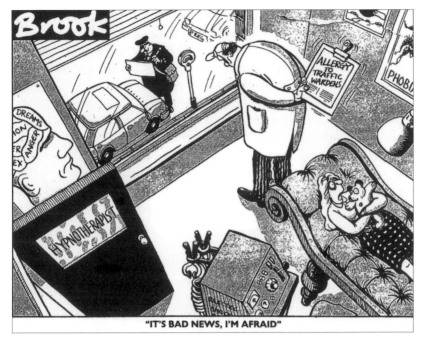

"IT'S BAD NEWS, I'M AFRAID"

The Sun, August 1996.

reaction', with the distinct irony that Glaxo constituted the world's leading manufacturer of anti-allergy medication.[129]

At the turn of the millennium, in a retrospective anthology of novel words that had been introduced to the English language during the course of the twentieth century, the publisher HarperCollins suggested that, although the term allergy had initially denoted only physical reactions to various external stimuli when it had been introduced by Clemens von Pirquet, during the course of the century it had 'gained figurative currency' as a form of aversion.[130] The notion of currency was apposite. By the dawn of the twenty-first century, allergy had become a rich cultural resource for expressing and exchanging social anxieties about the material and ideological determinants and consequences of environmental degradation, ecological imbalance and global disharmony. Allergy had also emerged as a convenient vehicle for exposing and explaining diverse modern forms of individual physiological, psychological and political antagonism. Significantly, the allegorical potency of allergy was rooted not only in its broader cultural and ecological applications but also in its original scientific meaning. For Clemens von Pirquet, allergy captured the manner in which internal bodily reactions, rather than merely external agents, shaped the manifestations of disease. Primarily indicative of a self-destructive pathological process, allergy was adopted both as a suitable metaphor for the self-inflicted damage being wrought by Western civilization and as a symbol of radical endeavours to resist the commercial values and biological hazards propagated by modern society. Perhaps more than any other condition, allergy embodied the biological, political and spiritual challenges faced by inhabitants of the post-modern world.

7
FUTURES

When will we be able to define the structures that determine, in the
secret volume of the body, the course of allergic reactions?

Michel Foucault, 1963[1]

On the eve of the new millennium, as the ideologies and structures of late
modernity were being systematically challenged and progressively disman-
tled, the English prize-winning novelist Jeff Noon deftly captured in a single
metaphor the multiple perils supposedly inherent in modern Westernized,
industrialized and commercialized lifestyles. Set in a futuristic urban society
struggling to resist the murderous intrusion of pollinating plants from the
world of dreams and apparently inspired both by childhood experiences of
hay fever and by an awareness of the AIDS epidemic, Noon's cyberpunk novel,
Pollen, first published in 1995, graphically charted the damage caused by
uncontrolled technological innovation, genetic manipulation, environmental
degradation, drug abuse, sexual licence and the gradual erosion of barriers
between species. In Noon's apocalyptic vision of the horrors awaiting the
post-modern world, hay fever constituted the archetypal disease of civilization, induced by modern modes of living but in turn responsible for generating bizarre obsessions with health, a lucrative market for both conventional
and alternative remedies, and sensational stories in the mass media.[2]

Noon was not alone in imagining future risks. In the late twentieth
century, many commentators echoed the fears expressed in 1982 by an
eminent British allergist, Maurice H. Lessof, that human beings were now
living 'in an allergy-prone world'.[3] Although epidemiological studies
revealed persistent geographical and social gradients in the prevalence of
allergic diseases, regular reports of soaring seasonal pollen counts and
sharply rising global levels of allergies encouraged Western clinicians, scientists and journalists to issue stringent warnings that, if modern trends
remained unchecked, 50 per cent of all Europeans would be suffering from
an allergy by 2015. Such speculations encouraged the UCB Institute of Allergy
to nominate allergy as 'the epidemic of the 21st century'.[4] The potential
impact of this explosion of allergies on health, happiness and longevity was
clear: allergic reactions could severely compromise the quality of life and, in
some instances, kill.

Significantly, anxieties about the proliferation of allergies in humans may have been exacerbated by growing evidence of the parallel spread of allergic diseases in animals. During the closing decades of the twentieth century, allergic reactions to a wide variety of common inhalants, insects and foods were implicated in equine diseases such as chronic obstructive pulmonary disease, urticaria, headshaking and sweet itch (the equine equivalent of eczema). Drawing on human models of diagnosis and treatment, equine allergy clinics not only offered tests to measure blood levels of IgE and to establish skin sensitivity to intradermal provocation with allergens, but also introduced courses of allergy neutralization treatment in order to desensitize horses.[5] The diffusion of allergy across species as well as across time and space, and the proliferation of commercial opportunities in the field of veterinary allergy, arguably served to accentuate apprehensions of impending global catastrophe.

Pessimistic forecasts of future hazards can be understood in different ways. On the one hand, contemporary fears that rising trends in allergy will eventually suffocate most of the global population can be regarded as a product of realistic calculations of the environmental risks being generated by modern industrial society. On the other hand, anxieties about a global epidemic of allergies can be construed as merely the reaffirmation of a familiar, and perhaps weary, critique of social and medical progress, in which cultural and political contingencies have manifestly moulded statistical figures and epidemiological patterns into objects of terror. Of course, contrasting discourses on trends in allergy should not be regarded as mutually exclusive. Multiple sensitivities to chemicals and foods can, at the same time, constitute severe, life-threatening immunological reactions to environmental pollution as well as potent manifestations of individual psychological disturbances and broader social, political and professional insurgency.

Allergists, patients, politicians and international health care agencies struggling to loosen the grip of allergy on modern societies have adopted conflicting strategies. Those who believe in the promise of medical progress have tended to retreat into the narrow domain of orthodox biomedicine and biostatistics. Emphasizing the role of professional knowledge and expert systems of diagnosis and management, scientists and clinicians have attempted to generate more expansive epidemiological studies of the social and geographical distribution of allergic diseases and to delve more deeply into the secret spaces and biochemical processes in the body that appear to define and drive allergic reactions. At the turn of the millennium, continuing commitment to Maurice Lessof's conviction that scientific methods could effectively 'separate fact from fiction' in the field of allergy,[6] together with tentative suspicions that acute asthma episodes were beginning to decline in the wake of modern treatment regimes,[7] served to promote more refined studies of the genes, antibodies, cells and intercellular mediators involved in allergic reactions as well as the formulation of innovative therapeutic approaches aimed at moderating or controlling harmful immunological reactivity.[8]

Of course, utopian dreams of the biomedical conquest of allergy are not new. In 1939 Warren Vaughan insisted that scientists would 'eventually solve the riddle of allergy'.[9] Three years later, Milton B. Cohen, who served as president of both American allergy societies before their merger in 1943 and was the architect of the American Allergy Foundation, and his wife suggested that if 'we are to succeed in eliminating the allergic state, our approach must be biochemical or biophysical', and urged their fellow allergists to push back relentlessly the 'frontiers of allergic prevention'.[10] However, striking evidence that allergies have been rising in spite of substantial advances in biomedical knowledge has led some allergists, clinical ecologists and environmental activists in particular to posit an alternative solution to the global plague of allergic diseases. Arguing that modern medicine, along with many other industries, has been largely responsible for generating new environmental illnesses, and drawing on romantic notions of a natural, but mythical, unpolluted past, a variety of alternative practitioners have persistently challenged the values and practices of Western society. By exposing what they regard as the 'spiritual bankruptcy' of orthodox medicine and modern lifestyles, alternative practitioners have attempted to reassert the importance of ecological balance and individual harmony in the battle against environmental desolation and disease.[11]

Neither optimistic bioscientific dreams of future freedom from disease nor despairing ecological dramatizations of impending environmental disaster accurately reflect the ambiguous place and meaning of allergy in the modern world. The remarkable efflorescence of allergies during recent decades has been the product of a complex interplay of socio-economic and cultural factors. Like many other chronic conditions, allergy is a malady of our own creating. At one level, this modern formulation of Thomas Beddoes's beliefs about the aetiology of tuberculosis in the early nineteenth century simply implies that allergic diseases constitute existential realities that are intimately related to the material processes of modern civilization and which are vulnerable to scientific dissection, epidemiological investigation and biochemical manipulation. At another level, the provocative notion that the modern world has created allergic diseases also suggests that allergy has flour-ished as an index of cultural anxiety, as a pathological concept closely shaped by the imaginative force of radical environmentalist critiques of modern commercial civilization and spiritual yearnings for individual solace.

As René Dubos was eager to point out in the 1950s and '60s, it is 'unwise to predict the future from the short perspective of the past decades'.[12] Nevertheless, Dubos was confident that neither narrow preoccupations with biomedicine nor broader programmes of social and spiritual reform offered realistic routes to health. 'There is overwhelming historical evidence', he wrote in 1961, 'that the evolution of diseases is influenced by many determining factors which are not as yet amenable to social or medical control, and may never be.'[13] For Dubos, patterns of health and disease were more closely fashioned by what he termed the 'creative emergent quality of human existence':[14]

> We must beware lest we create the illusion that health will be a birthright for all in the medical utopia, or a state to be reached passively by following the directives of physicians or by taking drugs bought at the corner store. In the real world of the future, as in the past, health will depend on a creative way of life, on the manner in which men respond to unpredictable challenges that continue to arise from an ever changing environment.[15]

So what does the real world of the future hold for allergy? In 1942 Milton and June Cohen whimsically proposed that medical advances often depended upon prior sensitization of a scientist's mind. The mid-nineteenth-century solution to the problems of post-operative sepsis, they argued, resulted from the fact that Joseph Lister (1827–1912) had, metaphorically, been sensitized by the work of Louis Pasteur (1822–1896). According to the Cohens, the future of allergy would be determined in a similar manner:

> Some day an allergist will appear whose mind has become sensitized by the problems of allergy. During his life-time an idea will be born in the laboratory of the physicist or the chemist. This idea will have to do with the workings of the living cell. It will act as an allergen. It will produce in the mind of the allergist an altered reactivity. As a result, our understanding of allergy may be revolutionized. The appearance of the allergic state may become no more than an occasional curiosity. The family of allergic diseases may become merely an interesting episode in medical history.[16]

This neat and symmetrical, but as yet unrealized, vision of future developments, in which allergy holds the key to its own fate, is striking not only for its belief in the redemptive powers of modern medicine but also for its rich resonance with Clemens von Pirquet's original expansive, but largely discarded, formulation of altered reactivity. As in so many other aspects of the history of allergy, however, the metaphor of allergic sensitization mobilized by Milton and June Cohen to predict future patterns of allergic disease immediately offers the possibility of alternative existential, intellectual and political trajectories. Unremitting exposure to the diverse biological and cultural manifestations of allergy as well as to the myriad allergens and irritants in the modern enviroment might serve not to sensitize, but eventually to desensitize, modern populations. As biological and psychological tolerance spreads, allergy may well retreat, leaving a vacuum to be filled by new diseases, fresh cultural obsessions and novel metaphors.

GLOSSARY

aerobiology the study of organisms and other biologically significant materials present in the atmosphere and their impact on animal, plant, and human systems

aetiology the cause of a disease or the study of causative factors in disease

allergen any substance capable of stimulating an allergic reaction

allergic alveolitis a form of hypersensitivity caused by exposure to dusts of animal and vegetable origin and leading to inflammation in the lungs

allergy a term introduced by Clemens von Pirquet in 1906 to denote any form of altered biological reactivity; subsequently narrowed to signify only particular forms of hypersensitivity

anaphylaxis a term introduced by Charles Richet and Paul Portier in 1902, meaning literally the 'absence of protection'; subsequently used more commonly to describe immediate, and sometimes fatal, allergic reactions, such as 'anaphylactic shock'

angioneurotic oedema a condition leading to swelling of the skin and mucosal surfaces and caused either by an inherited enzyme deficiency or by an allergic reaction

antibody a protein, or immunoglobulin, which binds specifically to an antigen

antigen any substance capable of stimulating an immune response

atopy a familial tendency to immediate Type I hypersensitivity reactions

autoimmunity a situation in which immune responses develop to self antigens, sometimes causing disease

bronchodilator a type of medication which relaxes bronchial smooth muscles and facilitates breathing

cardiotoxic harmful to the heart

complement a series of proteins in the blood which combine to facilitate defence against pathogens

corticosteroids a group of medicines, related to naturally occurring steroids, which possess anti-inflammatory properties

desensitization the process of inducing immunological tolerance by injecting increasing doses of an allergen; also known as allergen immunotherapy or therapeutic inoculation

emphysema a disease in which the alveoli in the lungs become damaged

eosinophilia an excess of certain white cells (eosinophils) in the blood

epidemiology the study of diseases in groups of people

histamine an inflammatory mediator, stored in mast cells and released on binding of an antigen to cell surface IgE

hyperpyraemia a theory of allergy which was first introduced by Francis Hare in 1905 and according to which the accumulation of certain irritants in the blood provokes dilatation of blood vessels

hypersensitivity a term introduced by Emil von Behring in 1894 to signify an exaggerated response to foreign substances with resultant tissue damage or death; subsequently categorized into four types according to the immunological mechanisms involved

idiosyncrasy a term commonly used in the nineteenth century to describe an unusual sensitivity to foreign substances such as dust, hay, feathers, animals and various foods

idiotype a unique antigen-binding site on an antibody

Immunoglobulin E (IgE) the immunoglobulin or antibody involved in Type I hypersensitivity reactions

immunochemistry the study of the chemistry of immunological processes, including antigen-antibody interactions

immunopathology the study of immune reactions which result in tissue injury

leukotriene an inflammatory mediator produced by certain white blood cells (macrophages)

pathogenesis the pathological processes by which a disease develops

status asthmaticus a severe and prolonged attack of asthma

urticaria a skin condition also known as nettle-rash

REFERENCES

Preface

1   Local Government Association, *Independent Commission on the Organisation of the School Year: The Rhythms of Schooling* (London, 2003).
2   'Hay fever as an educational handicap', *Medical Officer*, 118 (1967), p. 290; T. E. Roberts, 'Hay fever in adolescents', *Medical Officer*, 118 (1967), pp. 291–4; Brenda Sanderson, 'Hay fever and exams', *The Times* (14 July 1973), 13g; S. C. Littlewood, 'Hay fever during exams', *The Times* (21 July 1973), 13e; David Nicholson-Lord, 'Hay-fever bureau to back earlier exams', *The Times* (3 August 1983), 3a; Thomson Prentice, 'Hay fever blamed for poor exam results', *The Times* (2 May 1985), 3h.

Chapter 1: Histories

1   Thomas Beddoes, *Hygëia; or, Essays Moral and Medical on the Causes Affecting the Personal State of our Middling and Affluent Classes* (London, 1802), vol. II, p. 98.
2   Clemens von Pirquet, 'Allergie', *Münchener Medizinische Wochenschrift*, 30 (1906), pp. 1457–8.
3   Charles Richet, *L'Anaphylaxie* (Paris, 1912), p. 80: 'Pirquet et Schick ont appelé *allergie* ce phénomène de réaction de l'organisme a une substance étrangère: mais il ne me paraît pas nécessaire d-introduire ce mot conjointement avec le mot d'anaphylaxie.'
4   Béla Schick, 'Pediatrics in Vienna at the beginning of the century', *Journal of Pediatrics*, 50 (1957), pp. 114–24; Hans Selye, *The Stress of Life* (New York, 1956), p. 193.
5   Von Pirquet, 'Allergie'.
6   World Health Organization, 'The Prevention of Allergic Diseases', *Clinical Allergy*, 16 (1986), Supplement.
7   Royal College of Physicians, *Allergy: The Unmet Need* (London, 2003).
8   'The modern plague: special allergy issue', *Sunday Times Magazine* (19 October 1997).
9   Katherine Ott, *Fevered Lives: Tuberculosis in American Culture since 1870* (Cambridge, MA, 1996), p. 1.
10 F. F. Cartwright, *The English Pioneers of Anaesthesia* (Bristol, 1952).
11 Beddoes, *Hygëia*, p. 102.
12 Ibid., p. 98.
13 Roy Porter, 'Civilisation and disease: medical ideology in the Enlightenment', in

    Culture, Politics and Society in Britain, 1660–1800, ed. Jeremy Black and Jeremy Gregory (Manchester, 1991), pp. 154–83.

14   Charles E. Rosenberg, 'Pathologies of progress: the idea of civilization as risk', *Bulletin of the History of Medicine*, 72 (1998), pp. 714–30.

15   Porter, 'Civilisation and disease'.

16   Roy Porter and G. S. Rousseau, *Gout: The Patrician Malady* (New Haven, CT, 1998).

17   Ott, *Fevered Lives*, p. 1.

18   Rosenberg, 'Pathologies of progress', p. 716.

19   Charles E. Rosenberg, 'Introduction', in George Beard, *American Nervousness: Its Causes and Consequences* (1881) (New York, 1972).

20   Porter, 'Civilisation and disease', p. 160.

21   Rosenberg, 'Pathologies of progress'.

22   Ibid. See also Roy Porter, 'Diseases of civilization', in *Companion Encyclopedia of the History of Medicine*, ed. W. F. Bynum and Roy Porter (London, 1993), vol. I, pp. 584–600.

23   René Dubos, *The Dreams of Reason: Science and Utopias* (New York, 1961), p. 84.

24   Norbert Elias, *The Civilizing Process: Sociogenetic and Psychogenetic Investigations* (1939) (Oxford, 2000), p. xiv.

25   Albert Camus, *The Plague* (London, 1981), p. 207. On Hirszfeld and Fleck, see Peter Keating, 'Holistic bacteriology: Ludwik Hirszfeld's doctrine of serogenesis between the two world wars', in *Greater than the Parts: Holism in Biomedicine, 1920–1950*, ed. Christopher Lawrence and George Weisz (New York, 1998), pp. 283–302; Ilana Löwy, 'The immunological construction of self', in *Organism and the Origins of Self*, ed. Alfred I. Tauber (Dordrecht, 1991), pp. 43–75; Ilana Löwy, *Medical Acts and Medical Facts* (Cracow, 2000).

26   Rosenberg, 'Pathologies of progress', p. 723.

27   See, for example: Randolph M. Nesse and George C. Williams, *Evolution and Healing: The New Science of Darwinian Medicine* (Phoenix, AZ, 1996); Peter Radetsky, *Allergic to the Twentieth Century* (Boston, MA, 1997).

28   Radetsky, *Allergic to the Twentieth Century*, p. 18.

29   See Brian Inglis, *The Diseases of Civilisation* (London, 1981), pp. 227–8.

30   Porter and Rousseau, *Gout*, pp. 2–3.

31   James T. Patterson, *The Dread Disease: Cancer and Modern American Culture* (Cambridge, MA, 1987); Joan Austoker, *A History of the Imperial Cancer Research Fund, 1902–1986* (Oxford, 1986); Evelleen Richards, *Vitamin C and Cancer: Medicine or Politics?* (Basingstoke, 1991); David Cantor, 'Contracting cancer: the politics of commissioned histories', *Social History of Medicine*, 5 (1992), pp. 131–42; Patrice Pinell, *Naissance d'un fléau: histoire de la lutte contre le cancer en France, 1890–1940* (Paris, 1992); S. Robert Lichter and Stanley Rothman, *Environmental Cancer: A Political Disease?* (New Haven, CT, 1999).

32   Geoffrey Tweedale, *Magic Mineral to Killer Dust: Turner & Newall and the Asbestos Hazard* (Oxford, 2000); David Rosner and Gerald Markowitz, *Deadly Dust: Silicosis and the Politics of Occupational Disease in Twentieth-Century America* (Princeton, NJ, 1991); Alan Derickson, *Black Lung: Anatomy of a Public Health Disaster* (Ithaca, NY,

1998); Christopher C. Sellers, *Hazards of the Job: From Industrial Disease to Environmental Health Science* (Chapel Hill, NC, 1997); Christian Warren, *Brush with Death: A Social History of Lead Poisoning* (Baltimore, MD, 2000).

33 Ernest M. Gruenberg, 'The failures of success', *Millbank Memorial Fund Quarterly/Health and Society*, 55 (1977), pp. 3–24. For historical attention to chronic diseases in these terms, see James C. Riley, *Rising Life Expectancy: A Global History* (Cambridge, 2001); Gerald C. Grob, *The Deadly Truth: A History of Disease in America* (Cambridge, MA, 2002).

34 Alfred I. Tauber and Leon Chernyak, *Metchnikoff and the Origins of Immunology: From Metaphor to Theory* (Oxford, 1991); Alfred I. Tauber, *The Immune Self: Theory or Metaphor?* (Cambridge, 1994); A. M. Moulin and A. Cambrosio, eds, *Singular Selves: Historical Issues and Contemporary Debates in Immunology* (Amsterdam, 2000); Leslie Brent, *A History of Transplantation Immunology* (San Diego, CA, 1997); Arthur M. Silverstein, *A History of Immunology* (San Diego, CA, 1989); Pauline M. H. Mazumdar, ed., *Immunology, 1930–1980: Essays on the History of Immunology* (Toronto, 1989); Pauline M. H. Mazumdar, *Species and Specificity: An Interpretation of the History of Immunology* (Cambridge, 1995); Anne Marie Moulin, 'The immune system: a key concept for the history of immunology', *History and Philosophy of the Life Sciences*, 11 (1989) pp. 221–36; Anne Marie Moulin, *Le dernier langage de la médecine* (Paris, 1991); Ilana Löwy, 'The strength of loose concepts – boundary concepts, federative experimental strategies and disciplinary growth: the case of immunology', *History of Science*, 30 (1992), pp. 371–96; Alberto Cambrosio and Peter Keating, *Exquisite Specificity: The Monoclonal Antibody Revolution* (New York, 1995); Arthur M. Silverstein, *Paul Ehrlich's Receptor Immunology: The Magnificent Obsession* (San Diego, CA, 2002); Cay-Rüdiger Prüll, 'Part of a scientific master plan? Paul Ehrlich and the origins of his receptor concept', *Medical History*, 47 (2003), pp. 332–56; Thomas Söderqvist, *Science as Autobiography: The Troubled Life of Niels Jerne* (New Haven, CT, 2003); Scott Podolsky and Alfred I. Tauber, *The Generation of Diversity: Clonal Selection Theory and the Rise of Molecular Immunology* (Cambridge, MA, 1998).

35 The term was first used by Arrhenius in a series of lectures delivered at Berkeley in 1904 and was later incorporated in the title of his *Immunochemistry: The Application of the Principles of Physical Chemistry to the Study of the Biological Antibodies* (New York, 1907).

36 Löwy, 'The strength of loose concepts', p. 372.

37 Warwick Anderson, Myles Jackson and Barbara Gutmann Rosenkrantz, 'Toward an unnatural history of immunology', *Journal of the History of Biology*, 27 (1994), pp. 575–94. See also Moulin, 'The immune system', p. 236.

38 D. J. Bibel, *Milestones in Immunology: A Historical Exploration* (Madison, WI, 1988); Sheldon G. Cohen and Max Samter, eds, *Excerpts from Classics in Allergy* (Carlsbad, CA, 1982); Richard B. Gallagher et al., eds, *Immunology: The Making of a Modern Science* (London, 1995); J. Mazana and M. R. Ariño, 'Charles Robert Richet and some milestones in the history of allergies', *Journal of Investigative Allergology and Clinical Immunology*, 1 (1991), pp. 93–100; P. E. Richardson, J. E. Landry and S. G. Cohen, 'Immunologists honored by commemorative and special issues of postage

stamps', *Allergy Proceedings*, 14 (1993), pp. 429–38; L. Unger and M. C. Harris, 'Stepping stones in allergy', *Annals of Allergy*, 32 (1974), pp. 214–30, 266–78, 348–60; 33 (1975), pp. 50–64, 113–27, 182–8, 228–47, 299–311, 353–63; 34 (1975), pp. 60–69, 125–9, 185–200, 253–7, 336–7.

39 Hans Schadewaldt, *Geschichte der Allergie*, 4 vols (Munich, 1979–83).

40 Anderson, Jackson and Rosenkrantz, 'Toward an unnatural history'.

41 Quoted in Löwy, 'The immunological construction of self', p. 47.

42 Ott, *Fevered Lives*, p. 2.

43 Kathryn J. Waite, 'Blackley and the development of hay fever as a disease of civilization in the nineteenth century', *Medical History*, 39 (1995), pp. 186–96; M. B. Emanuel, 'Hay fever, a post industrial revolution epidemic: a history of its growth during the 19th century', *Clinical Allergy*, 18 (1988), pp. 295–304.

44 John Gabbay, 'Asthma attacked? Tactics for the reconstruction of a disease concept', in *The Problem of Medical Knowledge*, ed. Peter Wright and Andrew Treacher (Edinburgh, 1982), pp. 23–48; Carla C. Keirns, 'Better than nature: the changing treatment of asthma and hay fever in the United States, 1910–1945', *Studies in History and Philosophy of Biological and Biomedical Sciences*, 34 (2003), pp. 511–31.

45 Ilana Löwy, 'On guinea pigs, dogs and men: anaphylaxis and the study of biological individuality, 1902–1939', *Studies in History and Philosophy of Biological and Biomedical Sciences*, 34 (2003), pp. 399–424; E. M. Tansey, 'Henry Dale, histamine and anaphylaxis: reflections on the role of chance in the history of allergy', ibid., pp. 455–72; Ohad Parnes, '"Trouble from within": allergy, autoimmunity and pathology in the first half of the twentieth century', ibid., pp. 425–54; Kenton Kroker, 'Immunity and its other: the anaphylactic selves of Charles Richet', *Studies in History and Philosophy of Biological and Biomedical Sciences*, 30 (1999), pp. 273–96.

46 Gregg Mitman, 'Natural history and the clinic: the regional ecology of allergy in America', *Studies in History and Philosophy of Biological and Biomedical Sciences*, 34 (2003), pp. 491–510. See also: Gregg Mitman, 'Hay fever holiday: health, leisure and place in gilded-age America', *Bulletin of the History of Medicine*, 77 (2003), pp. 600–35; Gregg Mitman, 'What's in a weed? A cultural geography of *Ambrosia artemesiaefolia*', in *The Moral Authority of Nature*, ed. Lorraine Daston and Fernando Vidal (Chicago, 2003), pp. 438–65; Gregg Mitman, 'Geographies of hope: mining the frontiers of health in Denver and beyond, 1870–1965', *Osiris*, 19 (2004), pp. 93–111.

47 Anderson, Jackson and Rosenkrantz, 'Toward an unnatural history', p. 587.

48 CIBA-Broschüre, 'Steckt eine Allergie dahinter?' (1948), reproduced in Ulrich Meyer, *Steckt eine Allergie dahinter? Die Industrialisierung von Arzneimittel-Entwicklung, -Herstellung und -Vermarktung am Beispiel der Antiallergika* (Stuttgart, 2002).

49 Ulrich Beck, *Risk Society: Towards a New Modernity* (London, 1992), p. 19.

50 J. Harvey Black, 'The state of allergy', reprinted in *Journal of Allergy and Clinical Immunology*, 64 (1979), pp. 469–71.

51 Warren T. Vaughan, *Primer of Allergy* (St Louis, MO, 1939), pp. 29–40.

52 Warren T. Vaughan, *Strange Malady: The Story of Allergy* (New York, 1941), p. 7.

53 Roland Davies, 'Hayfever: is it on the increase?', *Medical Dialogue Weekly*, 236 (June 1989).

54 Gregg Mitman, Michelle Murphy and Christopher Sellers, 'Introduction: a cloud over history', in Mitman, Murphy and Sellers, eds, *Landscapes of Exposure: Knowledge and Illness in Modern Environments, Osiris: Special Issue*, 19 (2004), pp. 1–17 (p. 13).

55 Ott, *Fevered Lives*, p. 4.

Chapter 2: Strange Reactions

1 Clemens von Pirquet, 'Allergie', *Münchener Medizinische Wochenschrift*, 30 (1906), pp. 1457–8. An English translation of the article (by Carl Prausnitz) is reproduced in P.G.H. Gell and R.R.A. Coombs, *Clinical Aspects of Immunology* (Oxford, 1963), pp. 805–7.

2 Sheldon G. Cohen and Peter J. Bianchine, 'Hymenoptera, hypersensitivity and history', *Annals of Allergy, Asthma and Immunology*, 74 (1995), pp. 198–217.

3 Sheldon G. Cohen and Max Samter, eds, *Excerpts from Classics in Allergy* (Carlsbad, CA, 1992), pp. 8–9.

4 Ibid., pp. 10–11.

5 Jonathan Hutchinson, *The Pedigree of Disease: Being Six Lectures on Temperament, Idiosyncrasy and Diathesis* (London, 1884), p. 24.

6 Cohen and Bianchine, 'Hymenoptera, hypersensitivity and history'.

7 On drug idiosyncrasies, see Sir Humphry Rolleston, *Idiosyncrasies* (London, 1927), pp. 70–90.

8 John Floyer, *A Treatise of the Asthma* (London, 1698).

9 Morell Mackenzie, *Hay Fever and Paroxysmal Sneezing* (London, 1887), p. 10.

10 George M. Beard, *American Nervousness: Its Causes and Consequences* (New York, 1881), p. 7.

11 W. D. Foster, *A History of Medical Bacteriology and Immunology* (London, 1970), pp. 92–126; Alfred I. Tauber and Leon Chernyak, *Metchnikoff and the Origins of Immunology: From Metaphor to Theory* (New York, 1991); Ilana Löwy, '"The terrain is all": Metchnikoff's heritage at the Pasteur Institute, from Besredka's "antivirus" to Bardach's "orthobiotic serum"', in *Greater than the Parts: Holism in Biomedicine, 1920–1950*, ed. Christopher Lawrence and George Weisz (New York, 1998), pp. 257–82. For a more general discussion of the germ theory of disease, see Michael Worboys, *Spreading Germs: Disease Theories and Medical Practice in Britain, 1865–1900* (Cambridge, 2000); Nancy Tomes, *The Gospel of Germs: Men, Women, and the Microbe in American Life* (Cambridge, MA, 1998); K. Codell Carter, *The Rise of Causal Concepts of Disease* (Aldershot, 2003).

12 Foster, *A History of Medical Bacteriology*, pp. 101–5; Paul Weindling, 'From medical research to clinical practice: serum therapy for diphtheria in the 1890s', in *Medical Innovations in Historical Perspective*, ed. John Pickstone (London, 1992), pp. 72–83; F. J. Grundbacher, 'Behring's discovery of diphtheria and tetanus antitoxins', *Immunology Today*, 13 (1992), pp. 188–90.

13 Grundbacher, 'Behring's discovery'.

14 W. P. Dunbar, 'Etiology and specific therapy of hay fever', *Annals of Otology*,

Rhinology and Laryngology, 12 (1903), pp. 487–506.

15 Dr Risien Russell, 'The treatment of epilepsy', *British Medical Journal* (14 February 1903), p. 371.

16 For suggestions that the first officially documented death (of the son of the German doctor Paul Langerhans) occurred in 1896, see Anne Marie Moulin, *Le dernier langage de la médecine* (Paris, 1991), p. 143; Kenton Kroker, 'Immunity and its other: the anaphlyactic selves of Charles Richet', *Studies in History and Philosophy of Biological and Biomedical Sciences*, 30 (1999), pp. 273–96.

17 'The antitoxin treatment of diphtheria', *British Medical Journal* (4 May 1895), p. 987.

18 François Magendie, *Vorlesungen über das Blut* (Leipzig, 1839).

19 Arthur M. Silverstein, *A History of Immunology* (San Diego, CA, 1989), p. 216.

20 Charles Richet, *L'Anaphylaxie* (Paris, 1912); Charles Richet, 'Anaphylaxis: Nobel Lecture, 11 December 1913', reprinted in *Scandinavian Journal of Immunology*, 31 (1990), pp. 375–88. See also: Ilana Löwy, 'On guinea pigs, dogs and men: anaphylaxis and the study of biological individuality, 1902–1939', *Studies in History and Philosophy of Biological and Biomedical Sciences*, 34 (2003), pp. 399–424; Kroker, 'Immunity and its other'; J. Mazana and M. R. Ariño, 'Charles Robert Richet and some milestones in the history of allergies', *Journal of Investigative Allergology and Clinical Immunology*, 1 (1991), pp. 93–100; Charles D. May, 'The ancestry of allergy: being an account of the original experimental induction of hypersensitivity recognizing the contribution of Paul Portier', *Journal of Allergy and Clinical Immunology*, 75 (1985), pp. 485–95.

21 M. Arthus, 'Injections répétées de sérum de cheval chez le lapin', *C. R. Société de Biologie*, 55 (1903), pp. 817–20; M. Arthus, *De l'anaphylaxie à l'immunité* (Paris, 1921).

22 M. J. Rosenau and J. F. Anderson, 'A study of the cause of sudden death following the injection of horse serum', *Hygienic Laboratory Bulletin, No. 29, Public Health and Marine Hospital Services* (1906), p. 95.

23 J. Bordet, 'The Harben Lectures, 1913: Anaphylaxis – its importance and mechanism', *Journal of State Medicine*, 21 (1913), pp. 449–64.

24 Biographical details are taken from Richard Wagner, *Clemens von Pirquet: His Life and Work* (Baltimore, MD, 1968).

25 Ibid.

26 Von Pirquet's words in a letter to Gruber, written in 1903, quoted in Wagner, *Clemens von Pirquet*, p. 30.

27 M. Gruber and C. von Pirquet, 'Toxin and antitoxin', *Münchener Medizinische Wochenschrift*, 50 (1903), p. 1193. For discussion of the dispute between Ehrlich and Gruber and von Pirquet, see Cay-Rüdiger Prüll, 'Part of a scientific master plan? Paul Ehrlich and the origins of his receptor concept', *Medical History*, 47 (2003), pp. 332–56; Alberto Cambrosio, Daniel Jacobi and Peter Keating, 'Ehrlich's "beautiful pictures" and the controversial beginnings of immunological imagery', *Isis*, 84 (1993), pp. 662–99; Pauline M. H. Mazumdar, 'The antigen-antibody reaction and the physics and chemistry of life', *Bulletin of the History of Medicine*, 48 (1974), pp. 1–21; Pauline M. H. Mazumdar, 'The purpose of immunity: Landsteiner's interpretation of the human isoantibodies', *Journal of the History of Biology*, 8 (1975), pp. 115–33.

28 Clemens von Pirquet, 'On the theory of infectious diseases', unpublished paper deposited with the Imperial Academy of Sciences in Vienna in April 1903, cited in Wagner, *Clemens von Pirquet*, pp. 52–4.

29 Hutchinson, *The Pedigree of Disease*, p. 67. The book, published in 1884, was based on lectures delivered in 1881.

30 Ohad Parnes, '"Trouble from within": allergy, autoimmunity and pathology in the first half of the twentieth century', *Studies in History and Philosophy of Biological and Biomedical Sciences*, 34 (2003), pp. 425–54.

31 Ibid., pp. 430–33.

32 Ilana Löwy, 'The immunological construction of self', in *Organism and the Origins of Self*, ed. Alfred I. Tauber (Dordrecht, 1991), pp. 43–75; Ilana Löwy, *Medical Acts and Medical Facts* (Cracow, 2000).

33 C. von Pirquet and B. Schick, 'Zur theorie der inkubationszeit', *Wiener Klinische Wochenschrift*, 16 (1903), p. 1244.

34 C. von Pirquet and B. Schick, *Die Serumkrankheit* (Vienna, 1905).

35 C. von Pirquet and B. Schick, *Serum Sickness*, trans. B. Schick (1905) (Baltimore, MD, 1951), p. 119.

36 Von Pirquet, 'Allergie'.

37 Ibid.

38 Ibid.

39 Ibid.

40 Wagner, *Clemens von Pirquet*, pp. 73–120.

41 C. von Pirquet, *Allergy* (Chicago, 1911).

42 Ibid. See also Hutchinson, *The Pedigree of Disease*.

43 Von Pirquet, *Allergy*, pp. 13–19.

44 Ibid., p. 55.

45 Richet, *L'Anaphylaxie*, p. 80.

46 *Lancet*, I (1911), pp. 746–7.

47 Arthur F. Coca and Robert Cooke, 'On the classification of the phenomena of hypersensitiveness', *Journal of Immunology*, 8 (1923), pp. 163–82.

48 Charles Frederick Bolduan, *Immune Sera* (New York, 1908), p. 143. On Bolduan, see Herman O. Mosenthal, 'Charles F. Bolduan: his role in the attack on diabetes as a public health problem', *Diabetes*, 3 (1954), pp. 495–7.

49 Coca and Cooke, 'On the classification of the phenomena of hypersensitiveness'.

50 Von Pirquet, *Allergy*, p. 3.

51 Ibid., p. 4.

52 Richet, *L'Anaphylaxie*; A. Besredka, *Anaphylaxis and Anti-Anaphylaxis*, trans. S. Roodhouse Gloyne (London, 1919); Auguste Lumière, *Le problème de l'anaphylaxie* (Paris, 1924); R. Cranston Low, *Anaphylaxis and Sensitisation* (Edinburgh, 1924).

53 Bordet, 'The Harben Lectures'.

54 'Review of Charles Richet, *Anaphylaxis*, trans. J. Murray Bligh', *Lancet*, II (1913), p. 800.

55 Besredka, *Anaphylaxis and Anti-Anaphylaxis*, pp. 1–2.

56 Ludvig Hektoen, 'Allergy or anaphylaxis in experiment and disease', *Journal of the American Medical Association*, 58 (1912), pp. 1081–8.

57 B. P. Sormani, 'Prophylactic vaccination against hay fever', *Lancet*, I (1916), pp. 348–50.

58 A. G. Auld, 'Observations on peptone immunisation in asthma and other allergies', *Lancet*, I (1923), pp. 790–94; A. G. Auld, 'New peptone treatment in asthma and other allergies', *Lancet*, II (1932), pp. 67–8; Alexander Gunn Auld, *The Nature and Treatment of Asthma, Hay Fever and Migraine* (London, 1936), p. vii.

59 W. Storm van Leeuwen, *Allergic Diseases* (London, 1926); William W. Duke, *Allergy, Asthma, Hay Fever, Urticaria and Allied Manifestations of Reaction* (London, 1927).

60 See C. von Pirquet, 'Tuberkulindiagnose durch cutane Impfung', *Berliner Klinische Wochenschrift*, 20 (20 May 1907); C. von Pirquet, 'Die Allergieprobe zur Diagnose der Tuberkulose im Kindersalter', *Wiener Medizinische Wochenschrift*, 57 (1907), p. 1369; Clemens F. von Pirquet, 'Quantitative experiments with the cutaneous tuberculin reaction', *Journal of Pharmacology and Experimental Therapeutics*, 1 (1909), pp. 151–74. For a discussion of von Pirquet's work in this area, see Wagner, *Clemens von Pirquet*, pp. 66–72. For an example of the application of the test in England, see J. W. Bride, 'The tuberculin skin reaction (von Pirquet's)', *British Medical Journal* (14 May 1909), p. 1161.

61 Clemens Pirquet, 'Zur Geschichte der Allergie', *Wiener Medizinische Wochenschrift*, 23 (1927), pp. 745–48. The passage is translated in Wagner, *Clemens von Pirquet*, p. 69.

62 Arnold R. Rich, *The Pathogenesis of Tuberculosis*, 2nd edn (Oxford, 1951), pp. 509–70.

63 Wagner, *Clemens von Pirquet*, p. 205.

64 Arthur M. Silverstein, 'The historical origins of modern immunology', in *Immunology: The Making of a Modern Science*, ed. Richard B. Gallagher et al. (London, 1995), pp. 5–20.

65 Niels K. Jerne, 'The common sense of immunology', *Cold Spring Harbor Symposium on Quantitative Biology*, 41 (1977), pp. 1–4.

66 Von Pirquet, 'Allergie', pp. 1457–8; A. Wolff-Eisner, *Das Heufieber* (Munich, 1906); S. J. Meltzer, 'Bronchial asthma as a phenomenon of anaphylaxis', *Journal of the American Medical Association*, 55 (1910), pp. 1021–4; H. G. Adamson, 'Goulstonian lectures on modern views upon the significance of skin eruptions', *Lancet*, I (1912), pp. 969–75; Rolleston, *Idiosyncrasies*, pp. 83–90; G. Billard, 'Anaphylaxia in hay fever, nettle-rash and asthma', *Lancet*, II (1910), pp. 1208–9; Hektoen, 'Allergy or anaphylaxis'; Albert H. Rowe, *Food Allergy: Its Manifestations, Diagnosis and Treatment* (Philadelphia, 1932); Anon., 'Anaphylaxis and idiosyncrasy', *Lancet*, I (1914), p. 1696; A. T. Waterhouse, 'Bee-stings and anaphylaxis', *Lancet*, II (1914), p. 946; Von Pirquet, *Allergy*; Anon., 'The anti-anaphylactic treatment of infections', *British Medical Journal* (21 September 1918), p. 323; H. Batty Shaw, 'Hypersensitiveness', *Lancet*, I (1912), pp. 713–19.

67 R. G. Eccles, 'A Darwinian interpretation of anaphylaxis', *Medical Record*, 80 (1911), pp. 309–18; Rolleston, *Idiosyncrasies*, p. 84.

68 'Asthma and affections of the skin', *Lancet*, I (1928), p. 246.

69 Rolleston, *Idiosyncrasies*, pp. 104, 58–61; Billard, 'Anaphylaxia', p. 1208.

70 Anne Marie Moulin, 'The defended body', in *Medicine in the 20th Century*, ed. Roger Cooter and John Pickstone (Amsterdam, 2000), pp. 385–98.

71 John Freeman, 'An address on toxic idiopathies', *Lancet*, II (1920), pp. 229–35.

72 See the report of a paper read by John Freeman to the Nottingham Medico-Chirurgical Society on the 'Pathological mechanism of the asthma syndrome', *Lancet*, I (1928), pp. 288–90.

73 See the report of a paper read by C. P. Lapage to the Manchester Medical Society on 'Asthma in children', *Lancet*, II (1922), pp. 1332–3.

74 John Freeman, *Hay-Fever: A Key to the Allergic Disorders* (London, 1950).

75 Sir William Osler, *The Principles and Practice of Medicine*, 8th edn (New York, 1914), p. 627.

76 Rolleston, *Idiosyncrasies*, pp. 92–102. See also the report of a paper presented by Rolleston to a British Medical Association conference in 1921 in *Lancet*, II (1921), pp. 280–81. On the Vaccine Committee, see Linda Bryder, 'Public health research and the MRC', in *Historical Perspectives on the Role of the MRC*, ed. Joan Austoker and Linda Bryder (Oxford, 1989), pp. 59–81.

77 Rolleston, *Idiosyncrasies*, p. 58; Lapage, 'Asthma in children'.

78 *Lancet*, II (1909), p. 472; *Lancet*, II (1927), pp. 1085–6.

79 Rolleston, *Idiosyncrasies*, pp. 94–5; Arthur F. Hurst, 'An address on asthma', *Lancet*, I (1921), pp. 1113–17.

80 Hurst, 'An address on asthma', pp. 1115–16.

81 L. Noon, 'Prophylactic inoculation against hay fever', *Lancet*, I (1911), pp. 1572–3. See chapter Three for further discussion of the work of Noon and Freeman.

82 Bordet, 'The Harben Lectures'.

83 'What is allergy?', *Lancet*, II (1926), p. 1021.

84 Alexander Francis, *The Francis Treatment of Asthma* (London, 1932), p. 17.

85 'The Walker tests for asthma', *Lancet*, II (1922), pp. 526–7; Rolleston, *Idiosyncrasies*, p. 96. On Walker, see Francis M. Rackemann, 'Isaac Chandler Walker 1883–1950', *Transactions of the Association of American Physicians*, 64 (1951), pp. 23–4.

86 C. Prausnitz and H. Küstner, 'Studien über überempfindlichkeit', *Centralbl. für Bakteriologie*, 86 (1921), pp. 160–69.

87 Von Pirquet, 'Quantitative experiments with the cutaneous tuberculin reaction', pp. 155–6; Richet, 'Anaphylaxis: Nobel Lecture', pp. 384–5.

88 Rolleston, *Idiosyncrasies*, pp. 75–6.

89 S. Wyard, 'The phenomena of anaphylaxis', *Lancet*, I (1917), pp. 105–9.

90 Cambrosio, Jacobi and Keating, 'Ehrlich's "beautiful pictures"'; Mazumdar, 'The antigen-antibody reaction'; Mazumdar, 'The purpose of immunity'.

91 Leon Unger and M. Coleman Harris, 'Immunology, infectious diseases and allergy: the recent years', *Annals of Allergy*, 33 (1974), pp. 50–64.

92 Richet, *L'Anaphylaxie*, p. 236; Richet, 'Anaphylaxis: Nobel Lecture', p. 383. For an overview of the various theories, see Hektoen, 'Allergy or anaphylaxis'; Wyard, 'The phenomena of anaphylaxis'; Anon., 'Anaphylaxis', *British Medical Journal* (21 May 1920), pp. 1254–5.

93 Bordet, 'The Harben Lectures'.

94 Von Pirquet, *Allergy*, p. 17.

95 *Lancet*, II (1919), pp. 202–3.

96 E. M. Tansey, 'Henry Dale, histamine and anaphylaxis: reflections on the role of

chance in the history of allergy', *Studies in History and Philosophy of Biological and Biomedical Sciences*, 34 (2003), pp. 455–72.

97 H. H. Dale and P. P. Laidlaw, 'Further observations on the action of ß-iminazolylethylamine', *Journal of Physiology*, 43 (1911), pp. 182–95.

98 H. H. Dale, 'The anaphylactic reaction of plain muscle in the guinea-pig', *Journal of Pharmacology and Experimental Therapeutics*, 4 (1913), pp. 167–223.

99 H. H. Dale, 'Croonian Lectures on some chemical factors in the control of the circulation: Lecture III', *Lancet*, I (1929), pp. 1285–90.

100 Ibid., p. 1286.

101 Kroker, 'Immunity and its other'.

102 Freeman, *Hay-Fever*, p. 25. On differences between species, see Rolleston, *Idiosyncrasies*, pp. 45.

103 H. H. Dale, 'The biological significance of anaphylaxis', *Proceedings of the Royal Society*, 91 (1920), pp. 126–46; Dale, 'Croonian Lectures'.

104 Parnes, '"Trouble from within"'; Silverstein, *A History of Immunology*, pp. 160–89.

105 Carl Prausnitz, 'In quest of allergy', the Jenner Memorial Lecture delivered on 4 June 1959, the manuscript of which is in the Contemporary Medical Archives Centre, Wellcome Library for the History and Understanding of Medicine, GC/33/3.

106 Eccles, 'A Darwinian interpretation'.

107 Hektoen, 'Allergy or anaphylaxis', p. 1088.

108 Bordet, 'The Harben lectures', p. 464.

109 Richet, 'Anaphylaxis: Nobel Lecture'.

110 Ibid. See also Charles Richet, 'An address on ancient humorism and modern humorism', *British Medical Journal* (1 October 1910), pp. 921–6.

111 See chapter Three below.

112 Kroker, 'Immunity and its other'; Löwy, 'On guinea pigs, dogs and men'; Laura Otis, *Membranes: Metaphors of Invasion in Nineteenth-Century Literature, Science and Politics* (Baltimore, MD, 1999).

113 Löwy, 'On guinea pigs, dogs and men'.

114 Ibid., p. 418.

115 Wagner, *Clemens von Pirquet*.

116 Ibid., pp. 163–83.

117 Ibid., p. 197.

118 Ibid., pp. 102–7.

119 Von Pirquet, 'Zur Geschichte der Allergie', p. 748 (my translation).

120 C. Pirquet, 'Allergie des Lebensalters', *Wiener Klinische Wochenschrift*, 42 (1929), pp. 65–7. See also Wagner, *Clemens von Pirquet*, pp. 187–93.

121 Rolleston, *Idiosyncrasies*, pp. 13–14.

122 'Announcement', *Journal of Allergy*, 1 (1929), p. 1.

123 Arnold Rice Rich, 'Experimental pathological studies on the nature and role of bacterial allergy', *Lancet*, I (1933), pp. 521–5.

124 *Lancet*, I (1930), p. 1084.

Chapter 3: Allergy in the Clinic

1   John Freeman, 'An address on toxic idiopathies', *Lancet*, II (1920), pp. 229–35.
2   John Bostock, 'Case of a periodical affection of the eyes and chest', *Medico-Chirurgical Transactions*, 10 (1819), pp. 161–2.
3   On the early history of hay fever, see Samuel H. Hurwitz, 'Hay fever: a sketch of its early history', *Journal of Allergy*, 1 (1930), pp. 245–59; Arthur F. Coca, Matthew Walzer and August A. Thommen, *Asthma and Hay Fever in Theory and Practice* (Springfield, IL, 1931), pp. 487–515; Ronald Finn, 'John Bostock, hay fever and the mechanism of allergy', *Lancet*, II (1992), pp. 1453–5; M. B. Emanuel, 'Hay fever, a post-industrial revolution epidemic: a history of its growth during the nineteenth century', *Clinical Allergy*, 18 (1988), pp. 295–304; Kathryn J. Waite, 'Blackley and the development of hay fever as a disease of civilization in the nineteenth century', *Medical History*, 39 (1995), pp. 186–96; Gholam Ali Bungy et al., 'Razi's report about seasonal allergic rhinitis (hay fever) from the 10th century AD', *International Archives of Allergy and Immunology*, 110 (1996), pp. 219–24.
4   John Bostock, 'On the catarrhus aestivus or summer catarrh', *Medico-Chirurgical Transactions*, 14 (1828), pp. 437–46.
5   John Elliotson, 'Hay fever', *Lancet*, II (1830–31), pp. 370–33.
6   Walter Hayle Walshe, *A Practical Treatise on the Diseases of the Lungs* (London, 1871), p. 227.
7   Charles H. Blackley, *Experimental Researches on the Causes and Nature of Catarrhus Aestivus (Hay-Fever or Hay-Asthma)* (London, 1873), p. 5.
8   Gregg Mitman, 'Hay fever holiday: health, leisure and place in gilded age America', *Bulletin of the History of Medicine*, 77 (2003), pp. 600–35; Gregg Mitman, 'What's in a weed? A cultural geography of *Ambrosia artemesiaefolia*', in *The Moral Authority of Nature*, ed. Lorraine Daston and Fernando Vidal (Chicago, 2003), pp. 438–65.
9   W. C. Hollopeter, *Hay-Fever: Its Prevention and Cure* (New York and London, 1916), pp. 161–7. See also Mitman, 'What's in a weed?'.
10 'A remedy for hay fever', *Lancet*, I (1874), p. 740.
11 Philipp Phoebus, 'Hay asthma', *Lancet*, II (1859), p. 655; Philipp Phoebus, *Der Typische Frühsommerkatarrh* (Geissen, 1862).
12 Morrill Wyman, *Autumnal Catarrh (Hay Fever)* (New York, 1872). On Wyman, see Mitman, 'Hay fever holiday'; Waite, 'Blackley and the development of hay fever'.
13 George M. Beard, *Hay-fever; or, Summer Catarrh: Its Nature and Treatment* (New York, 1876); George M. Beard, *A Practical Treatise on Nervous Exhaustion (Neurasthenia)* (New York, 1880); George M. Beard, *American Nervousness: Its Causes and Consequences* (New York, 1881).
14 Beard, *American Nervousness*, p. 138.
15 Walshe, *A Practical Treatise*, p. 227.
16 Blackley, *Experimental Researches*, p. 153. A second edition of the book, with an expanded section on treatment, was published several years later: Charles Harrison Blackley, *Hay Fever: Its Causes, Treatment and Effective Prevention. Experimental Researches* (London, 1880).

17 Morrell Mackenzie, *Hay Fever and Paroxysmal Sneezing* (London, 1887). For contemporary reactions to Blackley, see Waite, 'Blackley and the development of hay fever', pp. 191–3.

18 Mackenzie, *Hay Fever*, p. 60.

19 'A remedy for hay fever'.

20 Beard, *Hay-fever*; W. Young, 'Hay fever', *Lancet*, II (1874), p. 145.

21 W. P. Dunbar, 'Etiology and specific therapy of hay fever', *Annals of Otology, Rhinology and Laryngology*, 12 (1903), pp. 487–506; W. P. Dunbar, 'The present state of our knowledge of hay fever', *Journal of Hygiene*, 13 (1905), pp. 105–48.

22 Blackley, *Experimental Researches*, pp. 154–62.

23 Blackley, *Experimental Researches*, pp. 198–9; Blackley, *Hay Fever*, pp. 246–53; Walshe, *A Practical Treatise*, pp. 228–9; Mackenzie, *Hay Fever*, pp. 60–64; Andrew Clark, 'The Cavendish Lecture on a speedy and sometimes successful method of treating hay-fever', *British Medical Journal*, I (1887), pp. 1255–7.

24 Blackley, *Experimental Researches*, pp. 199–201; Walshe, *A Practical Treatise*, p. 228; Mackenzie, *Hay Fever*, pp. 65–7.

25 Mitman, 'Hay fever holiday'.

26 Blackley, *Experimental Researches*, p. 201; Mackenzie, *Hay Fever*, p. 65.

27 Blackley, *Experimental Researches*, pp. 7, 155.

28 Beard, *American Nervousness*, pp. 188–9.

29 Clark, 'The Cavendish Lecture', p. 1255.

30 Blackley, *Experimental Researches*, p. 155.

31 Dunbar, 'Etiology and specific therapy'.

32 Blackley, *Experimental Researches*, p. 162.

33 Mitman, 'Hay fever holiday'.

34 Morell Mackenzie, *The Fatal Illness of Frederick the Noble* (London, 1888); H. R. Haweis, *Sir Morell Mackenzie, Physician and Operator* (London, 1893).

35 Mackenzie, *Hay Fever*, p. 9.

36 Ibid., p. 10.

37 In the early twentieth century, Osler insisted that hay fever was hereditary and more common in women than men. See Sir William Osler, *The Principles and Practice of Medicine*, 8th edn (New York, 1914), p. 612.

38 Mackenzie, *Hay Fever*, p. 10.

39 Ibid., pp. 10–11.

40 E. M. Forster, *Howards End* (1910) (London, 1965), p. 11.

41 Ibid., p. 122. See John Carey, *The Intellectuals and the Masses: Pride and Prejudice among the Literary Intelligentsia, 1880–1939* (London, 1992), pp. 18–19; Peter Widdowson, *E. M. Forster's Howards End: Fiction as History* (London, 1977).

42 Mackenzie, *Hay Fever*, p. 11. For a discussion of the role of scientific knowledge in the naturalization of political boundaries in this way, see Laura Otis, *Membranes: Metaphors of Invasion in Nineteenth-Century Literature, Science and Politics* (Baltimore, MD, 1999).

43 Raphael C. Panzani, 'Seneca and his asthma: the illnesses, life and death of a Roman stoic philosopher', *Journal of Asthma*, 25 (1988), pp. 163–74. On the early

history of asthma, see Edmund L. Keeney, 'The history of asthma from Hippocrates to Meltzer', *Journal of Allergy*, 35 (1964), pp. 215–26; John Gabbay, 'Asthma attacked? Tactics for the reconstruction of a diseases concept', in *The Problem of Medical Knowledge*, ed. Peter Wright and Andrew Treacher (Edinburgh, 1982), pp. 23–48; E. Stolkind, 'The history of bronchial asthma and allergy', *Proceedings of the Royal Society of Medicine*, 26 (1932–3), pp. 1120–26; Alex Sakula, 'A history of asthma', *Journal of the Royal College of Physicians*, 22 (1988), pp. 36–44; Sheldon C. Siegel, 'The history of asthma deaths from antiquity', *Journal of Allergy and Clinical Immunology*, 80 (1987), pp. 458–62; Ian Gregg, 'Some historical aspects of asthma', *Southampton Medical Journal* (1991), pp. 11–21.

44   Thomas Willis, *The Practice of Physick* (London, 1684), pp. 92–6; John Floyer, *A Treatise of the Asthma* (London, 1698).

45   On the introduction and reception of these diagnostic techniques, see Jacalyn Duffin, *History of Medicine: A Scandalously Short Introduction* (Toronto, 1999), pp. 191–211; Jacalyn Duffin, *To See with a Better Eye: A Life of R.T.H. Laennec* (Princeton, NJ, 1998); Noel Snell, 'Inhalation devices: a brief history', *Respiratory Disease in Practice* (Summer 1995), pp. 13–15.

46   Walshe, *A Practical Treatise*, pp. 543–56.

47   Henry Hyde Salter, *On Asthma: Its Pathology and Treatment* (London, 1860); Henry Hyde Salter, 'On the effects of local spasmodic influences on asthma', *Edinburgh Medical Journal*, 3 (1857–8), pp. 1092–3; Henry Hyde Salter, 'On some points in the treatment and clinical history of asthma', *Edinburgh Medical Journal*, 5 (1859–60), pp. 1109–15; Henry Hyde Salter, 'On the treatment of asthma by belladonna', *Lancet*, I (1869), pp. 152–3.

48   Walshe, *A Practical Treatise*, p. 543.

49   F. B. Michel et al., 'History of concepts of asthma in France', ACI *International*, 8 (1996), pp. 67–9.

50   John Gabbay, 'Asthma: a case study of the relationship between changing theoretical concepts of a disease and its treatment', unpublished dissertation, Cambridge, 1977, pp. 50–51. See also: John Millar, *Observations on the Asthma, and on the Hooping Cough* (London, 1769); Sheldon G. Cohen, 'Asthma among the famous', *Allergy and Asthma Proceedings*, 17 (1996), pp. 161–71.

51   Walshe, *A Practical Treatise*, pp. 554–5. On climate therapy, see Carla Keirns, 'Better than nature: the changing treatment of asthma and hay fever in the United States, 1910–1945', *Studies in History and Philosophy of Biological and Biomedical Sciences*, 34 (2003), pp. 511–31.

52   Salter, *On Asthma*, p. 194.

53   Ibid., pp. 161–204.

54   John Thorowgood, *Notes on Asthma: Its Nature, Forms and Treatment* (London, 1870); John Thorowgood, *Asthma and Chronic Bronchitis* (London, 1894).

55   Mina Curtiss, ed., *Letters of Marcel Proust* (London, 1950), pp. 271, 281.

56   Bernard Straus, *Maladies of Marcel Proust: Doctors and Disease in his Life and Work* (New York, 1980); Constantine J. Falliers, 'The literary genius and the many maladies of Marcel Proust', *Journal of Asthma*, 23 (1986), pp. 157–64.

57 Emanuel, 'Hay fever', p. 302.
58 Gerald N. Grob, *The Deadly Truth: A History of Disease in America* (Cambridge, MA, 2002), pp. 217–42.
59 Mitman, 'What's in a weed?', p. 438.
60 Leonard Colebrook, *Almroth Wright: Provocative Doctor and Thinker* (London, 1954); Zachary Cope, *Almroth Wright: Founder of Modern Vaccine-Therapy* (London, 1966); Michael Dunnill, *The Plato of Praed Street: The Life and Times of Almroth Wright* (London, 2000); Michael Worboys, 'Vaccine therapy and laboratory medicine in Edwardian England', in *Medical Innovations in Historical Perspective*, ed. John Pickstone (London, 1992), pp. 84–103; E. A. Heaman, *St Mary's: The History of a London Teaching Hospital* (Montreal, 2003).
61 Wai Chen, 'The laboratory as business: Sir Almroth Wright's vaccine programme and the construction of penicillin', in *The Laboratory Revolution in Medicine*, ed. Andrew Cunningham and Perry Williams (Cambridge, 1992), pp. 245–92.
62 Colebrook, *Almroth Wright*, pp. 135–6.
63 Ilana Löwy, 'Immunology and literature in the early twentieth century: *Arrowsmith* and *The Doctor's Dilemma*', *Medical History*, 32 (1988), pp. 314–32.
64 'Obituary: John Freeman', *Journal of Pathology and Bacteriology*, 85 (1963), pp. 243–7; 'Obituary: John Freeman', *International Archives of Allergy and Applied Immunology*, 20 (1962), pp. 314–15.
65 'Obituary: Leonard Noon', *St. Mary's Hospital Gazette*, 19 (March 1913), p. 44; John Freeman, 'Leonard Noon', *International Archives of Allergy and Applied Immunology*, 4 (1953), pp. 282–4. On Noon's work at the Lister, see his notebook in the Fleming Papers in the British Library, Add. 56223.
66 Freeman, 'Leonard Noon', p. 284.
67 Dunbar, 'Etiology and specific therapy'.
68 Leonard Noon, 'Prophylactic inoculation against hay fever', *Lancet*, I (1911), pp. 1572–3.
69 Ibid., p. 1573.
70 John Freeman, 'Further observations on the treatment of hay fever by the hypodermic inoculations of pollen vaccine', *Lancet*, II (1911), pp. 814–17.
71 Ibid., p. 815.
72 John Freeman, 'Vaccination against hay fever', *Lancet*, I (1914), pp. 1178–80.
73 Christopher Lawrence and George Weisz, 'Medical holism: the context', in *Greater than the Parts: Holism in Biomedicine, 1920–1950*, ed. Christopher Lawrence and George Weisz (Oxford, 1998), pp. 1–22.
74 H. Holbrook Curtis, 'The immunizing cure of hay-fever', *Medical News*, 77 (1900), pp. 16–18.
75 Alfred T. Schofield, 'A case of egg poisoning', *Lancet*, I (1908), p. 716.
76 John Freeman, 'An address on toxic idiopathies', *Lancet*, II (1920), pp. 229–35.
77 Freeman, 'Further observations', p. 814.
78 Sir Almroth Wright, 'Brief survey of the history and development of the Inoculation Department, St Mary's Hospital, W2' (no date), p. 7, located in St Mary's Hospital Archives, WF/MX3/6.

79 A. G. Haynes Lovell, 'The vaccine treatment of hay fever', *Lancet*, II (1912), p. 1716; B. P. Sormani, 'Prophylactic vaccination against hay fever', *Lancet*, I (1916), pp. 348–50; John Freeman, 'Prophylactic vaccination against hay fever', *Lancet*, I (1916), p. 552; Arthur F. Hurst, 'An address on asthma', *Lancet*, I (1921), pp. 1113–17; Arthur Latham, 'An address on some aspects of bronchial asthma', *Lancet*, I (1922), pp. 261–3; 'Hay fever reaction outfits', *Lancet*, I (1912), p. 1448.

80 Gregg Mitman, 'Natural history and the clinic: the regional ecology of allergy in America', *Studies in History and Philosophy of Biological and Biomedical Sciences*, 34 (2003), pp. 491–510 (p. 494). American studies were often reported in the British medical press. See 'Recent work on hay fever', *Lancet*, I (1916), pp. 872–3; 'The treatment of hay fever', *Lancet*, II (1922), pp. 678–9.

81 Mitman, 'Natural history and the clinic', p. 494. See also: K. K. Koessler, 'The specific treatment of hay fever by active immunization', *Illinois Medical Journal* (1914), pp. 120–27; Hollopeter, *Hay-Fever*, pp. 254–5.

82 Robert A. Cooke, 'The treatment of hay fever by active immunization', *Laryngoscope*, 25 (1915), pp. 108–12.

83 Max Samter, 'Allergy and clinical immunology: fifty years from now', *Journal of Allergy and Clinical Immunology*, 64 (1979), pp. 321–30.

84 Freeman, 'An address on toxic idiopathies', p. 235.

85 Sheldon G. Cohen, 'The American Academy of Allergy: an historical review', *Journal of Allergy and Clinical Immunology*, 64 (1979), pp. 332–466 (pp. 334, 377). On early paediatric allergy clinics, see Edward Scott O'Keefe, 'The history of paediatric allergy', in *The Allergic Child*, ed. Frederic Speer (New York, 1963), pp. 3–13.

86 Cohen, 'The American Academy of Allergy', pp. 333–41.

87 Ibid., pp. 342–52.

88 Ibid., pp. 353–62.

89 Ibid., pp. 375–90.

90 Francis M. Rackemann, *Clinical Allergy, particularly Asthma and Hay Fever: Mechanism and Treatment* (New York, 1931); Coca, Walzer and Thommen, *Asthma and Hay Fever in Theory and Practice*; Warren T. Vaughan, *Allergy and Applied Immunology* (St Louis, MO, 1934); Albert H. Rowe, *Food Allergy: Its Manifestations, Diagnosis and Treatment* (Philadelphia, 1931).

91 Arthur F. Coca and Robert A. Cooke, 'On the classification of the phenomena of hypersensitiveness', *Journal of Immunology*, 8 (1923), pp. 163–82.

92 Jack B. Anon, 'Otolaryngic allergy: the last half century', *Otolaryngic Allergy*, 25 (1992), pp. 1–12.

93 Cohen, 'The American Academy of Allergy', pp. 365–8.

94 Warren T. Vaughan, 'Minor allergy: its distribution, clinical aspects and significance', *Journal of Allergy*, 5 (1934), pp. 184–96. For objections to the notion of minor allergy, see the discussion of Vaughan's paper in ibid., pp. 211–12.

95 Mitman, 'Natural history and the clinic', p. 506.

96 Ibid., p. 503. For later concerns about the accuracy of pollen counts, see 'Pollen counts and the hay fever problem', *Science* (16 January 1953), pp. 64–5.

97 Mitman, 'Natural history and the clinic', p. 506.

98 'Statistics of hay fever', *Lancet*, II (1902), pp. 49–50.

99 W. Storm van Leeuwen, *Allergic Diseases: Diagnosis and Treatment of Bronchial Asthma, Hay-fever and other Allergic Diseases* (London, 1926); Hugo Kämmerer, *Allergische Diathese und Allergische Erkrankungen* (Munich, 1926); W. Storm van Leeuwen and H. Varekamp, 'On the tuberculin treatment of bronchial asthma and hay fever', *Lancet*, II (1921), pp. 1366–9; Byron H. Waksman, ed., *1939–1989: Fifty Years Progress in Allergy: A Tribute to Paul Kallós* (Basle, 1990).

100 Ronald Hare, *The Birth of Penicillin and the Disarming of Microbes* (London, 1970), pp. 83–4. For further details of this story, see the letter from A. W. Frankland, in the British Library, Add. 71717, fol. 17.

101 'Asthma research', *The Times* (26 October 1927), 10d; 'An Asthma Research Council', *The Times* (27 October 1927), 9d. Early records are kept at the National Asthma Campaign in London and include: Minute Books, 1927–36, 1941–75, 1975–80; Medical Advisory Committee Minutes, 1950–65; and minutes from the Finance and Social Functions Committee from the 1970s. Miscellaneous papers from the Asthma Research Council, including reports and correspondence 1927–53, are in the Public Record Office (PRO) FD1/2279. Published reports of progress for 1932, 1936 and 1938 are in the Wellcome Library for the History and Understanding of Medicine.

102 'Asthma research', *The Times* (19 December 1928), 14e; 'For sufferers from asthma', *The Times* (22 November 1930), 8d.

103 'Research into asthma', *Lancet*, I (1929), p. 36.

104 *The Times* (13 June 1936), 14f; (18 June 1936), 13b, 17d. Clive Shields, *Hay Fever with Special Reference to Treatment by Intranasal Ionization* (Oxford, 1937).

105 'Obituary: John Freeman', *Journal of Pathology and Bacteriology*, p. 245.

106 Details of Frankland's appointment are in *Minutes of the Meetings of the Council of the Inoculation Department, 1947–1955*, St Mary's Hospital Archives, WF/AD3/1, meeting on 29 April 1947.

107 *Annual Report of the Wright-Fleming Institute of Microbiology for 1955*, St Mary's Hospital Archives, WF/AD6/1, p. 1.

108 Freeman, *Hay-Fever*, pp. 267–83; A. W. Frankland, 'Aerobiology and allergy: an autobiography', *Aerobiologia*, 12 (1996), pp. 55–61.

109 John Freeman, 'The significance of idiopathic skin reactions', *Lancet*, II (1930), pp. 1197–9; Freeman, *Hay-Fever*, p. 26.

110 Parke, Davis & Company, *Vaccine and Serum Therapy* (London, 1935), p. 121.

111 John Freeman, '"Rush" inoculation, with special reference to hay-fever treatment', *Lancet*, I (1930), pp. 744–7.

112 Worboys, 'Vaccine therapy', p. 103.

113 Parke, Davis & Company, *Vaccine Therapy* (London, 1931); Parke, Davis & Company, *Vaccine and Serum Therapy* (London, 1935).

114 Details are in the *Annual Report of the Wright-Fleming Institute of Microbiology for the Year 1960*, St Mary's Hospital Archives, WF/AD6/2.

115 H. G. Lazell, *From Pills to Penicillin: The Beecham Story* (London, 1975), p. 166; C. L.

Bencard Ltd, *The Bencard Manual of Allergy* (London, 1956). Examples of the Bencard kits are in Blythe House Store at the National Museum of Science and Industry, 1981–488.

116 David Harley, 'Hay fever, I: A study of reagin-allergen mixtures', *British Journal of Experimental Pathology*, 14 (1933), pp. 171–9; David Harley, *Studies in Hay Fever and Asthma* (London, 1942); David Harley, 'Hay fever: its immunological mechanism, diagnosis and treatment', *British Medical Journal* (13 April 1935), pp. 754–6; David Harley, 'Asthma: immunological mechanism, diagnosis and treatment', *Lancet*, II (1936), pp. 367–70; John Freeman and W. H. Hughes, 'Biological polyvalency of antigens with special reference to hay-fever', *Lancet*, I (1938), pp. 941–3.

117 A. W. Frankland and R. Augustin, 'Prophylaxis of summer hay-fever and asthma', *Lancet*, I (1954), pp. 1055–7. Details of Rosa Augustin's work are in *Annual Reports of the Wright-Fleming Institute of Microbiology, 1950–1966*, St Mary's Hospital Archives, WF/AD6/1 and WF/AD6/2.

118 A. W. Frankland and R. H. Gorrill, 'Summer hay-fever and asthma treated with antihistaminic drugs', *British Medical Journal* (4 April 1953), pp. 761–4; A. W. Frankland, 'Locust sensitivity', *Annals of Allergy*, 11 (1953), pp. 445–53; A. W. Frankland, 'High and low dose pollen extract treatment in summer hay fever and asthma', *Acta Allergologica*, 9 (1955), pp. 183–7.

119 Erich Wittkower, 'Studies in hay-fever patients (the allergic personality)', *Journal of Mental Science*, 84 (1938), pp. 352–69.

120 Chase Patterson Kimball, 'Conceptual developments in psychosomatic medicine, 1939–69', *Annals of Internal Medicine*, 73 (1970), pp. 307–16; Dorothy Levenson, *Mind, Body, and Medicine: A History of the American Psychosomatic Society* (American Psychosomatic Society, 1994). For a discussion of Wittkower's work on eczema, see J. Barrie Murray, *Some Common Psychosomatic Manifestations* (London, 1951), pp. 88–9.

121 Erwin Pulay, *Allergic Man: Susceptibility and Hypersensitivity* (London, 1945), pp. 13, 97, 90, 10. See also: Erwin Pulay, *Ekzem and Urtikaria: Klinik, Pathogenese und Therapie* (Berlin, 1925); E. Pulay, A. P. Cawadias and P. Lansel, *Constitutional Medicine and Endocrinology*, 4 vols (London, 1944–7).

122 Hans Selye, *The Stress of Life* (New York, 1956), p. viii; Hans Selye, *The Story of the Adaptation Syndrome* (Montreal, 1952); Hans Selye, 'Allergy and the general adaptation syndrome', *International Archives of Allergy*, 3 (1952), pp. 267–78.

123 Pulay, *Allergic Man*, pp. 104–13.

124 John Bowlby, *Child Care and the Growth of Love* (London, 1953).

125 Flanders Dunbar, *Mind and Body: Psychosomatic Medicine* (London, 1947), pp. 174–96; Brian Inglis, *The Diseases of Civilisation* (London, 1981), pp. 218–26.

126 C. P. Taylor, *Allergy* (London, 1966); Anne Sexton, 'Man and Wife', in *Live or Die* (London, 1966), pp. 27–8. I am grateful to Jo Gill from Bath Spa University for alerting me to the work of Anne Sexton.

127 See Reg Smythe's Andy Capp cartoon in the *Daily Mirror* (11 March 1958).

128 John Morrison Smith, 'The recent history of the treatment of asthma: a personal view', *Thorax*, 38 (1983), pp. 244–53; A. Philip Magonet, *Hypnosis in Asthma* (London, 1955).

129 *Annual Report of the Medical Research Council, 1932–1933* (Cmd. 4503) (London, 1933–4), p. 104. See also the MRC records in PRO, FD1/2281.

130 Stephen Black, 'Inhibition of immediate-type hypersensitivity response by direct suggestion under hypnosis', *British Medical Journal* (6 April 1963), pp. 925–9; Stephen Black, 'Shift in dose-response curve of Prausnitz-Küstner reaction by direct suggestion under hypnosis', *British Medical Journal* (13 April 1963), pp. 990–92; Stephen Black, J. H. Humphrey and Janet S. F. Niven, 'Inhibition of Mantoux reaction by direct suggestion under hypnosis', *British Medical Journal* (22 June 1963), pp. 1649–52.

131 'Hypnosis may aid treatment of asthma', *The Times* (14 October 1968), 15a.

132 Linda Bryder, '"Wonderlands of buttercup, clover and daisies": tuberculosis and the open-air school movement in Britain, 1907–39', in *In the Name of the Child: Health and Welfare, 1880–1940*, ed. Roger Cooter (London, 1992), pp. 72–95; Frances Wilmot and Pauline Saul, *A Breath of Fresh Air: Birmingham's Open-Air Schools, 1911–1970* (Chichester, 1998).

133 Smith, 'The recent history', p. 247; 'Children saved by affection', *The Times* (1 November 1962), 13f.

134 M. M. Peshkin and H. S. Tuft, 'Rehabilitation of the intractable asthmatic child by the institutional approach', *Quarterly Review of Pediatrics*, 11 (1956), pp. 7–9. For an English account, see Aaron Lask, *Asthma: Attitude and Milieu* (London, 1966).

135 Philip Pinkerton and Corinna M. Weaver, 'Childhood asthma', in Oscar W. Hill, ed., *Modern Trends in Psychosomatic Medicine* 2 (London, 1970), p. 87.

136 Freeman, 'Vaccination against hay fever'.

137 Freeman, *Hay-Fever*, pp. 69–71; *Annual Report of the Wright-Fleming Institute of Microbiology for the Year 1957*, St. Mary's Hospital Archives, WF/AD6/2, p. 22.

138 John Freeman, 'Dangers and disappointments in hay-fever desensitization', *International Archives of Allergy*, 6 (1955), pp. 197–202.

139 Freeman, *Hay-Fever*, p. viii.

140 Details are in *Minutes of the Meetings of the Council of the Inoculation Department, 1947–1955*, St Mary's Hospital Archives, WF/AD3/1, meeting on 25 November 1948.

141 Freeman, *Hay-Fever*, p. xi.

142 For details of MRC funded projects, see the MRC archives in PRO, FD1/4741, FD1/2528–9, FD1/3624, FD1/2281–2, FD1/2279–85, FD1/4527–8, FD1/7150–66. See also *Annual Report of the Medical Research Council, 1954–1955* (Cmd. 9798) (London, 1955–6), pp. 18–20. For the MRC's emphasis on scientific data, see Katy Walker, '"A unique organisation with a unique purpose"? A reassessment of the pioneer Health Centre Peckham, 1926–50, a failed experiment in preventative medicine', MA dissertation, Exeter, 2003, pp. 16, 91–3. On Wright's relationship with the MRC, see A. Landsborough Thomson, *Half a Century of Medical Research* (London, 1973), vol. I, pp. 115–16.

143 B. P. Sormani, 'Prophylactic vaccination against hay fever', *Lancet*, I (1916), pp. 348–50; John Freeman, 'Prophylactic vaccination against hay fever', *Lancet*, I (1916), p. 532.

144 John Freeman, 'Treatment of hay-fever', *Lancet*, I (1927), pp. 940–41.

145 Cooke, 'The treatment of hay fever', p. 110.

146 Freeman, 'The significance of idiopathic skin reactions', p. 1198. Similar problems regarding commercial allergen preparations plagued American allergists – see Mitman, 'Natural history and the clinic'.

147 Committee on Safety of Medicines, 'Update: desensitising vaccines', *British Medical Journal* (1986), p. 948.

148 John Freeman, 'The significance of idiopathic skin reactions', *Lancet*, I (1930), pp. 1141–2; Thomas Nelson and Arthur D. Porter, 'Protein in asthma', *Lancet*, II (1931), pp. 1342–4.

149 Freeman, '"Rush" inoculation', p. 744.

150 Ibid., p. 746.

151 Robert A. Cooke et al., 'Serological evidence of immunity with coexisting sensitization in a type of human allergy (hay fever)', *Journal of Experimental Medicine*, 62 (1935), pp. 733–51.

152 John D. L. Fitzgerald and William B. Sherman, 'The specificity of blocking antibody induced by grass pollen extracts', *Journal of Allergy*, 20 (1949), pp. 286–91; Kenneth L. Burdon, 'On possible mechanisms of hyposensitization: some pertinent laboratory findings', *Annals of Allergy*, 25 (1967), pp. 483–95.

153 Cooke, 'The treatment of hay fever', p. 112.

154 David Harley, 'Reactions of the human skin to foreign sera', *Lancet*, I (1933), pp. 690–92; 'Prophylaxis and anaphylaxis', *Lancet*, II (1934), pp. 817–18; 'Association of Clinical Pathologists', *Lancet*, I (1942), p. 354; 'Patient's death at Guy's Hospital', *Lancet*, II (1954), pp. 188–9. See also the letter, dated 1 July 1954, and a card about the incident in St Mary's Hospital Archives, WF/AD21/1.

155 Freeman, 'Vaccination against hay fever'; David Harley, 'Asthma: immunological mechanisms, diagnosis and treatment', *Lancet*, II (1936), pp. 367–70.

156 See the illustration in Milton Millman, *Pardon My Sneeze . . . The Story of Allergy* (San Diego, CA, 1960), facing p. 3.

157 Charles W. Forward, *The Golden Calf: An Exposure of Vaccine-Therapy* (London, 1933), p. 8. See also Charles W. Forward, *The Food of the Future: A Summary of Arguments in Favour of a Non-Flesh Diet* (London, 1904).

158 A. J. Cronin, *The Citadel* (London, 1938), p. 285.

159 John A. Ryle, 'Observations on the abdominal and circulatory phenomena of allergy', *Lancet*, I (1935), pp. 1257–61.

160 Freeman, *Hay-Fever*, p. ix.

161 Arnold R. Rich, *The Pathogenesis of Tuberculosis*, 2nd edn (Oxford, 1951), pp. 511–12, 334–5. See also the comments on terminology in J. Pepys, 'Editorial: "clinical immunology" and the "practise of allergy"', *Clinical Allergy*, 1 (1971), pp. 1–7.

162 *Annual Reports of the Wright-Fleming Institute of Microbiology, 1950–1966*, in St Mary's Hospital Archives, WF/AD6/1 and WF/AD 6/2.

163 See the annual report for 1952 in *Annual Reports of the Wright-Fleming Institute of Microbiology, 1950–1955*, in St Mary's Hospital Archives, WF/AD 6/1, p. 12.

164 Further details are in the *Annual Reports of the Wright-Fleming Institute of Microbiology, 1950–1966*, WF/AD 6/1 and WF/AD 6/2. In 1953 the Department produced a fifteen-

minute educational film entitled *Hay Fever*, a copy of which is in the Wellcome Trust Medical Film and Video Library.

165 Ian Murray, 'Annual torture of hay fever sufferers', *The Times* (5 May 1976), 13a.

166 *Annual Report of the Wright-Fleming Institute of Microbiology for the Year 1962–63*, St Mary's Hospital Archives, WF/AD 6/2, p. 13.

167 J. Emberlin, M. Savage and S. Jones, 'Annual variations in grass pollen seasons in London, 1961–1990: trends and forecast models', *Clinical and Experimental Allergy*, 23 (1993), pp. 911–18; Frankland, 'Aerobiology'.

168 A. W. Frankland, 'A brief history of the Society', BSACI *News* (1997), pp. 9–11.

169 See the papers from the British Society for Immunology, Contemporary Medical Archives Centre, SA/BSI/A1/1 and SA/BSI/F1/1.

170 J. H. Humphrey and R. G. White, *Immunology for Students of Medicine* (Oxford, 1963); Brigitte A. Askonas, 'John Herbert Humphrey', *Biographical Memoirs of Fellows of the Royal Society* (1988), pp. 275–300.

171 *Advances in Immunology* first appeared in 1961 and early issues regularly contained reviews on allergy and autoimmunity.

172 Ilana Löwy, 'Biomedical research and the constraints of medical practice: James Bumgardner Murphy and the early discovery of the role of lymphocytes in immune reactions', *Bulletin of the History of Medicine*, 63 (1989), pp. 356–91.

173 Cohen, 'The American Academy of Allergy', pp. 408–12. Details of the European Academy are available on its website, www.eaaci.org.

174 See, for example, the discussion of the importance of further studies of hypersensitivity in World Health Organization, *Research in Immunology: Technical Report Series No. 286* (Geneva, 1964). See also chapter Four below.

175 See the various contributions to discussions at the WHO meeting convened in 1978, in the WHO Library, IMM/ALL/78.1.

176 Milton B. Cohen and June B. Cohen, *Your Allergy and What To Do About It* (London, 1942), p. 5.

177 Noël Coward, *Plays: One* (London, 1985).

178 Warren T. Vaughan, *Primer of Allergy* (St Louis, MO, 1939), p. 7; Warren T. Vaughan, *Strange Malady: The Story of Allergy* (New York, 1941).

179 R. A. Cooke and A. Vander Veer, 'Human sensitization', *Journal of Immunology*, 1 (1916), pp. 201–305.

180 Vaughan, 'Minor allergy'; B. Jimenez, 'A survey of sensitization in students of the University of Michigan', *Journal of the Michigan State Medical Society*, 33 (1934), pp. 310–12; W. C. Service, 'The incidence of major allergic diseases in Colorado Springs', *Journal of the American Medical Association*, 112 (1939), pp. 2034–7; Bret Ratner and David E. Silberman, 'Allergy: its distribution and the hereditary concept', *Annals of Allergy*, 9 (1952), pp. 1–20.

181 Vaughan, *Strange Malady*, pp. 7–8.

182 Vaughan, 'Minor allergy'. p. 194.

183 Cohen and Cohen, *Your Allergy*, p. 6.

184 Ratner and Silberman, 'Allergy', p. 17.

185 Vaughan, 'Minor allergy'. p. 194.

Chapter 4: The Global Economy of Allergy

1   World Health Organization (WHO), 'Global medium-term programme for noncommunicable disease prevention and control: Chapter v: Immunology', p. 3. This document is in the WHO Library, Geneva, IMM/80.1.

2   'Five die in Cuba asthma wave', *The Times* (27 September 1963), 12c; 'Tension-blamed for Negroes' asthma', *The Times* (26 July 1965), 8c. The role of cockroaches is discussed in Gregg Mitman, 'Cockroaches, housing and race: a history of asthma and urban ecology in America' (unpublished paper presented at a conference held at the University of Exeter, March 2005).

3   'Asthmatic child's education needs', *The Times* (26 March 1965), 6d.

4   John Morrison Smith, 'Death from asthma', *Lancet*, I (1966), p. 1042.

5   F. E. Speizer, R. Doll and P. Heaf, 'Observations on recent increase in mortality from asthma', *British Medical Journal* (10 February 1968), pp. 335–9.

6   W. H. W. Inman and A. M. Adelstein, 'Rise and fall of asthma mortality in England and Wales in relation to use of pressurised aerosols', *Lancet*, II (1969), pp. 279–85.

7   'Implications of increase in asthma deaths', *The Times* (13 August 1968), 7e; 'Alarm at asthma deaths', *The Times* (28 October 1968), 2a; 'Drug warning to asthma patients: care needed with aerosols', *The Times* (23 June 1967), 3e.

8   M. J. Greenberg, 'Isoprenaline in myocardial failure', *Lancet*, II (1965), pp. 442–3; M. J. Greenberg and A. Pines, 'Pressurized aerosols in asthma', *British Medical Journal* (4 March 1967), p. 563; Bryan Gandevia, 'Pressurized aerosols in asthma', *British Medical Journal* (13 May 1967), p. 441.

9   Speizer, Doll and Heaf, 'Observations on recent increase', p. 337.

10 CIBA Guest Symposium, 'Terminology, definitions and classification of chronic pulmonary emphysema and related conditions', *Thorax*, 14 (1959), pp. 286–99; J. G. Scadding, 'Meaning of diagnostic terms in broncho-pulmonary disease', *British Medical Journal* (7 December 1963), pp. 1425–30.

11 D. J. Pereira Gray, 'Gale Memorial Lecture 1979: Just a GP', *Journal of the Royal College of General Practitioners*, 30 (1980), pp. 231–9.

12 Roger Robinson, 'A paper that changed my practice: wheezy children', *British Medical Journal*, 302 (22 June 1991), p. 1516.

13 Speizer, Doll and Heaf, 'Observations on recent increase', p. 337.

14 Ibid. See also F. E. Speizer et al., 'Investigation into use of drugs preceding death from asthma', *British Medical Journal* (10 February 1968), pp. 339–43.

15 Inman and Adelstein, 'Rise and fall of asthma mortality'; Asthma Research Council Annual Report, *The Urgency of Asthma Research* (London, 1971); 'Reduction in asthma toll', *The Times* (21 March 1972), 4c.

16 Speizer, Doll and Heaf, 'Observations on recent increase'; Ian Gregg and John Batten, 'Sudden death in a young asthmatic', *British Medical Journal* (5 April 1969), pp. 29–30; Philip Pinkerton and Corinna M. Weaver, 'Childhood asthma', in *Modern Trends in Psychosomatic Medicine 2*, ed. Oscar W. Hill (London, 1970), pp. 97–8.

17 Paul D. Stolley, 'Asthma mortality: why the United States was spared an epidemic

of deaths due to asthma', *American Review of Respiratory Disease*, 105 (1972), pp. 883–90.

18   Richard Beasley, Neil Pearce and Julian Crane, 'International trends in asthma mortality', in *The Rising Trends in Asthma*, ed. Derek J. Chadwick and Gail Cardew (Chichester, 1997), pp. 140–50; G. Keating et al., 'Trends in sales of drugs for asthma in New Zealand, Australia and the United Kingdom, 1975–81', *British Medical Journal*, 289 (1984), pp. 348–51.

19   John Morrison Smith, 'The recent history of the treatment of asthma: a personal view', *Thorax*, 38 (1983), pp. 244–53; Sheldon C. Siegel, 'History of asthma deaths from antiquity', *Journal of Allergy and Clinical Immunology*, 80 (1987), pp. 458–62.

20   Department of Health, *Asthma: An Epidemiological Overview* (London, 1995). See also the information provided by the Lung & Asthma Information Agency (LAIA), Factsheets 92/1, 92/4, 93/6, 95/1, 96/2, 97/3, 99/1, 2002/1, available at http://www.sghms.ac.uk/depts/laia/laia.htm.

21   D. M. Fleming and D. L. Crombie, 'Prevalence of asthma and hay fever in England and Wales', *British Medical Journal*, 294 (1987), pp. 279–83; Mark N. Upton et al., 'Intergenerational 20 year trends in the prevalence of asthma and hay fever in adults: the Midspan family study surveys of parents and offspring', *British Medical Journal*, 321 (2000), pp. 88–92.

22   K. K. Eaton, 'The incidence of allergy – has it changed?', *Clinical Allergy*, 12 (1982), pp. 107–10.

23   Upton et al., 'Intergenerational 20 year trends'; Fleming and Crombie, 'Prevalence of asthma'.

24   Brent Taylor et al., 'Changes in the reported prevalence of childhood eczema since the 1939–45 war', *Lancet*, II (1984), pp. 1255–7.

25   James Meikle, 'Child eczema "has tripled since 1970s"', *Guardian* (23 December 2003).

26   LAIA, Factsheet 98/3, 'Hay fever'. See also: WHO, 'The prevention of allergic diseases', *Clinical Allergy*, 16 Supplement (1986), p. 13; UCB Institute of Allergy, *European Allergy White Paper: Allergic Diseases as a Public Health Problem* (Brussels, 1997).

27   Ann J. Woolcock and Jennifer K. Peat, 'Evidence for the increase in asthma world-wide', in *The Rising Trends in Asthma*, pp. 122–34; Ian Gregg, 'Epidemiological aspects', in *Asthma*, ed. T.J.H. Clark and S. Godfrey, 2nd edn (London, 1983), pp. 242–83; WHO, 'The prevention of allergic diseases'.

28   Roy Patterson and Anthony J. Ricketti, 'Allergy', *World Health* (November 1983), pp. 14–17; Chris Mihill, 'Asthma sufferers face "exploitation"', *Guardian* (10 December 1996).

29   Roland Davies, 'Hayfever: is it on the increase?', *Medical Dialogue Weekly*, 236 (June 1989); Gregg, 'Epidemiological aspects', p. 261; WHO, 'Report of a meeting on allergic diseases', *Clinical Allergy*, 10 (1980), pp. 1–20.

30   See de Weck's full report in the WHO archives, WHO 15/181/89.

31   WHO, 'Report of a meeting', pp. 2, 8.

32   WHO, 'Meeting on allergic diseases', WHO Library, IMM/ALL/78.1–78.6.

33   WHO, 'Report of a meeting', p. 15.

34   Ian Gregg, 'Epidemiological research in asthma: the need for a broad perspec-

tive', *Clinical Allergy*, 16 (1986), pp. 17–23; Gregg, 'Epidemiological aspects', p. 263.

35 Woolcock and Peat, 'Evidence for the increase', p. 124.

36 WHO, 'The prevention of allergic diseases', p. 7.

37 ISAAC Steering Committee, 'Worldwide variation in prevalence of symptoms of asthma, allergic rhinoconjunctivitis and atopic eczema: ISAAC', *Lancet*, 351 (1998), pp. 1225–32.

38 See, for example: Peter Townsend, Nick Davidson and Margaret Whitehead, eds, *Inequalities in Health: The Black Report and The Health Divide* (London, 1990); LAIA, Factsheet 98/3, 'Hay fever', and Factsheet 2000/3, 'Asthma and social class'; R. J. Hancox et al., 'Relationship between socioeconomic status and asthma: a longitudinal cohort study', *Thorax*, 59 (2004), pp. 376–80.

39 Irvin Broder et al., 'Epidemiology of asthma and allergic rhinitis in a total community, Tecumseh, Michigan', *Journal of Allergy and Clinical Immunology*, 53 (1974), pp. 127–38; Tari Haahtela et al., 'Skin prick test reactivity to common allergens in Finnish adolescents', *Allergy*, 35 (1980); Eaton, 'The incidence of allergy'; B. Wüthrich et al., 'Epidemiology of allergic rhinitis (pollinosis), in Switzerland', in *Excerpta Medica*, ed. B. Wüthrich and L. Jäger (Amsterdam, 1986), pp. 10–17.

40 'Asthma', *The Times* (15 January 1929), 13c.

41 Denis Herbstein, 'Hay fever's advantages are not to be sneezed at', *The Times* (1 July 1985), 11b.

42 Department of Health, *Asthma*, p. 3.

43 Jacqueline Hoare and Maggie Bruce, 'Prevalence of treated asthma and its management in general practice in England and Wales, 1994–1998', *Health Statistics Quarterly*, 17 (2003), pp. 15–22; Maxine Frith, 'Allergy in the UK: NHS Bill reaches an irritating £1bn', *Independent* (15 April 2004), pp. 14–15.

44 WHO, 'Report of a meeting', pp. 14–15.

45 'More asthma but progress towards control', *The Times* (4 April 1977), 2e.

46 Department of Health, *Asthma*, p. 24; Mike Thomas and David Price, 'Measuring and costing quality in asthma', *Costs and Options*, 25 (July 2002), pp. 3–8.

47 WHO, 'Report of a meeting', p. 14.

48 Claude A. Frazier, *Parents' Guide to Allergy in Children* (New York, 1973), p. ix.

49 WHO, 'Report of a meeting', p. 14.

50 WHO, 'The prevention of allergic diseases', p. 16.

51 UCB Institute of Allergy, *European Allergy White Paper*, p. 105.

52 WHO, 'The prevention of allergic diseases', p. 16. See also the travel report in the WHO archives dated 10/11/82, WHO 15/86/10/J.2.

53 WHO, 'Report of a meeting', p. 14.

54 WHO, Travel report, 10/11/82, WHO 15/86/10/J.2.

55 WHO, 'The prevention of allergic diseases', p. 16.

56 UCB Institute of Allergy, *European Allergy White Paper*.

57 Dr Hugh Jolly, 'Seeing asthma as a nuisance rather than a debilitating disease', *The Times* (23 April 1975), 10e; G. W. Farndon, 'Asthma problem', *The Times* (14 January 1970), 11f.

58 'Asthma: need for urgent action', *The Times* (18 June 1976), 16e; Dr E. Sherwood Jones, 'Asthma deaths', *The Times* (13 July 1976), 15g; Annabel Ferriman, 'Cards drive to reduce asthma toll', *The Times* (12 August 1981), 2c; Jenny Bryan, 'Asthma: don't just rely on the hospital', *The Times* (23 February 1983), 11a.

59 National Asthma Campaign, 'Parliament puts asthma on the agenda', NAC website, http://www.asthma.org.uk/news, 8 May 2003.

60 For the latest guidelines, see Scottish Intercollegiate Guidelines Network and The British Thoracic Society, *British Guidelines on the Management of Asthma* (2003).

61 National Heart, Lung and Blood Institute, *Guidelines for the Diagnosis and Management of Asthma: Expert Panel Report* (Bethesda, 1991).

62 WHO, *The First Ten Years of the World Health Organization* (Geneva, 1958); Paul Weindling, ed., *International Health Organisations and Movements, 1918–1939* (Cambridge, 1995); Javed Siddiqi, *World Health and World Politics* (Carolina, LA, 1995).

63 'Communication of the Director-General on Immunology', 1 May 1963, WHO ACMR 5/4; Howard Goodman, 'WHO's first research unit: immunology', *World Health* (December 1983), pp. 14–15.

64 WHO, *Research in Immunology*, WHO Technical Report Series No. 286 (Geneva, 1964), p. 4.

65 Ibid., pp. 22–37; Scientific Group on Immuno-prophylaxis and Therapy, 'Notes on draft agenda', 18 January 1962, WHO Immun/14.

66 Dr A. D. Ado, 'The teaching of allergology', in WHO Imm/EC.3/WP/66.12.

67 WHO, *Teaching of Immunology in the Medical Curriculum*, WHO Technical Report Series No. 358 (Geneva, 1967), pp. 15–19.

68 Ibid., pp. 23–5. A copy of the memorandum, which was originally prepared for the Royal Commission on Medical Education in 1966, is also in the BSI archives in the Contemporary Medical Archives Centre, Wellcome Library, SA/BSI/A 1/4.

69 WHO, *Clinical Immunology*, WHO Technical Report Series No. 496 (Geneva, 1972), pp. 28–35.

70 'Five years of research on immunology', WHO *Chronicle*, 24 (1970), pp. 153–61; WHO, 'Programme Review: Immunology' (1969), WHO EB45/26.

71 For details of the contracts, see WHO 15/181/28, 15/181/66, 15/181/67, 15/181/75.

72 Details are in WHO 15/181/89, memorandum dated 23 February 1976.

73 WHO documents relating to this committee as well as copies of the newsletters are in WHO 15/82/2/J.1–4.

74 B. Cinader, 'The origins and early years of IUIS', *Immunology Today*, 13 (1992), pp. 323–6. Bernard Cinader, who died in 2001, was a leading immunologist in Canada and first president of the IUIS. The first international congresses organized by the IUIS were held in the United States in 1971 and in England in 1974. On further activities of the IUIS and WHO, see letters and other documents in WHO 15/82/2/J.1–4 and WHO 15/86/13/J.1–2.

75 Anne Marie Moulin, 'The immune system: a key concept for the history of immunology', *History and Philosophy of Life Sciences*, 11 (1989), pp. 221–36.

76 The report is in WHO 15/181/89.

77 The papers are in WHO 15/86/10/J.1.

78 See Howard Goodman's report of the discussion in WHO 15/86/10/J.1.

79 'Programme review: immunology', WHO EB45/26.

80 WHO, *Clinical Immunology*; WHO, 'Report of a meeting', pp. 2–3.

81 WHO, 'Report of a meeting'; WHO IMM/ALL/78.1; WHO, 'The prevention of allergic diseases'; Travel report, 10/11/82, WHO 15/86/10/J.2.

82 WHO, 'Global medium-term programme for noncommunicable disease prevention and control: immunology', WHO IMM/80.1.

83 WHO, 'Global medium-term programme: immunology', WHO CDS (IMM)/MTP/83.1, p. 4.

84 WHO, *Manual of the International Statistical Classification of Diseases, Injuries and Causes of Death* (Geneva, 1957), vol. I, p. xxi. See also WHO, *The First Ten Years*, pp. 278–88.

85 WHO, *Research in Immunology*, p. 29.

86 WHO, *Manual of the International Statistical Classification of Diseases* (1957).

87 See the comments in WHO HS/ICD/29.

88 See the reports of discussions and recommendations in WHO HS/IUCD/50, WHO HS/ICD/50 Add. 11, WHO HS/ICD/74.65. The WHO committees responsible were the Sub-Committee on Classification of Diseases and the Expert Committee on Health Statistics. See also WHO, *Manual of the International Statistical Classification of Diseases, Injuries and Causes of Death* (Geneva, 1967), vol. I.

89 Arthur F. Coca and Robert A. Cooke, 'On the classification of the phenomena of hypersensitiveness', *Journal of Immunology*, 8 (1923), pp. 163–82.

90 Arnold R. Rich, *The Pathogenesis of Tuberculosis* (Oxford, 1951), pp. 335–41.

91 Ibid., p. 341.

92 P.G.H. Gell and R.R.A. Coombs, eds, *Clinical Aspects of Immunology* (Oxford, 1963), p. 317.

93 Ibid., pp. 320–23.

94 According to Gell and Coombs, Type IV hypersensitivity was mediated by 'specifically modified mononuclear cells containing a substance or mechanism capable of responding specifically to allergen deposited at a local site' – ibid., p. 323.

95 M. W. Chase, 'The cellular transfer of cutaneous hypersensitivity to tuberculin', *Proceedings of the Society for Experimental Biology and Medicine*, 59 (1945), p. 134; Gell and Coombs, *Clinical Aspects*, p. 323.

96 J. Pepys, 'Editorial: "Clinical immunology" and the "practise of allergy"', *Clinical Allergy*, 1 (1971), pp. 1–7; Patterson and Ricketti, 'Allergy'; Fred Karush and Herman N. Eisen, 'A theory of delayed hypersensitivity', *Science*, 136 (1962), pp. 1032–9.

97 Gell and Coombs, *Clinical Aspects*, p. 319.

98 See Coombs' comments in E. M. Tansey et al., eds, 'Self and non-self: a history of autoimmunity', in *Wellcome Witnesses to Twentieth Century Medicine* (London, 1997), vol. I, pp. 46–7.

99 William Cookson, 'The alliance of genes and environment in asthma and allergy', *Nature*, 402 Supplement (1999), B5–11; M. Peakman and D. Vergani, *Basic and Clinical Immunology* (New York, 1997), p. 132.

100 P.G.H. Gell and R.R.A. Coombs, eds, *Clinical Aspects of Immunology*, 2nd edn (Oxford, 1968), pp. 432–42.

101 Kenneth C. Hutchin, *Allergy* (London, 1961), p. 18. See also 'Medicine: prevention of bee-sting allergy', *The Times* (12 June 1974), 18e.

102 Thomas B. Thomasi, 'The discovery of secretory IgA and the mucosal immune system', *Immunology Today*, 13 (1992), pp. 416–18.

103 'Immunoglobulin E, a new class of human immunoglobulin', *Bulletin of the World Health Organization*, 38 (1968), pp. 151–2. The Committee responsible for validating the status of IgE was the WHO Committee on the Nomenclature for Human Immunoglobulins.

104 M. H. Lessof, 'Food intolerance and the scientific trap', *Clinical and Experimental Allergy*, 23 (1993), pp. 971–2.

105 'Immediate hypersensitivity', *Lancet*, II (1973), p. 1364. See also *Lancet*, II (1981), p. 506.

106 The specific test used was the radioallergosorbent test or RAST.

107 William T. Knicker, 'Editorial: is the choice of allergy skin testing versus *in vitro* determination of specific IgE no longer a scientific issue?', *Annals of Allergy*, 62 (1989), pp. 373–4.

108 T. G. Merrett et al., 'Circulating IgE levels in the over-seventies', *Clinical Allergy*, 10 (1980), pp. 433–9; Robert A. Barbee et al., 'Distribution of IgE in a community population sample: correlations with age, sex and allergen skin test reactivity', *Journal of Allergy and Clinical Immunology*, 68 (1981), pp. 106–11; 'Report on a National Institute of Allergy and Infectious Diseases-sponsored workshop on the genetics of total immunoglobulin E levels in humans', *Journal of Allergy and Clinical Immunology*, 67 (1981), pp. 167–70; R. A. Thompson and A. G. Bird, 'How necessary are specific IgE antibody tests in allergy diagnosis?', *Lancet*, I (1983), pp. 169–73.

109 Ohad Parnes, '"Trouble from within": allergy, autoimmunity and pathology in the first half of the twentieth century', *Studies in History and Philosophy of Biological and Biomedical Sciences*, 34 (2003), pp. 425–54. The term 'trouble from within' was introduced by Warren T. Vaughan in *Strange Malady: The Story of Allergy* (New York, 1941), p. 191.

110 See the allergy testing kits advertised by Boots Company PLC in their booklet *Living with Allergy: Your Guide to Diagnosing and Managing your Allergy* (Nottingham, n.d.), or the tests for specific IgG-mediated intolerance available through the York Nutritional Laboratory and advertised in a booklet produced by Lloydspharmacy, *Food Intolerance Testing* (Coventry, n.d.).

111 Smith, 'The recent history'. See also David Jack, 'Drug treatment of bronchial asthma, 1948–1995: years of change', *International Pharmacy Journal*, 10 (1996), pp. 50–52.

112 H. Herxheimer, 'Atropine cigarettes in asthma and emphysema', *British Medical Journal* (15 August 1959), pp. 167–71.

113 See the advertisement for Germolene in *Woman's Pictorial* (18 July 1936), p. 46.

114 R.A.L. Brewis, ed., *Classic Papers in Asthma*, vol. II (1991), 'Introduction'.

115 'Lhude Sing Tishu', *The Times* (22 June 1938), 17d.

116 The Bayer Products Company, *Chronic Bronchitis, Asthma and Hay Fever* (Surbiton, 1963).

117 Brewis, *Classic Papers*, 'Introduction'.

118 British Felsol Company, *Asthma – The Medical Profession and Felsol* (n.p., n.d.).

119 Brewis, *Classic Papers*, 'Introduction'; Charles D. May, 'History of the introduction of theophylline into the treatment of asthma', *Clinical Allergy*, 4 (1974), pp. 211–17.

120 Miles Weatherall, 'Drug therapies', in *Companion Encyclopedia of the History of Medicine*, ed. W. F. Bynum and Roy Porter (London, 1993), vol. II, pp. 915–38; Jonathan Liebenau, *Medical Science and Medical Industry: The Formation of the American Pharmaceutical Industry* (Basingstoke, 1987); Judy Slinn, 'Research and development in the UK pharmaceutical industry from the nineteenth century to the 1960s', in *Drugs and Narcotics in History*, ed. Roy Porter and Mikuláš Teich (Cambridge, 1995), pp. 168–86.

121 Liebenau, *Medical Science and Medical Industry*.

122 Noel Snell, 'Inhalation devices: a brief history', *Respiratory Disease in Practice* (Summer 1995), pp. 13–15.

123 On Parke, Davis & Company, see chapter Three above. On American companies, see Gregg Mitman, 'Natural history and the clinic: the regional ecology of allergy in America', *Studies in History and Philosophy of Biological and Biomedical Sciences*, 34 (2003), pp. 491–510; Louis Galambos and Jane Eliot Sewell, *Networks of Innovation: Vaccine Development at Merck, Sharp & Dohme, and Mulford* (Cambridge, 1995).

124 Alain de Weck's report is in WHO 15/181/89.

125 'Controlled trial of effects of cortisone acetate in chronic asthma', *Lancet*, II (1956), pp. 798–803; 'Controlled trial of effects of cortisone acetate in status asthmaticus', *Lancet*, II (1956), pp. 803–6. See also the MRC records from these trials in PRO FD1/7156 and 7157.

126 Ulrich Meyer, *Steckt eine Allergie dahinter?: Die Industrialisierung von Arzneimittel-Entwicklung, -Herstellung und -Vermarktung am Beispiel der Antiallergika* (Stuttgart, 2002), pp. 52–62.

127 D. Bovet and A.-M. Staub, 'Action protectrice des éthers phénoliques au cours de l'intoxication histaminique', *Comptes Rendus des Séances de la Société de Biologie*, 124 (1937) , pp. 547–8.

128 A. W. Frankland and R. H. Gorrill, 'Summer hay-fever and asthma treated with antihistaminic drugs', *British Medical Journal* (4 April 1953), pp. 761–4.

129 'Allen & Hanburys Limited: home and oversea sales expansion', *The Times* (20 December 1955), 12d. For a history of Allen & Hanburys, see Geoffrey Tweedale, *At the Sign of the Plough: 275 Years of Allen & Hanburys and the British Pharmaceutical Industry, 1715–1990* (London, 1990).

130 C. L. Bencard Ltd, *The Bencard Manual of Allergy* (London, 1956), p. 46.

131 P. H. Howarth and S. T. Holgate, 'Comparative trial of two non-sedative H_1 antihistamines, terfenadine and astemizole, for hay fever', *Thorax*, 39 (1984), pp. 668–72; 'Advance in treatment of hay fever', *The Times* (3 March 1982), 2a.

132 C. Kellaway and E. Trethewie, 'The liberation of a slow reacting smooth muscle-stimulating substance in anaphylaxis', *Quarterly Journal of Experimental Physiology*,

30 (1940), p. 121; 'Pharmacology: asthma agent made', *The Times* (26 February 1980), 14c; Pearce Wright, 'Effective relief from hay fever likely', *The Times* (23 June 1984), 10d.

133   Thomas Stuttaford, 'Asthmatics move into class of their own', *The Times* (10 February 1998), 16c; Thomas Stuttaford, 'Pill helps to prevent asthma', *The Times* (28 January 1999), 20a.

134   Pamela W. Ewan, 'Hay fever', *Journal of the Royal College of Physicians*, 23 (1989), pp. 68–76.

135   J. R. Murray, 'The history of corticosteroids', *Acta Dermato-Venereologica*, 69 (Supplement, 1989), pp. 4–6; Brewis, *Classic Papers*, 'Introduction'; Viviane Quirke, 'Making British cortisone: Glaxo and the development of corticosteroids in Britain in the 1950s–1960s', *Studies in History and Philosophy of Biological and Biomedical Sciences*, 36 (2005), pp. 645–74.

136   Hugh Jolly, 'What to do about eczema', *The Times* (18 June 1975), 7e; Quirke, 'Making British cortisone'; R. P. T. Davenport-Hines and Judy Slinn, *Glaxo: A History to 1962* (Cambridge, 1992).

137   H. Morrow Brown, G. Storey and W.H.S. George, 'Beclomethasone dipropionate: a new steroid aerosol for the treatment of allergic asthma', *British Medical Journal* (4 March 1972), pp. 585–90.

138   Tweedale, *At the Sign of the Plough*, pp. 215–16; Jack, 'Drug treatment'.

139   Jonathan Brostoff, 'Hayfever and corticosteroids', *Lancet*, I (1975), p. 1424. For a similar discussion in America, see Leon Unger and M. Coleman Harris, 'Stepping stones in allergy', *Annals of Allergy*, 34 (1975), pp. 194–5.

140   See the comments in WHO IMM/ALL/78.1 to the effect that neither Becotide nor Intal were available in Indonesia in the late 1970s.

141   Brewis, *Classic Papers*, 'Introduction'; Jack, 'Drug treatment'.

142   D. Hartley et al., 'New class of selective stimulants of ß-adrenergic receptors', *Nature*, 219 (1968), pp. 861–2; R. T. Brittain et al., 'Alpha-[(t-butylamino)methyl]-4-hydroxy-m-xylene-alpha^1, alpha^3-diol (AH.3365): a selective ß-adrenergic stimulant', *Nature*, 219 (1968), pp. 862–3.

143   '30 years of Ventolin: text for island display, GWHW, Greenford'. I am grateful to Sarah Flynn, archivist at GlaxoWellcome until 2000, for supplying a copy of this document from the company's Heritage Archives.

144   Smith, 'The recent history', pp. 251–2.

145   See, for example: Sarah M. Dennis et al., 'Regular inhaled salbutamol and asthma control: the TRUST randomised trial', *Lancet*, 355 (2000), pp. 1675–9; Scottish Intercollegiate Guidelines Network and The British Thoracic Society, *British Guidelines*.

146   William Golding, *Lord of the Flies* (Harmondsworth, 1960), p. 9; 'Asthma "can be beaten"', *The Times* (30 October 1980), 3c; BBC, 'A Breath of Fresh Air?' (First Sight, 1998).

147   J.B.L. Howell and R.E.C. Altounyan, 'A double-blind trial of disodium cromoglycate in the treatment of allergic bronchial asthma', *Lancet*, II (1967), pp. 539–42; R.E.C. Altounyan, 'Inhibition of experimental asthma by a new compound – disodium cromoglycate "Intal"', *Acta Allergologica*, 22 (167), p. 487.

148 I am grateful to Alan Edwards, a colleague of Altounyan's, for many of the details presented here. Altounyan's exploits are also commemorated in a film, *Hair Soup* (Yorkshire TV, 1992), produced by his daughter, Barbara. See also: U. Meyer, 'From khellin to sodium cromoglycate: a tribute to the work of Dr R.E.C. Altounyan, 1922–1987', *Pharmazie*, 57 (2002), pp. 62–9; A. M. Edwards and J.B.L. Howell, 'The chromones: history, chemistry and clinical development: a tribute to the work of Dr R.E.C. Altounyan', *Clinical and Experimental Allergy*, 30 (2000), pp. 756–74.

149 J. Pepys and A. W. Frankland, eds, *Disodium Cromoglycate in Allergic Airways Disease* (London, 1970).

150 Andrew Goodrick-Clarke, 'Fisons withdrawal of anti-asthma drug cuts £10m off shares value', *The Times* (13 January 1981), 15f.

151 Ibid. On public interest in the introduction of Rynacrom, see John Roper, 'New drug on prescription for hay fever relief', *The Times* (2 June 1971), 1a.

152 Amer Fasihi, 'A look at the worldwide asthma market', *Pharmaceutical Journal*, 255 (1995), p. 692. See also Cookson, 'The alliance of genes'.

153 Martin Burrow, 'Dose of GSK looks worthwhile', *The Times* (15 February 2002), 28a.

154 Charles W. Forward, *The Golden Calf: An Exposure of Vaccine-Therapy* (London, 1933), p. 8; A. J. Cronin, *The Citadel* (London, 1938).

155 Sheldon G. Cohen, 'The American Academy of Allergy: an historical review', *Journal of Allergy and Clinical Immunology*, 64 (1979), pp. 340, 395.

156 Alan Hamilton, 'Hay fever season has a late start', *The Times* (13 June 1978), 4g.

157 John Sutherland, 'Where there's mucus . . . there's brass', *Guardian* G2 (14 June 2001), 16c; Mihill, 'Asthma sufferers face "exploitation"'.

158 John Naish, 'Allergies: don't they make you sick!', *The Times Weekend* (10 May 2003), 1a.

159 Alexander Stalmatski, *Freedom from Asthma: Buteyko's Revolutionary Treatment* (London, 1997), p. 13.

160 Research at St Mary's, for example, was supported by Parke, Davis & Company, Beechams, and Pfizer during the twentieth century. The UCB Institute of Allergy in Brussels was funded by UCB Pharma, and companies such as Schering, Fisons, CIBA and Nestlé offered financial assistance for symposia.

161 See, for example: Bencard, *The Bencard Manual of Allergy*; Parke, Davis & Company, *Vaccine & Serum Therapy* (London, 1935); and Warner-Lambert's booklet, *All About Allergies*. In addition, the Lung & Asthma Information Agency received funds from Allen & Hanburys, Zeneca, and Merke Sharpe and Dohme and research coordinated by the British Lung Foundation was supported by Allen & Hanburys.

162 'History and profile of the Hoover Company', available on the Hoover website, http://www.hoover.com/dbPages/history.asp.

163 Joseph A. Amato, *Dust: A History of the Small and Invisible* (Berkeley, CA, 2000), p. 80.

164 I am grateful to Colin Taylor of Medivac and Mike Rhodes of HEALTHe Limited for information about the history of their companies. For examples of the range of products available, see www.healthy-house.co.uk, www.medivac.co.uk, and the brochures produced by Allerayde, Allergy Control Products.

165 The phrase appears on the cover of an Allerayde brochure.

166 Nancy Tomes, *The Gospel of Germs: Men, Women, and the Microbe in American Life* (Cambridge, MA, 1998).

167 Mihill, 'Asthma sufferers face "exploitation"'. I am grateful to Colin Taylor for generously sharing his own experiences relating to legal disputes concerning VAT charges on Medivac's products. For a fictional treatment of these issues, see Mark Wallington, *Happy Birthday Shakespeare* (London, 2000).

168 'Hypersensitiveness to silk', *Lancet*, I (1923), p. 498; 'Chronic eczema produced by wheat-flour', *Lancet*, II (1923), p. 28; Dr Prosser White, 'Baker's eczema: a clinical and experimental inquiry', *Lancet*, II (1924), p. 859.

169 Paul Brodeur, 'A reporter at large: the enigmatic enzyme', *New Yorker* (16 January 1971), pp. 42–74 (p. 42).

170 Rachel Carson, *Silent Spring* (1962) (Boston, 1994), pp. 238–9.

171 M.L.H. Flindt, 'Pulmonary disease due to inhalation of derivatives of Bacillus subtilis containing proteolytic enzyme', *Lancet*, I (1969), pp. 1177–81; J. Pepys et al., 'Allergic reactions of the lungs to enzymes of Bacillus subtilis', *Lancet*, I (1969), pp. 1181–4. See also: M.L.H. Flindt, 'Respiratory hazards from papain', *Lancet*, I (1978), pp. 430–32; M.L.H. Flindt, 'Allergy to alpha-amylase and papain', *Lancet*, I (1979), p. 1408; M.L.H. Flindt, 'Variables affecting the outcome of inhalation of enzyme dusts', *Annals of Occupational Hygiene*, 26 (1982), pp. 647–55; M.L.H. Flindt, 'Health and safety aspects of working with enzymes', *Process Biochemistry*, 13 (1978); Michael Flindt, 'Biological washing powders as allergens', *British Medical Journal*, 310 (1995), p. 195.

172 Brodeur, 'A reporter at large', p. 42. See Flindt's account of the disputes in Michael L. H. Flindt, 'Biological miracles and misadventures: identification of sensitization and asthma in enzyme detergent workers', *American Journal of Industrial Medicine*, 29 (1996), pp. 99–110.

173 Brodeur, 'A reporter at large', pp. 53, 68–74.

174 WHO, 'Report of a meeting'; WHO, 'The prevention of allergic diseases'.

175 'Occupational asthma', *The Times* (9 March 1982), 8f; P.A.B. Raffle et al., eds, *Hunter's Diseases of Occupations* (London, 1987), pp. 222–3.

176 '£200,000 award for crippled cook', *The Times* (10 October 2000), 6; '£157,000 for asthma nurse', *Guardian* (18 April 2000), 10e; 'Asthma case nurse awarded £157,000', *The Times* (18 April 2000), 3d.

177 Gell and Coombs, *Clinical Aspects of Immunology* (1963), pp. 514–34; 'Non-disclosure of allergy to hairdresser: Ingham v. Emes', *The Times* (23 June 1955), 14e.

178 'Non-disclosure of allergy to hairdresser'.

179 Dr T. Traherne and Frank Preston, eds, *Healthy Minds and Bodies* (London, 1956), p. 232.

180 Ibid. For recent examples, see the 'sensitive skin' range marketed by Marks & Spencer and the range of products available from Almay Hypoallergenic.

181 Women's Environmental Network, *Getting Lippy: Cosmetics, Toiletries and the Environment* (London, December 2003), p. 1.

182 P. Cadby, 'The producer's view: do we worry about adverse effects?', in *Fragrances: Beneficial and Adverse Effects*, ed. P. J. Frosch, J. D. Johansen and I. R. White (Berlin,

1998), pp. 193–6.

183 Louise Costa, 'In the news: understanding fragrance and health – 5 myths', *Human Ecologist Supplement*, 2 (1999).

184 Stephen Antczak and Gina Antczak, *Cosmetics Unmasked* (London, 2001); Theron G. Randolph and Ralph W. Moss, *An Alternative Approach to Allergies* (New York, 1980), p. 68.

185 'Dermatologic Challenged' (Whichonline, February 2004); Department of Trade and Industry, *A Guide to the Cosmetic Products (Safety) Regulations* (London, 1998).

186 Craig Clarke, 'Mother died in allergic fit "after using hair dye"', *The Times* (22 January 2001), 11a; Oliver Wright, 'Woman died after allergic reaction to hair colouring', *The Times* (9 May 2001), 5a.

187 Salmon R. Halpern et al., 'Development of childhood allergy in infants fed breast, soy, or cow milk', *Journal of Allergy and Clinical Immunology*, 51 (1973), pp. 139–51.

188 I am grateful to Dr Pierre Guesry for discussing the development of hypoallergenic formula milk during a trip to the Nestlé Research Center in Lausanne in 2002. See also Dietrich Reinhardt and Eberhard Schmidt, eds, *Food Allergy*, Nestlé Nutrition Workshop Series, vol. XVII (New York, 1988).

189 Ben F. Feingold, *Why Your Child is Hyperactive* (New York, 1974). I am grateful to Matthew Smith for alerting me to Feingold's work. I am also grateful to Ben Crowther, J. Sainsbury plc, letter dated 3 May 2000, for information relating to British interest in additives. See also: Gregg, 'Epidemiological research in asthma', p. 21; Susan Lewis, 'Cut down the colouring, cut down on asthma', *The Times* (2 August 1983), 11h; Robin Young, 'Food additive link to tantrums in 25% of toddlers', *The Times* (25 October 2002), 15a.

190 David Hide, 'Fatal anaphylaxis due to food', *British Medical Journal*, 307 (27 November 1993), p. 1427; E.S.K. Assem et al., 'Anaphylaxis induced by peanuts', *British Medical Journal*, 307 (26 May 1990), p. 1377; Kieron L. Donovan and J. Peters, 'Vegetable-burger allergy: all was nut as it appeared', *British Medical Journal*, 307 (26 May 1990), p. 1378; Tony Smith, 'Allergy to peanuts', *British Medical Journal*, 307 (26 May 1990), p. 1354; Pamela W. Ewan, 'Clinical study of peanut and nut allergy in 62 consecutive patients', *British Medical Journal*, 312 (1996), pp. 1074–8; Clare Thompson, 'One bite and he dies', *Sunday Times Magazine* (19 October 1997), pp. 24–8; Simon de Bruxelles, 'Nuts led to death of allergic scientist', *The Times* (21 November 1997), 5h; Tina Burchill, 'The rise of killer food', *The Times* T2 (22 January 2002), 10; Steve L. Taylor and Susan L. Hefle, 'Ingredient and labeling issues associated with allergenic foods', *Allergy*, 56 (2001), Supplement 67, pp. 64–9.

191 Trevor Rous and Alan Hunt, 'Governing peanuts: the regulation of the social bodies of children and the risks of food allergies', *Social Science and Medicine*, 58 (2004), pp. 825–36.

192 Committee on Toxicity of Chemicals in Food, Consumer Products and the Environment, *Peanut Allergy* (London, 1998).

193 Details are available from The Anaphylaxis Campaign, PO Box 149, Fleet, Hampshire, GU13 9XU. I am grateful to David Reading for sending me relevant literature.

194 Personal communication from Ben Crowther, who generously explained the

evolution of Sainsbury's policies on allergy and provided copies of the company's information booklets. I am also grateful to R. D. Bullock, Technical Manager at Thorntons, and Gail Williamson, Customer Service Manager at Tesco for sending me material. McDonald's restaurants provide a guide, entitled *Our Food*, which includes information on allergies. For British government advice, see Ministry of Agriculture, Fisheries and Food, *Food Allergy and Other Unpleasant Reactions to Food* (London, 1995).

195 The figures come from a survey by Mintel in February 2003, available on http://reports.mintel.com. The figures were also disseminated on the BBC website in March 2003, http://news.bbc.co.uk/1/hi/health/2842611.stm.

196 Sir Macfarlane Burnet, *The Integrity of the Body* (Cambridge, MA, 1962), p. 142. See also Gell and Coombs, eds, *Clinical Aspects of Immunology* (1963), pp. 448–96.

197 WHO, 'Report of a meeting', p. 9; WHO, 'The prevention of allergic diseases', p. 32.

198 Patterson and Ricketti, 'Allergy', p. 16. For an early English case, see R. C. Bell, 'Sudden death following injection of procaine penicillin', *Lancet*, I (1954), pp. 13–17.

Chapter 5: Civilization and Disease

1 René Dubos, *The Dreams of Reason: Science and Utopias* (New York, 1961), p. 71.

2 Ian Gregg, 'Epidemiological research in asthma: the need for a broad perspective', *Clinical Allergy*, 16 (1986), pp. 17–23. On links between globalization and health, see Kelley Lee, ed., *Health Impacts of Globalization* (Basingstoke, 2003); Christine McMurray and Roy Smith, *Diseases of Globalization: Socioeconomic Transitions and Health* (London, 2001).

3 Kenneth C. Hutchin, *Allergy* (London, 1961), pp. 11–13.

4 G. Payling Wright, *An Introduction to Pathology*, 2nd edn (London, 1954), p. 136.

5 Dubos, *The Dreams of Reason*, p. 69.

6 George Cheyne, *The English Malady: or, a Treatise of Nervous Diseases of All Kinds* (London, 1733); Thomas Trotter, *An Essay Medical, Philosophical and Chemical on Drunkenness and its Effects on the Human Body* (London, 1804); Thomas Trotter, *A View of the Nervous Temperament* (London, 1807).

7 Charles H. Blackley, *Experimental Researches on the Causes and Nature of Catarrhus Aestivus* (London, 1873), p. 162.

8 Charles E. Rosenberg, 'Pathologies of progress: the idea of civilization as risk', *Bulletin of the History of Medicine*, 72 (1998), pp. 714–30.

9 Gregg, 'Epidemiological research in asthma'; Jean-Francois Bach, 'The effect of infections on susceptibility to autoimmune and allergic diseases', *New England Journal of Medicine*, 347 (2002), pp. 911–20.

10 World Health Organization (WHO), 'The prevention of allergic diseases', *Clinical Allergy*, 16 Supplement (1986), p. 26.

11 D. M. Fleming and D. L. Crombie, 'Prevalence of asthma and hay fever in England and Wales', *British Medical Journal*, 294 (1987), pp. 279–83.

12 W. C. Spain and Robert A. Cooke, 'Studies in specific hypersensitiveness: the

familial occurrence of hay fever and bronchial asthma', *Journal of Immunology*, 9 (1924), pp. 521–69.

13 Ian Gregg, 'Epidemiological aspects', in T.J.H. Clark and S. Godfrey, eds, *Asthma*, 2nd edn (London, 1983), pp. 242–83.

14 M. J. Morris et al., 'HLA-A, B and C and HLA-DR antigens in intrinsic and allergic asthma', *Clinical Allergy*, 10 (1980), pp. 173–9; W.O.C.M. Cookson et al., 'Maternal inheritance of atopic IgE responsiveness on chromosome 11q', *Lancet*, 340 (1992), pp. 381–4; Julian M. Hopkin, 'Atopy and genetics', *Journal of the Royal College of Physicians of London*, 24 (1990), pp. 159–60; William Cookson, *The Gene Hunters: Adventures in the Genome Jungle* (London, 1994), pp. 123–42.

15 Herbert S. Kaufman and John R. Hobbs, 'Immunoglobulin deficiencies in an atopic population', *Lancet*, II (1970), pp. 1061–3; C. R. Stokes, Brent Taylor and M. W. Turner, 'Association of house-dust and grass-pollen allergies with specific IgA antibody deficiency', *Lancet*, II (1974), pp. 485–8; M. J. Morris et al., 'HLA-A, B and C and HLA-DR antigens'.

16 'Medicine: hope of early action to check hay fever', *The Times* (22 December 1972), 15e; 'Immunology: deficiency and allergy', *The Times* (5 September 1974), 16a; Mark Henderson, 'Asthma inherited', *The Times* (22 October 2001). For recent references to family history as a 'strong risk factor', see UCB Institute of Allergy, *European Allergy Update* (Brussels, 1999), p. 14.

17 Heinz J. Wittig et al., 'Risk factors for the development of allergic disease: analysis of 2,190 patient records', *Annals of Allergy*, 41 (1978), pp. 84–8.

18 William G. Rothstein, *Public Health and the Risk Factor: A History of an Uneven Medical Revolution* (Rochester, NY, 2003), p. 3.

19 Christopher Sellers, 'Discovering environmental cancer: Wilhelm Heuper, post-World War II epidemiology and the vanishing clinician's eye', *American Journal of Public Health*, 87 (1997), pp. 1824–35; Gerald N. Grob, *The Deadly Truth: A History of Disease in America* (Cambridge, MA, 2002), pp. 251–5; Trevor Rous and Alan Hunt, 'Governing peanuts: the regulation of the social bodies of children and the risks of food allergies', *Social Science and Medicine*, 58 (2004), pp. 825–36.

20 Lester Breslow, 'Risk factor intervention for health maintenance', *Science*, 200 (1978), pp. 908–12.

21 Sonja Olin Lauritzen, 'Lay voices on allergic conditions in children: parents' narratives and the negotiation of a diagnosis', *Social Science and Medicine*, 58 (2004), pp. 1299–1308.

22 Ulrich Beck, *Risk Society: Towards a New Modernity*, trans. Mark Ritter (London, 1992), p. 21. See also: Ulrich Beck, 'The naturalistic fallacy of the ecological movement', in *The Polity Reader in Social Theory*, ed. Anthony Giddens et al. (Cambridge, 1994), pp. 342–6; Ulrich Beck, 'Risk society and the provident state', in *Risk, Environment and Modernity: Towards a New Ecology*, ed. Scott Lash, Bronislaw Szersynski and Brian Wynne (London, 1996), pp. 27–43. On the role of risk in the new public health, see Alan Petersen and Deborah Lupton, *The New Public Health: Health and Self in the Age of Risk* (London, 2000).

23 Beck, *Risk Society*, p. 19.

24 Ibid.

25 Ibid., p. 17.

26 R. Szibor et al., 'Pollen analysis reveals murder season', *Nature*, 395 (1998), pp. 449–50.

27 Gregg Mitman, 'What's in a weed? A cultural geography of *Ambrosia artemesiaefolia*', in *The Moral Authority of Nature*, ed. Lorraine Daston and Fernando Vidal (Chicago, 2003), pp. 438–65.

28 Marilyn Manson, 'Diamonds and pollen' (on Disposable Teens, UK, 2000); The Divine Comedy, 'The pop singer's fear of the pollen count' (UK, 1999); Jeff Noon, *Pollen* (London, 1995).

29 Roland Davies, 'Hayfever: is it on the increase?', *Medical Dialogue Weekly*, 236 (June 1989); WHO, 'Report of a meeting on allergic diseases', *Clinical Allergy*, 10 (1980), pp. 12–13; Gregg, 'Epidemiological research in asthma', pp. 20–1.

30 See, for example, Max Samter and Oren C. Durham, eds, *Regional Allergy of the United States, Canada, Mexico and Cuba* (Springfield, IL, 1955).

31 R. R. Davies and L. P. Smith, 'Weather and the grass pollen content of the air', *Clinical Allergy*, 3 (1973), pp. 95–108; M. S. McDonald and B. J. O'Driscoll, 'Aerobiological studies based in Galway: a comparison of pollen and spore counts over two seasons of widely differing weather conditions', *Clinical Allergy*, 10 (1980), pp. 211–15.

32 Pamela W. Ewan, 'Hay fever: a report of the Royal College of Physicians', *Journal of the Royal College of Physicians of London*, 23 (1989), pp. 68–76.

33 Mitman, 'What's in a weed?'.

34 W. C. Hollopeter, *Hay-Fever: Its Prevention and Cure* (New York, 1916), pp. 161–7.

35 Eric Caulton, 'Ragweed (*Ambrosia* spp.): the super allergenic urban weed', BAF *News* (May 1999), pp. 3–4; Jonathan Brostoff and Linda Gamlin, *Hayfever* (Glasgow, 1994), pp. 130–31.

36 UCB Institute of Allergy, *European Allergy Update*, pp. 45–6.

37 D. J. Pearson, D.L.J. Freed and Geoffrey Taylor, 'Respiratory allergy and the month of birth', *Clinical Allergy*, 7 (1977), pp. 29–33; J. Morrison Smith and V. H. Springett, 'Atopic disease and month of birth', *Clinical Allergy*, 9 (1979), pp. 153–7.

38 F. Björkstén and I. Suoniemi, 'Dependence of immediate hypersensitivity on the month of birth', *Clinical Allergy*, 6 (1976), pp. 165–71; F. Björkstén, I. Suoniemi and V. Koski, 'Neonatal birch-pollen contact and subsequent allergy to birch pollen', *Clinical Allergy*, 10 (1980), pp. 585–91; Luisa Businco et al., 'Month of birth and grass pollen or mite sensitization in children with respiratory allergy: a significant relationship', *Clinical Allergy*, 18 (1988), pp. 269–74.

39 Kaufman and Hobbs, 'Immunoglobulin deficiencies'; Stokes, Taylor and Turner, 'Association of house-dust and grass-pollen allergies'; Gregg, 'Epidemiological aspects', p. 271; 'Immunology: deficiency and allergy', *The Times* (5 September 1974), 16a.

40 Ewan, 'Hay fever', p. 74; J. Emberlin, M. Savage and S. Jones, 'Annual variations in grass pollen seasons in London, 1961–1990: trends and forecast models', *Clinical and Experimental Allergy*, 23 (1993), pp. 911–18.

41   Sheldon G. Cohen and Peter J. Bianchine, 'Hymenoptera, hypersensitivity and history', *Annals of Allergy, Asthma and Immunology*, 74 (1995), pp. 198–221.

42   William Frew, 'Rapidly fatal result from the sting of a wasp', *British Medical Journal* (18 January 1896), p. 145; Dr R. Lynn Heard, 'Wasp sting', *British Medical Journal* (15 February 1896), pp. 447–8; F. H. Cooke, 'Fatal case of wasp sting', *British Medical Journal* (5 November 1898), p. 1429; T. Wilson Parry, 'A case of urticaria following immediately on wasp-sting', *Lancet*, II (1901), pp. 1120–21; 'The poison of the bee', *Lancet*, II (1904), p. 644; 'Wasp and bee stings', *Lancet*, II (1904), p. 843; Dr G. Harvey Low, 'Wasp stings', *British Medical Journal* (1907), p. 1112.

43   Parry, 'A case of urticaria', p. 1121.

44   A. T. Waterhouse, 'Bee-stings and anaphylaxis', *Lancet*, II (1914), p. 946.

45   M. Loveless and W. Fackler, 'Wasp venom allergy and immunity', *Annals of Allergy*, 14 (1956), p. 347.

46   'Insect stings', *Lancet*, II (1959), p. 501; H. Morrow Brown, 'Injectable adrenaline for bee stings', *Lancet*, II (1980), p. 1082.

47   Tony Smith, 'Insect allergies: the annual nightmare', *The Times* (19 June 1974), 8a; 'Medicine: the prevention of bee-sting allergy', *The Times* (12 June 1974), 18e.

48   Howard S. Rubenstein, 'Bee-sting diseases: Who is at risk? What is the treatment?', *Lancet*, I (1982), pp. 496–9; H. S. Rubenstein, 'Allergists who alarm the public: a problem in medical ethics', *Journal of the American Medical Association*, 243 (1980), pp. 793–4.

49   R. Urbanek et al., 'Bee stings', *Lancet*, I (1982), pp. 798–9. See also chapter Six.

50   A. W. Frankland, 'Locust sensitivity', *Annals of Allergy*, 11 (1953), pp. 445–53; 'Locusts cause asthma deaths', *Asthma Magazine* (January–March 2004), pp. 8–9; Olaf D. Cuthbert et al., '"Barn allergy": asthma and rhinitis due to storage mites', *Clinical Allergy*, 9 (1979), pp. 229–36; M. O. Gad El Rab and A. B. Kay, 'Widespread immunoglobulin E-mediated hypersensitivity in the Sudan to the "green nimitti" midge, *Cladotanytarsus lewisi* (diptera: Chironomidae)', *Journal of Allergy and Clinical Immunology*, 66 (1980), pp. 190–97; Ke Chen, Yuanfan Liao and Jintan Zhang, 'The major aeroallergens in Guangxi, China', *Clinical Allergy*, 18 (1988), pp. 589–96; S. M. McHugh et al., 'Evidence of hypersensitivity to chironomid midges in an English village community', *Clinical Allergy*, 18 (1988), pp. 275–85.

51   W. Storm van Leeuwen, *Allergic Diseases: Diagnosis and Treatment of Bronchial Asthma, Hay-Fever and Other Allergic Diseases* (Philadelphia, 1925). On research at St Mary's on this, see the *Annual Reports of the Wright-Fleming Insitute of Microbiology* for 1950, 1956 and 1957, in St Mary's Hospital Archives, WF/AD6/1 and 2. See also R. Voorhorst, *Basic Facts of Allergy* (Leiden, 1962), pp. 240–44.

52   P.G.H.Gell and R.R.A. Coombs, *Clinical Aspects of Immunology* (Oxford, 1963), pp. 400–03; D. J. Hendrick, Jennifer A. Faux and R. Marshall, 'Budgerigar-fancier's lung: the commonest form of allergic alveolitis in Britain', *British Medical Journal* (8 July 1978), pp. 81–4; J. L. Malo and R. Paquin, 'Incidence of immediate sensitivity to *Aspergillus fumigatus* in a North American asthmatic population', *Clinical Allergy*, 9 (1979), pp. 377–84; S. R. Benatar, G. A. Keen and W. Du Toit Naude, 'Aspergillus hypersensitivity in asthmatics in Cape Town', *Clinical Allergy*, 10

(1980), pp. 285–91; A. El-Hefny et al., 'Extrinsic allergic broncho-alveolitis in children', *Clinical Allergy*, 10 (1980), pp. 651–8; D.R.H. Vernon and Fay Allan, 'Environmental factors in allergic bronchopulmonary aspergillosis', *Clinical Allergy*, 10 (1980), pp. 217–27.

53 Thomas Stuttaford, 'Should we fear "flying rats"?', *The Times* T2 (20 November 2003), 13a.

54 Ibid.

55 Peter Brimblecombe, *The Big Smoke: A History of Air Pollution in London since Medieval Times* (London, 1987).

56 Ibid.; Stephen Mosley, *The Chimney of the World: A History of Smoke Pollution in Victorian and Edwardian Manchester* (Cambridge, 2001); Adam Markham, *A Brief History of Pollution* (London, 1994); J. Clarence Davies III, *The Politics of Pollution* (Indianapolis, IN, 1970); John McNeill, *Something New Under the Sun: An Environmental History of the Twentieth Century* (London, 2000); Harold Platt, *Shock Cities: The Environmental Transformation and Reform of Manchester and Chicago* (Chicago, 2005) .

57 Bill Luckin, 'Death and survival in the city: approaches to the history of disease', *Urban History Yearbook* (1980), pp. 53–62; Bill Luckin, 'Town, country and metropolis: the formation of an air pollution problem in London, 1800–1870', in *Energy and the City in Europe: From Preindustrial Wood-shortage to the Oil Crisis of the 1970s*, ed. Dieter Schott (Stuttgart, 1997), pp. 77–92; Bill Luckin and Graham Mooney, 'Urban history and historical epidemiology: the case of London, 1860–1920', *Urban History*, 24 (1997), pp. 37–55; Bill Luckin, 'Review essay: versions of the environmental', *Journal of Urban History*, 24 (1998), pp. 510–23. See 'Fogs', *Nature*, 21 (12 February 1880), pp. 355–6; 'Fog fatality in London', *British Medical Journal* (14 February 1880), p. 254; 'Influence of fog on the London death-rate', *Lancet*, I (1882), p. 283.

58 Mosley, *The Chimney of the World*; Mark Jackson, 'Cleansing the air and promoting health: the politics of pollution in post-war Britain', in *Medicine, the Market and the Mass Media: Producing Health in the Twentieth Century*, ed. Virginia Berridge and Kelly Loughlin (London, 2005), pp. 219–41.

59 Davies, *The Politics of Pollution*, p. 33; McNeill, *Something New Under the Sun*, pp. 68–70.

60 'Asthma Research Council', *Lancet*, I (1928), pp. 561–2.

61 Mosley, *The Chimney of the World*; Devra Davis, *When Smoke Ran Like Water: Tales of Environmental Deception and the Battle Against Pollution* (New York, 2002).

62 Brimblecombe, *The Big Smoke*, pp. 165–6; McNeill, *Something New Under the Sun*, pp. 64–75.

63 For a reconstruction of events, see *Killer Fog* (Channel 4, 1999); William Wise, *Killer Smog: The World's Worst Air Pollution Disaster* (Chicago, 1968).

64 *The Times* (12 December 1952), 9e; *The Times* (6 February 1953), 7d; *Parliamentary Debates*, 515 (1953), col. 845; *Parliamentary Debates*, 518 (1953), col. 202.

65 Roy Parker, 'The struggle for clean air', in *Change, Choice and Conflict in Social Policy*, ed. Phoebe Hall et al. (London, 1975), pp. 371–409; Eric Ashby and Mary Anderson, *The Politics of Clean Air* (Oxford, 1981).

66 *Committee on Air Pollution – Interim Report* (London, HMSO, 1953, Cmd. 9011).

67 *Committee on Air Pollution – Report* (London, HMSO, 1954, Cmd. 9322), paras. 12–18.

68 *Interim Report*, para. 41.
69 Brimblecombe, *The Big Smoke*; Parker, 'The struggle for clean air'.
70 Peter Ackroyd, *London: The Biography* (London, 2000), p. 438.
71 Ministry of Health, *Reports on public health and medical subjects No. 95: mortality and morbidity during the London fog of December 1952* (London, 1954); Royal College of Physicians, *Air Pollution and Health* (London, 1970).
72 Harvey W. Phelps, Gerald W. Sobel and Neal E. Fisher, 'Air pollution asthma among military personnel in Japan', *Journal of the American Medical Association*, 175 (1961), pp. 990–93; Harvey W. Phelps and Shigeo Koike, '"Tokyo-Yokohama asthma": the rapid development of respiratory distress presumably due to air pollution', *American Review of Respiratory Diseases*, 86 (1962), pp. 55–63.
73 Inge F. Goldstein and Eric M. Dulberg, 'Air pollution and asthma: search for a relationship', *Journal of the Air Pollution Control Association*, 31 (1981), pp. 370–6.
74 R. Jeffrey Smith, 'Utilities choke on asthma research', *Science*, 212 (1981), pp. 1251–4.
75 Robert C. Ziegenfus, 'Air quality and health', in *Public Health and the Environment: The United States Experience*, ed. Michael R. Greenberg (New York, 1987), pp. 139–72.
76 *World Conference on Smoking and Health: A Summary of Proceedings* (1967); Royal College of Physicians, *Smoking and Health Now* (London, 1971); Department of Health and Social Security, *Smoking and Health* (London, 1971).
77 H. Ross Anderson, 'Air pollution and trends in asthma', in *The Rising Trends in Asthma*, ed. Derek J. Chadwick and Gail Cardew (New York, 1997), pp. 190–203; LAIA, Factsheet 93/5.
78 N. Künzli et al., 'Public health impact of outdoor and traffic-related air pollution: a European assessment', *Lancet*, 356 (2000), pp. 795–801; Jon G. Ayres, 'Meteorology and respiratory disease', *Update* (15 March 1990), pp. 596–605; Linda Gamlin, 'The big sneeze', *New Scientist*, 126 (1990), pp. 37–41.
79 E. Von Mutius et al., 'Prevalence of asthma and allergic disorders among children in United Germany: a descriptive comparison', *British Medical Journal*, 305 (1992), pp. 1395–99; A. Wardlaw, ed., 'Air pollution and allergic disease: report of a working party of the British Society for Allergy and Clinical Immunology', *Clinical and Experimental Allergy*, 25, Supplement 3 (1995); Jill Warner, *Allergic Diseases and the Indoor Environment* (London, 2000).
80 Committee on the Medical Effects of Air Pollution, *Asthma and Outdoor Air Pollution* (London, 1995); Wardlaw, ed., 'Air pollution and allergic disease'.
81 Wardlaw, ed., 'Air pollution and allergic disease', p. 10.
82 'Exhausted' (BBC TV, 1993).
83 James Chapman, 'Dangers in the air', *Daily Mail* (6 March 2002), 31a; Steve Connor and Mark Austin, 'Rural air pollution is worse than in cities', *Sunday Times* (26 October 1997), 12a. See also the work of the 'Don't choke Britain' campaign, launched initially in 1991, http://www.lga.gov.uk/dcb/home.htm.
84 Beck, *Risk Society*, pp. 30, 26.
85 Anderson, 'Air pollution', pp. 190–91. See also chapter Six.
86 Nancy Tomes, *The Gospel of Germs: Men, Women, and the Microbe in American Life* (Cambridge, MA, 1998).

87 Alison Haggett, '"The remorseful battle against invasion from the germ world": a cultural history of home hygiene in the post-war British home, 1945–1960', MA dissertation, Exeter, 2003.

88 Ziegenfus, 'Air quality and health'; Theron G. Randolph and Ralph W. Moss, *An Alternative Approach to Allergies* (New York, 1980), p. 69.

89 World Health Organization, *Health Aspects Related to Indoor Air Quality* (Geneva, 1979).

90 Voorhorst, *Basic Facts of Allergy*, pp. 221–2; Leon Unger and M. Coleman Harris, 'Stepping stones in allergy', *Annals of Allergy*, 33 (October 1974), p. 233.

91 John Freeman, *Hay-Fever: A Key to the Allergic Disorders* (London, 1950), p. 58.

92 Voorhorst, *Basic Facts of Allergy*, p. 221.

93 Unger and Harris, 'Stepping stones in allergy' (October 1974), pp. 237–41.

94 Warner, *Allergic Diseases*, pp. 5, 15.

95 Chris Ayres, 'Designer cats will be nothing to sneeze at', *The Times* (28 June 2001), 1b.

96 R. Voorhorst et al., 'The house dust mite (Dermatophagoides pteronyssinus) and the allergens it produces: identity with the house-dust allergen', *Journal of Allergy*,39 (1967), pp. 325–39.

97 Hermann Dekker, 'Asthma und milben', *Münchener Medizinische Wochenschrift*, 75 (1928), pp. 515–16.

98 K. Maunsell, A. M. Hughes and D. C. Wraith, 'Mite asthma: cause and management', *Practitioner*, 205 (1970), pp. 779–83; G. Biliotti et al., 'Mites and house dust allergy', *Clinical Allergy*, 2 (1972), pp. 109–13; A. Margaret Hughes and Kate Maunsell, 'A study of a population of house dust mite in its natural enviroment', *Clinical Allergy*, 3 (1973), pp. 127–31; M. E. Blythe, 'Some aspects of the ecological study of the house dust mites', *British Journal of Diseases of the Chest*, 70 (1976), pp. 3–31; 'House dust a cause of hay fever', *The Times* (18 May 1971), 2a; 'Implications of increase in asthma deaths', *The Times* (13 August 1968), 7e.

99 Smith and Springett, 'Atopic disease and month of birth'; Businco et al., 'Month of birth and grass pollen or mite sensitization'.

100 David Ordman, 'The evolution in South Africa of the concept of "climate asthma" and of the associated climate patterns', *South African Medical Journal*, 44 (1970), pp. 1236–40; David Ordman, 'The incidence of "climate asthma" in South Africa: its relation to the distribution of mites', *South African Medical Journal*, 45 (1971), pp. 739–43.

101 F. Th. Spieksma, P. Zuidema and M. J. Leupen, 'High altitude and house-dust mites', *British Medical Journal* (9 January 1971), pp. 82–4.

102 Maunsell, Hughes and Wraith, 'Mite asthma'; 'Bedmaking may cause asthma', *The Times* (30 March 1968), 5e.

103 Warner, *Allergic Diseases*, p. v; J. Neville Bartlett, *Carpeting the Millions: The Growth of Britain's Carpet Industry* (Edinburgh, 1978).

104 Bartlett, *Carpeting the Millions.*

105 Warner, *Allergic Diseases*, p. vi.

106 Ziegenfus, 'Air quality and health', p. 159; Thomas A. Platts-Mills et al., 'The role

of domestic allergens', in *Rising Trends in Asthma*, pp. 173–85; Stephen Mosley, 'Fresh air and foul: the role of the open fireplace in ventilating the British home, 1837–1910', *Planning Perspectives*, 18 (2003), pp. 1–21.

107 A. P. Smith, 'Hyposensitization with Dermatophagoides pteronyssinus antigen: trial in asthma induced by house dust', *British Medical Journal* (23 October 1971), pp. 204–6; M. F. d'Souza et al., 'Hyposensitization with *Dermatophagoides pteronyssinus* in house dust allergy: a controlled study of clinical and immunological effects', *Clinical Allergy*, 3 (1973), pp. 177–93; John Gaddie, Craig Skinner and K.N.V. Palmer, 'Hyposensitisation with house dust mite vaccine in bronchial asthma', *British Medical Journal* (4 September 1976), pp. 561–2; Pamela W. Ewan et al., 'Effective hyposensitization in allergic rhinitis using a potent partially purified extract of house dust mite', *Clinical Allergy*, 18 (1988), pp. 501–8.

108 M. E. Blythe et al., 'Study of mites in three Birmingham hospitals', *British Medical Journal* (11 January 1975), pp. 62–4; V.R.M. Rao et al., 'A comparison of mite populations in mattress dust from hospital and from private houses in Cardiff, Wales', *Clinical Allergy*, 5 (1975), pp. 209–15.

109 A. J. Dorward et al., 'Effect of house dust mite avoidance measures on adult atopic asthma', *Thorax*, 43 (1988), pp. 98–102; Thomas A. E. Platts-Mills et al., 'Reduction in bronchial hyperreactivity during prolonged allergen avoidance', *Lancet* (25 September 1982), pp. 675–8; S. Kalra et al., 'Airborne house dust mite antigen after vacuum cleaning', *Lancet*, 336 (1990), p. 449.

110 'Development of a new British asthma vaccine', *The Times* (10 July 1972), 4e.

111 For the range of preparations available, see Colin Taylor, *Fight the Mite: A Practical Guide to House Dust Mite Allergy* (Wilmslow, 1992).

112 Carla Keirns, 'Better than nature: the changing treatment of asthma and hay fever in the United States, 1910–1945', *Studies in History and Philosophy of Biological and Biomedical Sciences*, 34 (2003), pp. 511–31; Van Leeuwen, *Allergic Diseases*, p. 113.

113 Doris J. Rapp and A. W. Frankland, *Allergies: Questions and Answers* (London, 1976), p. 249.

114 Keirns, 'Better than nature'; Tomes, *The Gospel of Germs*.

115 Tomes, *The Gospel of Germs*; Haggett, 'The remorseful battle'.

116 Alison Davies, 'Natural born winners', *Sunday Express Magazine* (30 July 2000), pp. 38–9; 'Building the future', *Asthma Magazine* (January–March, 2004), pp. 22–5.

117 Blythe, 'Some aspects of the ecological study'; Gregg, 'Epidemiological aspects', p. 274.

118 Tomes, *The Gospel of Germs*; Keirns, 'Better than nature'.

119 Rapp and Frankland, *Allergies*, p. 139.

120 F. Carswell et al., 'House dust mite in Bristol', *Clinical Allergy*, 12 (1982), pp. 533–45.

121 See chapter Three.

122 J. E. Gereda et al., 'Relation between house-dust endotoxin exposure, type 1 T-cell development, and allergen sensitisation in infants at high risk of asthma', *Lancet*, 355 (2000), pp. 1680–83.

123 Alexandra Frean, 'Dust can help to prevent asthma', *The Times* (12 May 2000), 12e.

124 S. B. Lehrer, R. M. Karr and J. E. Salvaggio, 'Analysis of green coffee bean and

castor bean allergens using RAST inhibition', *Clinical Allergy*, 11 (1981), pp. 357–66; D. Ordman, 'An outbreak of bronchial asthma in South Africa, affecting more than 200 persons, caused by castor bean dust from an oil-processing factory', *International Archives of Allergy*, 7 (1955), pp. 10–24.

125 See, for example, the survey of modern British lifestyles carried out by Mintel, 'Cash rich, time for . . . ? How convenience has changed the nation' (March 2004), available at http://reports.mintel.com.

126 Platts-Mills et al., 'The role of domestic allergens', p. 181; Peta Bee, 'Exotic reaction to a piece of fruit', *The Times* T2 (30 March 2004), 10a; Joanna Moorhead, 'Forbidden fruit', *Guardian* G2 (24 June 2003), 8a; Caroline Walker and Geoffrey Cannon, *The Food Scandal* (London, 1984); Richard A. Cone and Emily Martin, 'Corporeal flows: the immune system, global economies of food, and new implications for health', in *The Visible Woman: Imaging Technologies, Gender and Science*, ed. Paula A. Treichler, Lisa Cartwright and Constance Penley (New York, 1998), pp. 321–59.

127 N. Hijazi, B. Abalkhail and A. Seaton, 'Diet and childhood asthma in a society in transition: a study in urban and rural Saudi Arabia', *Thorax*, 55 (2000), pp. 775–9; Tim Radford, 'Junk food blamed for rise in asthma cases', *Guardian* (22 August 2000), 5a.

128 C. G. Grulee and H. N. Sanford, 'The influence of breast and artificial feeding on infantile eczema', *Journal of Pediatrics*, 9 (1936), pp. 223–5.

129 Wittig et al., 'Risk factors'.

130 C. Astarita et al., 'An epidemiological study of atopy in children', *Clinical Allergy*, 18 (1988), pp. 341–50.

131 Syed H. Arshad et al., 'Effect of allergen avoidance on development of allergic disorders in infancy', *Lancet*, 339 (1992), pp. 1493–7; Malcolm R. Sears et al., 'Long-term relationship between breastfeeding and development of atopy and asthma in children and young adults: a longitudinal study', *Lancet*, 360 (2002), pp. 901–07; Peter D. Sly and Patrick G. Holt, 'Breast is best for preventing asthma and allergies – or is it?', *Lancet*, 360 (2002), pp. 887–8.

132 Benjamin Burrows, Michael D. Liebowitz and Robert A. Barbee, 'Respiratory disorders and allergy skin-test reactions', *Annals of Internal Medicine*, 84 (1976), pp. 134–9.

133 Bjørn Lomborg, *The Skeptical Environmentalist: Measuring the Real State of the World* (Cambridge, 2003), p. 187.

134 Jill A. Warner et al., 'Prenatal origins of asthma and allergy', in *Rising Trends in Asthma*, pp. 220–32; Fernando D. Martinez, 'Maternal risk factors in asthma', ibid., pp. 233–43; David J. P. Barker, ed., *Fetal and Infant Origins of Adult Disease* (London, 1992).

135 Rosenberg, 'Pathologies of progress'; Roy Porter, 'Diseases of civilization', in *Companion Encyclopedia of the History of Medicine*, ed. W. F. Bynum and Roy Porter (London, 1993), vol. I, pp. 584–600.

136 David P. Strachan, 'Hay fever, hygiene and household size', *British Medical Journal*, 299 (1989), pp. 1259–60.

137 Ibid.

138 Ibid.
139 Freeman, *Hay-Fever*, p. 164.
140 'IgE, parasites and allergy', *Lancet* (24 April 1976), p. 894.
141 Freeman, *Hay-Fever*, p. 164.
142 Bach, 'The effect of infections'.
143 David P. Strachan, 'Family size, infection and atopy: the first decade of the "hygiene hypothesis"', *Thorax*, 55 Supplement (2000), s2–10.
144 Claire Infante-Rivard et al., 'Family size, day-care attendance and breastfeeding in relation to the incidence of childhood asthma', *American Journal of Epidemiology*, 153 (2001), pp. 653–8; Ian Murray, 'Nursery babies beat allergies', *The Times* (5 February 1999), 5a; Cherry Norton, 'Clean children run a higher risk of asthma', *Sunday Times* (1 March 1998), 5a; Simon Crompton, 'Too clean for our own good?', *The Times* T2 (4 April 2000), p. 13.
145 Sarah Scrivener et al., 'Independent effects of intestinal parasite infection and domestic allergen exposure on risk of wheeze in Ethiopia: a nested case-control study', *Lancet*, 358 (2001), pp. 1493–9; Maria Yazdanbakhsh, Peter G. Kremsner and Ronald van Ree, 'Allergy, parasites and the hygiene hypothesis', *Science*, 296 (2002), pp. 490–94; 'IgE, parasites and allergy'.
146 Johan S. Alm et al., 'Atopy in children of families with an anthroposophic lifestyle', *Lancet*, 353 (1999), pp. 1485–8; P. Cullinan et al., 'Early prescriptions of antibiotics and the risk of allergic disease in adults: a cohort study', *Thorax*, 59 (2004), pp. 11–15.
147 Paolo Maria Matricardi and Sergio Bonini, 'Mimicking microbial "education" of the immune system: a strategy to revert the epidemic trend of atopy and allergic asthma?', *Respiratory Research*, 1 (2000), pp. 129–32; Graham A. W. Rook and John L. Stanford, 'Give us this day our daily germs', *Immunology Today*, 19 (1998), pp. 113–16; Marko Kalliomäki et al., 'Probiotics in primary prevention of atopic disease: a randomised placebo-controlled trial', *Lancet*, 357 (2001), pp. 1076–9; Maxine Frith, 'Allergy in the UK: NHS bill reaches an irritating £1bn', *Independent* (15 April 2004), pp. 14–15.
148 'Electric allergy', *Sunday Times* (27 August 2000), 28h; Allan Hall, 'Kohl's wife kills herself because of allergy to sun', *The Times* (6 July 2001), 15a; M. R. Allansmith and R. N. Ross, 'Ocular allergy', *Clinical Allergy* 18 (1988), pp. 1–13.
149 Royal College of Physicians, *Allergy: The Unmet Need* (London, 2003), pp. xiv, 71, 93; A. W. Frankland, 'Latex allergy', *Journal of Nutritional and Environmental Medicine*, 9 (1999), pp. 313–21; A. W. Frankland, 'Latex-allergic children', *Pediatric Allergy and Immunology*, 10 (1999), pp. 152–9.
150 Moorhead, 'Forbidden fruit'; Bee, 'Exotic reaction to a piece of fruit'.
151 Asthma UK, *Living on a Knife Edge* (London, 2004), p. 8.
152 Claude Thérond, *L'Allergie: illusion ou réalité biologique?* (Paris, 1964).
153 'New treatment for allergies', *The Times* (23 May 1966), 15e; Milton Millman, *Pardon my Sneeze: The Story of Allergy* (San Diego, CA, 1960). See also chapter Three.
154 Beck, *Risk Society*, pp. 24–34.
155 Warren T. Vaughan, 'Minor allergy: its distribution, clinical aspects and signifi-

cance', *Journal of Allergy*, 5 (1934), pp. 184–96.

156 Claude A. Frazier, *Parents' Guide to Allergy in Children* (New York, 1973), p. 279; Iris R. Bell, *Clinical Ecology: A New Medical Approach to Environmental Illness* (Bolinas, CA, 1982), pp. 26–9.

157 For further discussion, see chapter Six.

158 Bronwen Murison, 'A sensitive subject', *World Medicine* (20 March 1982), pp. 50–6; 'Sterile home for allergy sufferer', *The Times* (5 February 1982), 2a; Craig Seton, 'Singer with "total allergy" returning', *The Times* (18 October 1982), 3c; 'Allergy woman expected today', *The Times* (19 October 1982), 2d; Craig Seton, 'Allergy woman flies home', *The Times* (20 October 1982), 2d; Craig Seton, 'Allergy flat unsuitable, friend says', *The Times* (21 October 1982), 2a; Craig Seton, 'Police are to investigate Sheila Rossall £65,000 allergy fund', *The Times* (22 October 1982), 3a.

159 'I am allergic to the 21st century', *Sunday Express* (8 February 2004), 54a; Peter Foster, 'Boy allergic to nearly all food', *The Times* (19 January 1998), 3b; Peter Radetsky, *Allergic to the Twentieth Century* (Boston, MA, 1997); Steve Kroll-Smith and H. Hugh Floyd, *Bodies in Protest: Environmental Illness and the Struggle over Medical Knowledge* (New York, 1997); Michelle Murphy, 'Sick buildings and sick bodies: the materialization of an occupational illness in late capitalism', PhD thesis, Harvard University, 1998; Michelle Murphy, 'The "elsewhere within here" and environmental illness; or, how to build yourself a body in a safe space', *Configurations*, 8 (2000), pp. 87–120.

160 Seton, 'Allergy woman flies home'.

161 Royal College of Physicians, *Allergy: Conventional and Alternative Concepts* (London, 1992), pp. 29–31; L. M. Howard and S. Wessely, 'Psychiatry in the allergy clinic: the nature and management of patients with non-allergic symptoms', *Clinical and Experimental Allergy*, 25 (1995), pp. 503–14.

162 'When the canaries stop singing' (Otmoor Productions, 1991); 'Allergic to the twentieth century' (Horizon, 1993); 'Why buildings make you sick' (Horizon, 1989).

163 *Safe*, directed by Todd Haynes (Tartan Video, 1996); Matthew Gandy, 'Allergy and allegory in Todd Haynes' [*Safe*]', in *Screening the City*, ed. Mark Shiel and Tony Fitzmaurice (London, 2003), pp. 239–61.

164 Radetsky, *Allergic to the Twentieth Century*, p. 18.

165 Steven N. Austad, correspondence, *New York Times* (3 October 1997).

166 Malcolm Gladwell, 'The Pima paradox', *New Yorker* (2 February 1998), pp. 44–57.

167 Lomborg, *The Skeptical Environmentalist*, pp. 3–42.

168 Dubos, *Dreams of Reason*, p. 77.

169 Beck, *Risk Society*, p. 37.

Chapter 6: Resisting Modernity

1 Anne Marie Moulin, *Le dernier langage de la médecine* (Paris, 1991), p. 11. I am grateful to Anne Marie for accepting my crude translation from her elegant French.

2   James L. Halliday, *Psychosocial Medicine: A Study of the Sick Society* (London, 1948). For similar concerns expressed elsewhere at this time, see Flanders Dunbar, *Mind and Body: Psychosomatic Medicine* (New York, 1947).

3   Ibid., p. 180.

4   Sheldon Krimsky, *Hormonal Chaos: The Scientific and Social Origins of the Environmental Endocrine Hypothesis* (Baltimore, MD, 2000); Theron G. Randolph and Ralph W. Moss, *An Alternative Approach to Allergies* (New York, 1980), pp. 60–61.

5   Prince Charles, 'We have become allergic to our western way of life', *Guardian* (28 February 2004), 24b.

6   Ibid.

7   Christopher Sellers, 'Body, place and the state: the makings of an "environmentalist" imaginary in the post-world war II US', *Radical History Review*, 74 (1999), pp. 31–64.

8   Roy Porter, 'Diseases of civilization', in *Companion Encyclopedia of the History of Medicine*, ed. W. F. Bynum and Roy Porter (London, 1993), vol. I, pp. 584–600 (p. 599). See also Rosalind Coward, *The Whole Truth: The Myth of Alternative Health* (London, 1989).

9   René Dubos, *Mirage of Health: Utopias, Progress, and Biological Change* (New York, 1959), p. 23.

10 René Dubos, *The Dreams of Reason: Science and Utopias* (New York, 1961), p. 71.

11 Ulrich Beck, 'The naturalistic fallacy of the ecological movement', in *the Polity Reader in Social Theory*, ed. Anthony Giddens et al. (Cambridge, 1994), pp. 342–6.

12 Dubos, *Mirage of Health*, p. 105.

13 Asthma UK, *Living on a Knife Edge* (London, 2004), p. 5; Daloni Carlisle, 'Breath of life – and hope', *Guardian* G2 (13 August 1996), 9; Wendy Wallace, 'Take a deep breath . . .', *Guardian* G2 (7 October 1997), 16.

14 Asthma UK, *Living on a Knife Edge*, p. 21; C. P. van Schayk et al., 'Underdiagnosis of asthma: is the doctor or the patient to blame? The DIMCA project', *Thorax*, 55 (2000), pp. 562–5; Robert J. Adams, Brian J. Smith and Richard E. Ruffin, 'Factors associated with hospital admissions and repeat emergency department visits for adults with asthma', *Thorax*, 55 (2000), pp. 566–73.

15 Royal College of Physicians, *Allergy: The Unmet Need* (London, 2003), p. 19.

16 Sheldon G. Cohen, 'The American Academy of Allergy: an historical review', *Journal of Allergy and Clinical Immunology*, 64 (1979), pp. 399–405; Thomas E. Van Metre, 'The advancement of the knowledge and practice of allergy', *Journal of Allergy and Clinical Immunology*, 64 (1979), pp. 235–41; Craig T. Norback, *The Allergy Encyclopedia* (New York, 1981).

17 Further information about Asthma UK and LAIA can be obtained from their websites: www.asthma.org.uk; www.sghms.ac.uk/depts/laia/laia.htm.

18 Information on Allergy UK is available at www.allergyfoundation. com.

19 Royal College of Physicians, *Allergy*, p. 19; see also the booklets and advice published by the National Eczema Society at www.eczema.org.

20 For popular advice books, see Allan Knight, *Asthma and Hay Fever* (London, 1981); Mark Levy, Sean Hilton and Greta Barnes, *Asthma at your Fingertips* (London,

1993); Jonathan Brostoff and Linda Gamlin, *Hayfever* (London, 1993); Jon Ayres, *Understanding Asthma* (1995); Jennifer Hay, *Allergies: Questions You Have . . . Answers You Need* (New York, 1997).

21 Department of Health, *Specialised Services for Allergy (all ages) – Definition No. 17* (2002), www.dh.gov.uk/PolicyandGuidance/HealthandSocialCareTopics.

22 Royal College of Physicians, *Allergy*, p. xi.

23 Ibid., pp. 28–31.

24 Anjana Ahuja, 'Gasping for action', *The Times* T2 (9 June 2003), 10a; Nigel Hawkes, 'NHS can't cope with millions of allergy patients', *The Times* (26 June 2003), 9a; Sarah Bosley, 'Allergy reaction to food and surroundings affects 1 in 3 – and the NHS just can't cope', *Guardian* (26 June 2003), 6a; Tina Burchill, 'Poor reactions to allergies', *The Times* T2 (27 April 2004), 10a.

25 R. Voorhorst, 'Allergology: past, present and future', *Annals of Allergy*, 40 (1978), pp. 206–10.

26 Stephen I. Wasserman, 'The allergist in the new millennium', *Journal of Allergy and Clinical Immunology*, 105 (2000), pp. 3–8.

27 Kjell Aas, 'Adequate clinical trials of immunotherapy', *Allergy*, 37 (1982), pp. 1–14. See also chapter Three.

28 Sherwin A. Gillman et al., 'Venom immunotherapy: comparison of "rush" vs "conventional" schedules', *Annals of Allergy*, 45 (1980), pp. 351–4; 'New treatment for allergies', *The Times* (23 May 1966), 15e.

29 J. Pepys, 'Editorial: "clinical immunology" and the "practise of allergy"', *Clinical Allergy*, 1 (1971), pp. 1–7.

30 David A. Rands, 'Anaphylactic reaction to desensitisation for allergic rhinitis and asthma', *British Medical Journal*, 281 (1980), p. 854; Anon., 'Man died after injection of drug for asthma', *The Times* (24 January 1973), 2d.

31 Pamela W. Ewan, 'Anaphylactic reaction to desensitisation', *British Medical Journal*, 281 (1980), p. 1069.

32 A. W. Frankland, 'Anaphylactic reaction to desensitisation', *British Medical Journal*, 281 (1980), p. 1429.

33 Aas, 'Adequate clinical trials'; Lawrence M. Lichtenstein, Martin D. Valentine and Philip S. Norman, 'A reevaluation of immunotherapy for asthma', *American Review of Respiratory Diseases*, 129 (1984), pp. 657–9.

34 I.W.B. Grant, 'Does immunotherapy have a role in the treatment of asthma?', *Clinical Allergy*, 16 (1986), pp. 7–10.

35 H. Mosbech and B. Weeke, 'Does immunotherapy have a role in the treatment of asthma?', *Clinical Allergy*, 16 (1986), pp. 10–16.

36 'Correspondence: the great debate: immunotherapy and asthma', *Clinical Allergy*, 16 (1986), pp. 269–77 (pp. 275–6); 'Correspondence', *Clinical Allergy*, 16 (1986), pp. 179–80.

37 'CSM update: desensitising vaccines', *British Medical Journal*, 293 (1986), p. 948.

38 A. J. Frew, 'Injection immunotherapy', *British Medical Journal*, 307 (1993), pp. 919–23.

39 Philip S. Norman and Thomas E. Van Metre, 'The safety of allergen immunotherapy', *Journal of Allergy and Clinical Immunology*, 85 (1990), pp. 522–5.

40   H.-J. Malling, ed., 'Immunotherapy: position paper', *Allergy*, 43 Supplement 6
     (1988); Jean Bousquet and François-B. Michel, 'Specific immunotherapy', *Allergy*,
     43 Supplement (1988), pp. 16–22; A. B. Kay, 'Allergen injection immunotherapy
     (hyposensitization) on trial', *Clinical and Experimental Allergy*, 19 (1989), pp. 591–6;
     Frew, 'Injection immunotherapy'; Jean Bousquet, Adnan Hejjaoui and François-
     B. Michel, 'Specific immunotherapy in asthma', *Journal of Allergy and Clinical
     Immunology*, 86 (1990), pp. 292–305; 'Position statement: the waiting period after
     allergen skin testing and immunotherapy', *Journal of Allergy and Clinical Immunology*,
     85 (1990), pp. 526–7; H.-J. Malling and B. Weeke, eds, 'Position paper:
     immunotherapy', *Allergy*, 48 Supplement 14 (1993).
41   See correspondence on immunotherapy and hay fever in *British Medical Journal*,
     302 (1991), pp. 530–31; Frew, 'Injection immunotherapy', p. 919.
42   'Current status of allergen immunotherapy (hyposensitization): memorandum
     from a WHO/IUIS meeting', *Bulletin of the World Health Organization*, 67 (1989),
     pp. 263–72.
43   Bousquet, Hejjaoui and Michel, 'Specific immunotherapy in asthma', p. 292.
44   M. H. Lessof, 'Food intolerance and the scientific trap', *Clinical and Experimental
     Allergy*, 23 (1993), pp. 971–2.
45   Theodore Dalrymple, 'Streaming eyes? Tiredness? You're suffering an allergy to
     the madding crowd', *The Times* (26 June 2003), 20a.
46   Noemi Eiser, 'Desensitisation today: a specialist procedure with few indications',
     British Medical Journal, 300 (1990), pp. 1412–13. See also the comments in Pamela
     W. Ewan et al., 'Effective hyposensitization in allergic rhinitis using a potent
     partially purified extract of house dust mite', *Clinical Allergy*, 18 (1988), pp. 501–8.
47   A. B. Kay and M. H. Lessof, *Allergy: Conventional and Alternative Concepts* (London,
     1992), p. 27.
48   Alyson L. Huntley, Adrian White and Edzard Ernst, 'Complementary medicine
     for asthma', *Focus on Alternative and Complementary Therapies*, 5 (2000), pp. 111–16.
49   Royal College of Physicians, *Allergy*, p. xi.
50   E. Ernst, 'Herbal medicine: where is the evidence?', *British Medical Journal*, 321
     (2000), pp. 395–6.
51   Mike Saks, *Orthodox and Alternative Medicine: Politics, Professionalization and Health
     Care* (London, 2003); Roy Porter, *Quacks: Fakers and Charlatans in English Medicine*
     (Stroud, 2001); Brian Inglis, *Fringe Medicine* (London, 1964); Coward, *The Whole
     Truth*.
52   P. A. Davis et al., 'Acupuncture in the treatment of asthma: a critical review',
     Allergologia et Immunopathologia, 26 (1998), pp. 263–71; Lai Xinsheng, 'Observation
     on the curative effect of acupuncture on type I allergic diseases', *Journal of Traditional
     Chinese Medicine*, 13 (1993), pp. 243–8; Huntley, White and Ernst, 'Complementary
     medicine'; Robina Dam, 'How good are the healers?', *Sunday Times Magazine* (19
     October 1997), pp. 70–73; Mark Henderson, 'Herbs "no cure for asthma"', *The
     Times* (24 October 2000), 14f; Luisa Dillner, 'Gentle remedies', *Guardian* G2 (22
     August 2000), pp. 8–9; Jenny Hope, 'The real alternative', *Daily Mail* (18 August
     2000), 35a; Dr John Briffa, 'Alternatively speaking', *Daily Mail* (1 June 1998), 40b;

Simon Birch, 'A hard cure to pinpoint', *Guardian* G2 (11 August 1998), 15a; Anne Woodham, 'Herbal relief for hay fever', *The Times* T2 (22 January 2002), 11a; Amber Cowan, 'Not to be sneezed at', *The Times* T2 (15 January 2005), 9a; Catherine Steven, *The Natural Way: Hay Fever* (Longmead, Dorset, 1999); Joseph P. Hou and Youyu Jin, *The Healing Power of Chinese Herbs and Medicinal Recipes* (New York, 2005); Richard A. Cone and Emily Martin, 'Corporeal flows: the immune system, global economies of food and new implications for health', in *The Visible Woman: Imaging Technologies, Gender and Science*, ed. Paula A. Treichler, Lisa Cartwright and Constance Penley (New York, 1998), pp. 321–59; Harry Benjamin, *Everybody's Guide to Nature Cure* (1936) (Wellingborough, 1961), pp. 244–6, 308–9.

53 Alexander Stalmatski, *Freedom from Asthma: Buteyko's Revolutionary Treatment* (London, 1997); Ian Murray, 'What to do if you get asthma: stop breathing', *The Times Weekend* (15 August 1998), 8a.

54 Royal College of Physicians, *Allergy*, p. 35; Jane Alexander, 'Herbal hope for itchy skin', *The Times* T2 (23 January 2001), 14a.

55 Royal College of Physicians, *Allergy*; Ernst, 'Herbal medicines'; Luisa Dillner, 'Alternative allergy treatments need clinical trials', *British Medical Journal*, 304 (18 April 1992), p. 1003.

56 Stalmatski, *Freedom from Asthma*, p. 13; Theron G. Randolph and Ralph W. Moss, *An Alternative Approach to Allergies* (New York, 1980), pp. 215–22.

57 T. G. Randolph, 'Concepts of food allergy important in specific diagnosis', *Journal of Allergy*, 21 (1950), pp. 471–7; T. G. Randolph, H. J. Rinkel and M. Zeller, *Food Allergy* (Springfield, IL, 1951).

58 Randolph and Moss, *An Alternative Approach*, p. 6; T. G. Randolph, *Human Ecology and Susceptibility to the Chemical Environment* (Springfield, IL, 1962).

59 Randolph and Moss, *An Alternative Approach*, pp. 4–8. See also Theron G. Randolph, *Environmental Medicine: Beginnings and Bibliographies of Clinical Ecology* (Colorado, 1987).

60 Richard Mackarness, *Not All in the Mind* (London, 1976); Russell C. G. Binns, 'Allergic to everyday living', *The Times* (8 January 1982), 7a.

61 Randolph and Moss, *An Alternative Approach*; Iris R. Bell, *Clinical Ecology: A New Medical Approach to Environmental Illness* (Bolinas, CA, 1982).

62 Bell, *Clinical Ecology*, pp. 30–37.

63 Steve McNamara, 'Environmental illness', reprinted in Randolph, *Environmental Medicine*, pp. 283–94.

64 Randolph and Moss, *An Alternative Approach*, pp. 178–211.

65 Gregg Mitman, *The State of Nature: Ecology, Community and American Social Thought, 1900–1950* (Chicago, 1992).

66 F.W.E. Hare, *The Food Factor in Disease* (London, 1905); Randolph, *Environmental Medicine*, pp. 80–89.

67 Alfred T. Schofield, 'A case of egg poisoning', *Lancet*, I (1908), p. 716; 'Asthma and urticaria due to an ice-cream', *Lancet*, II (1909), pp. 1227–8; Arthur F. Hurst, 'An address on asthma', *Lancet*, I (1921), pp. 1113–17; Arthur Latham, 'An address on some aspects of bronchial asthma', *Lancet*, I (1922), pp. 261–3; 'White wine

anaphylaxis', *Lancet*, I (1926), p. 214; 'Digestive anaphylaxis', *Lancet*, I (1926), pp. 1050–51; 'The aetiology of eczema', *Lancet*, II (1926), p. 28; John A. Ryle, 'Observations on the abdominal and circulatory phenomena of allergy', *Lancet*, I (1935), pp. 1257–61.

68 Albert H. Rowe, *Food Allergy: Its Manifestations, Diagnosis and Treatment* (Philadelphia, 1931).

69 Randolph, *Environmental Medicine*, pp. 96–8.

70 Arthur F. Coca, *Familial Nonreaginic Food Allergy* (Springfield, IL, 1943); Arthur F. Coca, *The Pulse Test for Allergy* (London, 1959).

71 Randolph, *Environmental Medicine*, pp. 89–98; Mackarness, *Not All in the Mind*, p. 27.

72 'Food allergy', *Lancet*, II (1963), p. 207.

73 Mackarness, *Not All in the Mind*, p. 47.

74 Hans Selye, *The Stress of Life* (New York, 1956); Hans Selye, *The Story of the General Adaptation Syndrome* (Montreal, 1952); Hans Selye, 'Allergy and the general adaptation syndrome', *International Archives of Allergy*, 3 (1952), pp. 267–78.

75 Selye, *The Stress of Life*, pp. 87–9.

76 Mackarness, *Not All in the Mind*; Randolph and Moss, *An Alternative Approach*.

77 F. Walter, 'The evolution of environmental sensitivity 1750–1950', in *The Silent Countdown: Essays in European Environmental History*, ed. P. Brimblecombe and C. Pfister (Berlin, 1990), pp. 231–47.

78 John McNeill, *Something New Under the Sun: An Environmental History of the Twentieth Century* (London, 2000), pp. 309–10, 337; John Sheail, *An Environmental History of Twentieth-Century Britain* (Basingstoke, 2002); Jeremy Black, *Modern British History since 1900* (Basingstoke, 2000), pp. 61–5.

79 S. Robert Lichter and Stanley Rothman, *Environmental Cancer: A Political Disease* (New Haven, CT, 1999), p. 9.

80 Rachel Carson, *Silent Spring* (Boston, MA, 1962); Linda Lear, *Rachel Carson: Witness for Nature* (New York, 1997); 'Obituary: Miss Rachel Carson', *The Times* (16 April 1964); C. W. Hume, 'An American Prophetess', *Nature* (13 April 1963), p. 117.

81 McNeill, *Something New Under the Sun*, pp. 339–40; Lichter and Rothman, *Environmental Cancer*, pp. 1–22.

82 Lichter and Rothman, *Environmental Cancer*, p. 9.

83 Black, *Modern British History*, p. 64.

84 Tim Jackson, *Material Concerns: Pollution, Profit and Quality of Life* (London, 1996).

85 World Health Organization, *Health Hazards of the Human Environment* (Geneva, 1972).

86 Lichter and Rothman, *Environmental Cancer*, pp. 9–19.

87 Randolph and Moss, *An Alternative Approach*, p. 201.

88 Ibid., pp. 186–7.

89 See, for example: Martin J. Walker, *Dirty Medicine* (London, 1994); Doris J. Rapp, *Our Toxic World: a Wake Up Call* (Environmental Medical Research, 2004).

90 Binns, 'Allergic to everyday living'.

91 Randolph and Moss, *An Alternative Approach*, p. 221; Mackarness, *Not All in the Mind*, p. 11; Ivan Illich, *Medical Nemesis: The Expropriation of Health* (London, 1975).

92 Klara Miller, 'Psychoneurological aspects of food allergy', in *Stress, the Immune System and Psychiatry*, ed. B. Leonard and K. Miller (London, 1995), pp. 185–206.

93 Royal College of Physicians, *Allergy*, pp. 29–33.

94 Michelle Murphy, 'The "elsewhere within here" and environmental illness; or, how to build yourself a body in a safe space', *Configurations*, 8 (2000), pp. 87–120.

95 Deborah M. Barnes, 'Nervous and immune system disorders linked in a variety of diseases', *Science*, 232 (1986), pp. 160–61; Miller, 'Psychoneurological aspects'.

96 Richard Mackarness, *Chemical Victims* (London, 1980). For references to the hazards of our 'chemical-oriented society' and the promotion of dianetics, see 'What is the purification programme?', on the Scientology website at www.scientology.org. See also: Annabelle Thorpe, 'Looks lovely but it might kill me', *The Times* (29 April 2000), 16a; Goldie Gibbons, 'An egg could kill my sons', *The Times* T2 (13 August 2002), 14a; Angela Neustatter, 'Feed me and it might kill me', *The Times* (12 June 2004), 19a; 'I am allergic to the 21st century', *Daily Mail* (8 February 2004), pp. 54–5.

97 Murphy, 'The "elsewhere within here"', p. 87.

98 Steve Kroll-Smith and H. Hugh Floyd, *Bodies in Protest: Environmental Illness and the Struggles over Medical Knowledge* (New York, 1997), p. 3.

99 Royal College of Physicians, *Allergy*, p. 52.

100 Ibid., p. 56.

101 L. M. Howard and S. Wessely, 'Psychiatry in the allergy clinic: the nature and management of patients with non-allergic symptoms', *Clinical and Experimental Allergy*, 25 (1995), pp. 503–14.

102 Peta Bee, 'Are food allergies a fantasy?', *The Times* T2 (27 June 2000), 15a; Eleanor Bailey, 'Bad reactions', *The Times Style* (29 October 1995), 20; Susan Clark, 'The allergy-free diet', *The Times* T2 (15 August 2000), 15.

103 John Naish, 'Allergies: don't they make you sick', *The Times Weekend* (10 May 2003), 1a; Bee, 'Are food allergies a fantasy?'.

104 Randolph and Moss, *An Alternative Approach*, p. 15.

105 Naish, 'Allergies'; Randolph and Moss, *An Alternative Approach*, p. 221.

106 Royal College of Physicians, *Allergy*, pp. 3–6.

107 Mark Peakman and Diego Vergani, *Basic and Clinical Immunology* (New York, 1997), p. 132.

108 William Cookson, 'The alliance of genes and environment in asthma and allergy', *Nature*, 42 Supplement (1999), B5–11.

109 Randolph and Moss, *An Alternative Approach*, p. 17.

110 Mackarness, *Not All in the Mind*, p. 26.

111 Ronald Finn and H. Newman Cohen, 'Food allergy: fact or fiction?', *Lancet* (25 February 1978), pp. 426–8; Jan de Vries, *Viruses, Allergies and the Immune System* (Edinburgh, 1988); Jonathan Brostoff and Linda Gamlin, *The Complete Guide to Food Allergy and Intolerance* (London, 1998), pp. 5–10.

112 Jules Bordet, 'The Harben Lectures, 1913: Anaphylaxis – its importance and mechanism', *Journal of State Medicine*, 21 (1913), pp. 449–64.

113 Carl Prausnitz, 'In quest of allergy', the Jenner Memorial Lecture delivered on 4

June 1959, the manuscript of which is in the Contemporary Medical Archives Centre, GC/33/3. See also A. W. Frankland, 'Chairman's introduction', in *Factors Affecting Sensitivity to Allergens*, ed. H.O.J. Collier (Stoke Poges, 1981), pp. 9–11.

114 Margie Profet, 'The function of allergy: immunological defense against toxins', *Quarterly Review of Biology*, 66 (1991), pp. 23–62.

115 Ibid.

116 Polly Matzinger, 'The danger model: a renewed sense of self', *Science*, 296 (2002), pp. 301–5; E. Cohen, 'My self as an other: on autoimmunity and "other" paradoxes', *Medical Humanities*, 30 (2004), pp. 7–11.

117 Cohen, 'The American Academy of Allergy', p. 326.

118 Elmer W. Fisherman, 'Does the allergic diathesis influence malignancy?', *Journal of Allergy*, 31 (1960), pp. 74–8; Roger Gabriel, Brenda M. Dudley and William D. Alexander, 'Lung cancer and allergy', *British Journal of Clinical Practice*, 26 (1972), pp. 202–4.

119 'Asthma', *The Times* (19 November 1934), 13c.

120 'Asthma and human excellence', *Journal of Asthma*, 23 (1986), p. 211.

121 Peta Bee, 'Are food allergies a fantasy?', *The Times T2* (27 June 2000), 15a.

122 Milton Millman, *Pardon My Sneeze: The Story of Allergy* (San Diego, CA, 1960), pp. 1–2.

123 Kenneth C. Hutchin, *Allergy* (London, 1961), p. 14.

124 Pepys, 'Editorial'.

125 Hans Selye, *Stress Without Distress* (New York, 1974), p. 11.

126 Dalrymple, 'Streaming eyes?'.

127 For examples of such broad popular usage, see John Russell Taylor, 'A slight case of allergy', *The Times* (10 February 1968), 19a; Royal College of Physicians, *Allergy: Conventional and Alternative Concepts*, p. 2; Vanora Bennett, 'Natural habitat', *The Times: Television and Radio* (20 July 2002), 30a.

128 'Delors attacks German "allergy"', *The Times* (23 June 1997), 14e.

129 John Jay, 'Allergic reaction', *The Sunday Times: Business* (26 April 1998), 3a.

130 'A century of words', *Collins Gem English Dictionary: 1902–2002 Centenary Edition* (London, 2002), pp. 1, 5–6.

Chapter 7: Futures

1 Michel Foucault, *The Birth of the Clinic: An Archaeology of Medical Perception*, trans. A. M. Sheridan (London, 1973), p. 3. This work was originally published as Michel Foucault, *Naissance de la clinique* (Paris, 1963).

2 Jeff Noon, *Pollen* (London, 1995); http://www.jeffnoon.com/novelnotes.htm.

3 M. H. Lessof, 'Introduction: advances in allergy', *Clinical Allergy*, 12 (1982), Supplement, pp. 1–3.

4 UCB Institute of Allergy, *European Allergy Update* (Brussels, 1999), facing p. 57; Sarah Boseley, 'The allergy epidemic: by 2015 half of us may be carrying one of these', *Guardian* (10 February 2004), 1a; James Meikle, 'Britain tops asthma league', *Guardian* (17 February 2004), 9a; Robin Yapp, 'Shocking asthma toll on

British children', *Daily Mail* (22 December 2003), 1a; Deborah Hutton, 'Deep breath', *Sunday Times Style* (22 February 2004), pp. 36–7; Barbara Davies, 'As pollen count soars across UK', *Daily Mirror* (16 June 2003), 6b.

5   J. R. Mansfield et al., 'Treatment of equine allergic diseases with allergy neutralization: a field study', *Journal of Nutritional and Environmental Medicine*, 8 (1998), pp. 329–4. I am grateful to React Equine Allergy Clinic in Dorking, England, for providing material on horse allergies.

6   Lessof, 'Introduction', p. 3.

7   R. S. Sunderland and D. M. Fleming, 'Continuing decline in acute asthma episodes in the community', *Archives of Disease in Childhood*, 89 (2004), pp. 282–5; R. MacFaul, 'Trends in asthma hospitalisation: is this related to prevention inhaler use?', *Archives of Disease in Childhood*, 89 (2004), pp. 1158–60.

8   See, for example, the new approaches to vaccination being developed by Peptide Therapeutics or new strategies to combat peanut allergies: Nigel Hawkes, 'An end to allergy danger?', *The Times* (7 November 1995), 16c; Christine Gorman, 'Fighting over peanuts', *Time* (24 March 2003), p. 59. I am grateful to Dr Lawrence Garland, Director of Research and Development at Peptide Therapeutics in Cambridge, for sending me details of the company's research.

9   Warren T. Vaughan, *Primer of Allergy* (St Louis, MO, 1939), p. 8.

10   Milton B. Cohen and June B. Cohen, *Your Allergy and What To Do About It* (London, 1942), pp. 151–3.

11   For an extensive discussion of these issues, see Rosalind Coward, *The Whole Truth: The Myth of Alternative Health* (London, 1989).

12   René Dubos, *The Dreams of Reason: Science and Utopias* (New York, 1961), p. 66.

13   Ibid.

14   René Dubos, *Mirage of Health: Utopias, Progress, and Biological Change* (New York, 1959), p. 24.

15   Dubos, *The Dreams of Reason*, p. 96.

16   Cohen and Cohen, *Your Allergy*, pp. 156–7.

BIBLIOGRAPHY

Amato, Joseph A., *Dust: A History of the Small and Invisible* (Berkeley, CA, 2000)

Anderson, Warwick, Myles Jackson and Barbara Gutmann Rosenkrantz, 'Toward an unnatural history of immunology', *Journal of the History of Biology*, 27 (1994), pp. 575–94

Ashby, Eric, and Mary Anderson, *The Politics of Clean Air* (Oxford, 1981)

Beck, Ulrich, *Risk Society: Towards a New Modernity* (London, 1992)

Bibel, D. J., *Milestones in Immunology: A Historical Exploration* (Madison, WI, 1988)

Brimblecombe, Peter, *The Big Smoke: A History of Air Pollution in London since Medieval Times* (London, 1987)

Brostoff, Jonathan, and Linda Gamlin, *Hayfever* (Glasgow, 1994)

Chadwick, Derek J., and Gail Cardew, eds, *The Rising Trends in Asthma* (Chichester, 1997)

Chen, Wai, 'The laboratory as business: Sir Almroth Wright's vaccine programme and the construction of penicillin', in *The Laboratory Revolution in Medicine*, ed. Andrew Cunningham and Perry Williams (Cambridge, 1992), pp. 245–92

Cohen, Sheldon G., and Peter J. Bianchine, 'Hymenoptera, hypersensitivity, and history', *Annals of Allergy, Asthma and Immunology*, 74 (1995), pp. 198–217

Cohen, Sheldon G., and Max Samter, eds, *Excerpts from Classics in Allergy* (Carlsbad, 1982)

Cone, Richard A., and Emily Martin, 'Corporeal flows: the immune system, global economies of food, and new implications for health', in *The Visible Woman: Imaging Technologies, Gender and Science*, ed. Paula A. Treichler, Lisa Cartwright and Constance Penley (New York, 1998), pp. 321–59

Coward, Rosalind, *The Whole Truth: The Myth of Alternative Health* (London, 1989)

Davis, Devra, *When Smoke Ran Like Water: Tales of Environmental Deception and the Battle Against Pollution* (New York, 2002)

Dubos, René, *Mirage of Health: Utopias, Progress, and Biological Change* (New York, 1959)

—, *The Dreams of Reason: Science and Utopias* (New York, 1961)

Edwards, A. M., and J.B.L. Howell, 'The chromones: history, chemistry and clinical development: a tribute to the work of Dr R.E.C. Altounyan', *Clinical and Experimental Allergy*, 30 (2000), pp. 756–74

Elias, Norbert, *The Civilizing Process: Sociogenetic and Psychogenetic Investigations* (1939) (Oxford, 2000)

Emanuel, M. B., 'Hay fever, a post industrial revolution epidemic: a history of its growth during the 19th century', *Clinical Allergy*, 18 (1988), pp. 295–304

Foster, W. D., *A History of Medical Bacteriology and Immunology* (London, 1970)

Foucault, Michel, *The Birth of the Clinic: An Archaeology of Medical Perception* (1963), trans. A. M. Sheridan (London, 1973)

Gabbay, John, 'Asthma attacked? Tactics for the reconstruction of a disease concept', in

The Problem of Medical Knowledge, ed. Peter Wright and Andrew Treacher (Edinburgh, 1982), pp. 23–48

Gallagher, Richard B. et al., eds, *Immunology: The Making of a Modern Science* (London, 1995)

Gandy, Matthew, 'Allergy and allegory in Todd Haynes' [*Safe*]', in *Screening the City*, ed. Mark Shiel and Tony Fitzmaurice, (London, 2003), pp. 239–61

Grob, Gerald C., *The Deadly Truth: A History of Disease in America* (Cambridge, MA, 2002)

Heaman, E. A., *St Mary's: The History of a London Teaching Hospital* (Montreal, 2003)

Inglis, Brian, *The Diseases of Civilisation* (London, 1981)

Jackson, Mark, 'Between scepticism and wild enthusiasm: the chequered history of allergen immunotherapy', in *Singular Selves: Historical Issues and Contemporary Debates in Immunology*, ed. Anne-Marie Moulin and Alberto Cambrosio (Amsterdam, 2000), pp. 155–64

—, 'Allergy: the making of a modern plague', *Clinical and Experimental Allergy*, 31 (2001), pp. 1665–71

—, 'Allergy and history', *Studies in History and Philosophy of Biological and Biomedical Sciences*, 34C (2003), pp. 383–98

—, 'John Freeman, hay fever and the origins of clinical allergy in Britain, 1900–1950', *Studies in History and Philosophy of Biological and Biomedical Sciences*, 34C (2003), pp. 473–90

—, 'Cleansing the air and promoting health: the politics of pollution in post-war Britain', in *Medicine, the Market and the Mass Media: Producing Health in the Twentieth Century*, ed. Virginia Berridge and Kelly Loughlin (London, 2005), pp. 219–41

Keirns, Carla C., 'Better than nature: the changing treatment of asthma and hay fever in the United States, 1910–1945', *Studies in History and Philosophy of Biological and Biomedical Sciences*, 34 (2003), pp. 511–31

Krimsky, Sheldon, *Hormonal Chaos: The Scientific and Social Origins of the Environmental Endocrine Hypothesis* (Baltimore, MD, 2000)

Kroker, Kenton, 'Immunity and its other: the anaphylactic selves of Charles Richet', *Studies in History and Philosophy of Biological and Biomedical Sciences*, 30 (1999), pp. 273–96

Kroll-Smith, Steve, and H. Hugh Floyd, *Bodies in Protest: Environmental Illness and the Struggle over Medical Knowledge* (New York, 1997)

Lawrence, Christopher, and George Weisz, eds, *Greater than the Parts: Holism in Biomedicine, 1920–1950* (New York, 1998).

Lear, Linda, *Rachel Carson: Witness for Nature* (New York, 1997)

Lichter, S. Robert, and Stanley Rothman, *Environmental Cancer: A Political Disease* (New Haven, CT, 1999)

Lomborg, Bjørn, *The Skeptical Environmentalist: Measuring the Real State of the World* (Cambridge, 2003)

Löwy, Ilana, 'On guinea pigs, dogs, and men: anaphylaxis and the study of biological individuality, 1902–1939', *Studies in History and Philosophy of Biological and Biomedical Sciences*, 34 (2003), pp. 399–424

Luckin, Bill, 'Town, country and metropolis: the formation of an air pollution problem in London, 1800–1870', in *Energy and the City in Europe: From Preindustrial Wood-shortage to the Oil Crisis of the 1970s*, ed. Dieter Schott (Stuttgart, 1997), pp. 77–92

Mazumdar, Pauline M. H., ed., *Immunology 1930–1980: Essays on the History of Immunology* (Toronto, 1989)

—, *Species and Specificity: An Interpretation of the History of Immunology* (Cambridge, 1995)

—, 'The purpose of immunity: Landsteiner's interpretation of the human isoantibodies', *Journal of the History of Biology*, 8 (1975), pp. 115–33

—, 'The antigen-antibody reaction and the physics and chemistry of life', *Bulletin of the History of Medicine*, 48 (1974), pp. 1–21

McNeill, John, *Something New Under the Sun: An Environmental History of the Twentieth Century* (London, 2000)

Meyer, Ulrich, *Steckt eine Allergie dahinter?: Die Industrialisierung von Arzneimittel-Entwicklung, -Herstellung und -Vermarktung am Beispiel der Antiallergika* (Stuttgart, 2002)

—, 'From khellin to sodium cromoglycate: a tribute to the work of Dr R.E.C. Altounyan (1922–1987)', *Pharmazie*, 57 (2002), pp. 62–9

Mitman, Gregg, *The State of Nature: Ecology, Community, and American Social Thought, 1900–1950* (Chicago, 1992)

—, 'Natural history and the clinic: the regional ecology of allergy in America', *Studies in History and Philosophy of Biological and Biomedical Sciences*, 34 (2003), pp. 491–510

—, 'Hay fever holiday: health, leisure, and place in gilded-age America', *Bulletin of the History of Medicine*, 77 (2003), pp. 600–35

—, 'What's in a weed? A cultural geography of *Ambrosia artemesiaefolia*', in *The Moral Authority of Nature*, ed. Lorraine Daston and Fernando Vidal (Chicago, 2003), pp. 438–65

—, 'Geographies of hope: mining the frontiers of health in Denver and beyond, 1870–1965', *Osiris*, 19 (2004), pp. 93–111

Mosley, Stephen, *The Chimney of the World: A History of Smoke Pollution in Victorian and Edwardian Manchester* (Cambridge, 2001)

Moulin, Anne Marie, 'The immune system: a key concept for the history of immunology', *History and Philosophy of the Life Sciences*, 11 (1989), pp. 221–36

—, *Le dernier langage de la médecine* (Paris, 1991)

—, 'The defended body', in *Medicine in the 20th Century*, ed. Roger Cooter and John Pickstone (Amsterdam, 2000), pp. 385–98

Murphy, Michelle, 'The "elsewhere within here" and environmental illness; or, how to build yourself a body in a safe space', *Configurations*, 8 (2000), pp. 87–120

Nesse, Randolph M., and George C. Williams, *Evolution and Healing: The New Science of Darwinian Medicine* (Phoenix, AZ, 1996)

Parker, Roy, 'The struggle for clean air', in *Change, Choice and Conflict in Social Policy*, ed. Phoebe Hall et al. (London, 1975), pp. 371–409

Parnes, Ohad, '"Trouble from within": allergy, autoimmunity and pathology in the first half of the twentieth century', *Studies in History and Philosophy of Biological and Biomedical Sciences*, 34 (2003), pp. 425–54

Platt, Harold, *Shock Cities: The Environmental Transformation and Reform of Manchester and Chicago* (Chicago, 2005)

Porter, Roy, 'Civilisation and disease: medical ideology in the Enlightenment', in *Culture, Politics and Society in Britain, 1660–1800*, ed. Jeremy Black and Jeremy Gregory

(Manchester, 1991), pp. 154–83

—, 'Diseases of civilization', in *Companion Encyclopedia of the History of Medicine*, ed. W. F. Bynum and Roy Porter (London, 1993), vol. I, pp. 584–600

Radetsky, Peter, *Allergic to the Twentieth Century* (Boston, MA, 1997)

Rosenberg, Charles E., 'Pathologies of progress: the idea of civilization as risk', *Bulletin of the History of Medicine*, 72 (1998), pp. 714–30

Rothstein, William G., *Public Health and the Risk Factor: A History of an Uneven Medical Revolution* (Rochester, NY, 2003)

Saks, Mike, *Orthodox and Alternative Medicine: Politics, Professionalization and Health Care* (London, 2003)

Schadewaldt, Hans, *Geschichte der Allergie*, 4 vols (Munich, 1979–83)

Sellers, Christopher, 'Body, place and the state: the makings of an "environmentalist" imaginery in the post-world war II US', *Radical History Review*, 74 (1999), pp. 31–64

Siegel, Sheldon C., 'History of asthma deaths from antiquity', *Journal of Allergy and Clinical Immunology*, 80 (1987), pp. 458–62

Silverstein, Arthur M., *A History of Immunology* (San Diego, CA, 1989)

Slinn, Judy, 'Research and development in the UK pharmaeutical industry from the nineteenth century to the 1960s', in *Drugs and Narcotics in History*, ed. Roy Porter and Mikulás Teich (Cambridge, 1995), pp. 168–86

Snell, Noel, 'Inhalation devices: a brief history', *Respiratory Disease in Practice* (Summer 1995), pp. 13–15

Söderqvist, Thomas, Craig Stillwell and Mark Jackson, 'Immunity and immunology', in *Cambridge History of Science*, ed. John V. Pickstone and Peter Bowler, vol. VI (in preparation)

Straus, Bernard, *Maladies of Marcel Proust: Doctors and Disease in his Life and Work* (New York, 1980)

Tansey, E. M., 'Henry Dale, histamine and anaphylaxis: reflections on the role of chance in the history of allergy', *Studies in History and Philosophy of Biological and Biomedical Sciences*, 34 (2003), pp. 455–72

—, et al., eds, 'Self and non-self: a history of autoimmunity', in *Wellcome Witnesses to Twentieth Century Medicine*, vol. I (London, 1997)

Tomes, Nancy, *The Gospel of Germs: Men, Women, and the Microbe in American Life* (Cambridge, MA, 1998)

Tweedale, Geoffrey, *At the Sign of the Plough: 275 Years of Allen & Hanburys and the British Pharmaceutical Industry, 1715–1990* (London, 1990)

Wagner, Richard, *Clemens von Pirquet: His Life and Work* (Baltimore, MD, 1968)

Waite, Kathryn J., 'Blackley and the development of hay fever as a disease of civilization in the nineteenth century', *Medical History*, 39 (1995), pp. 186–96

Walker, Martin J., *Dirty Medicine* (London, 1994)

Wilmot, Frances, and Pauline Saul, *A Breath of Fresh Air: Birmingham's Open-Air Schools, 1911–1970* (Chichester, 1998)

Worboys, Michael, *Spreading Germs: Disease Theories and Medical Practice in Britain, 1865–1900* (Cambridge, 2000)

ACKNOWLEDGEMENTS

The production of this book inevitably owes a great deal to the advice, support and inspiration of others. Most fundamentally, I am indebted to the Wellcome Trust for funding the research on which the book is based. I have also benefited immensely from the constructive guidance of staff at a number of libraries and archives. In particular, I would like to thank: staff at the Contemporary Medical Archives Centre in the Wellcome Library for the History and Understanding of Medicine for making available the records of the British Society for Immunology and the personal papers of Carl Prausnitz; Kevin Brown for leading me through the archives of the Inoculation Department and Allergy Clinic at St Mary's Hospital; Alice Nicholls for introducing me to the collections on allergy housed in the National Museum of Science and Industry; Sarah Flynn, archivist at the GlaxoWellcome Heritage Archives, for sending me material relating to the development of salbutamol and beclomethasone; Carole Modis and Panayiotis Massaoutis for revealing the library and archive holdings of the World Health Organization in Geneva; staff in the Moody Medical Library at the University of Texas Medical Branch in Galveston, Texas; Miriam Gutierrez-Perez of the Wellcome Medical Photographic Library, Sarah Sykes of the Science and Society Picture Library at the Science Musuem, Jane Newton from the Centre for the Study of Cartoons and Caricature at the University of Kent, Katherine Elworthy of The Advertising Archives, and Tom Watkins from the Science Photo Library, for providing many of the illustrations; and Robert Ford and Caroline Huxtable in the inter-library loan section of the University of Exeter Library for procuring obscure journal articles and books from all corners of the world with remarkable speed and good humour.

I am also grateful to Dr Pierre Guesry of the Nestlé Research Center in Lausanne for explaining the central scientific, as well as political, problems associated with the development of hypoallergenic formula milk during the 1970s and '80s, and to Mike Rhodes of HEALTHe Limited and Colin Taylor of Medivac Healthcare Limited for sharing their vast experience of the technical world of allergen avoidance and control. In addition, I have appreciated the generous information about their allergy policies and products provided by Sainsbury's, Thorntons, Tesco and Peptide Therapeutics. I am equally indebted to Pat Grassi for translating critical passages of German and to Catherine Mills, Claire Keyte and Amy Burdis for uncovering diverse references in the records and annual reports of the Medical Research Council, retrieving articles from medical journals and The Times, and alerting me to material on the web. I would also like to thank Richard Jackson for converting some of the illustrations from electronic to suitable print form. Part of chapter Three was first published as 'John Freeman, hay fever and the origins of clinical allergy in Britain, 1900–1950', in Studies in History and

Philosophy of Biological and Biomedical Sciences, 34 (2003), pp. 473–90. I am grateful to the editors of that journal for their kind permission to reproduce the relevant sections.

At a more personal level, I am grateful to Jeremy Black not only for providing the initial contact with Michael Leaman at Reaktion Books but also for his friendship and advice over recent years. I am also grateful to Michael Leaman himself for his confidence in the project and for waiting patiently for the final manuscript. In addition, I would like to thank Tony Woods and his colleagues in the History of Medicine section at the Wellcome Trust for their support and friendship, Ian Gregg, Bill Frankland, Alan Edwards, Michael Flindt, and the late George Feinberg for sharing with me their insights into, and enthusiasm for, the history of allergy and immunology over many years, and various colleagues around the world for generously exchanging work and ideas, particularly John Burnham, Chester Burns, Elsbeth Heaman, Rhodri Hayward, Carla Keirns, Ilana Löwy, Gregg Mitman, Anne Marie Moulin, Ohad Parnes, John Pickstone, Viviane Quirke, Chris Sellers, Judy Slinn, Thomas Söderqvist, Tilli Tansey and Mick Worboys.

Finally, I owe my greatest debt of gratitude to Siobhán, Ciara, Riordan and Conall, whom I love all alike. This book, however, is dedicated especially to Siobhán, who freed me from the rags of time.

PHOTO ACKNOWLEDGEMENTS

The author and publishers wish to express their thanks to the following sources of illustrative material and/or permission to reproduce it:

Photos courtesy of the Advertising Archives, London: pp. 68, 101, 128; photos courtesy of the Centre for the Study of Cartoons and Caricature, Templeman Library, University of Kent, Canterbury: pp. 88 (© Mirrorpix, 1958; reproduced by permission of Mirrorpix), 144 (© Solo Syndication, Limited, 2002, reproduced by permission of Solo Syndication), 155 (© Solo Syndication, Limited, 1970, reproduced by permission of Solo Syndication), 182 (© Solo Syndication, Limited, 2002, reproduced by permission of Solo Syndication), 183 (© Stanley Franklin/NI Syndication Limited, 1982, reproduced by permission of NI Syndication Ltd), 214 (© Rick Brookes/ NI Syndication Limited, 1996, reproduced by permission of NI Syndication Ltd); photo Clendening History of Medicine Library (Clendening Library Portrait Collection), University of Kansas Medical Center, Kansas City: p. 33; image Crown copyright, reproduced by kind permission of the Lung and Asthma Information Agency: p. 105 (from the Lung & Asthma Information Agency Factsheet 92/1 – 'Trends in asthma mortality in the elderly' http//:www.laia.ac.uk – last accessed February 2004); image from P.G.H. Gell and R.R.A. Coombs, *Clinical Aspects of Immunology* (Oxford: Blackwell Scientific Publications, 1963, p. 321, reproduced by kind permission of Blackwell Publishing Ltd): p. 122; photo Science Photo Library: p. 83; photo courtesy of the United States Patent and Trademark Office: p. 140; photos Wellcome Library, London: pp. 6, 32 (from Charles Richet's autobiographical text in L. R. Grote, *Die Medizin der Gegenwart in Selbstdarstellungen Sonderchruck*, vol. 7, Leipzig, 1928), 42, 71.

INDEX

racial predisposition 51–2, 104
see also class; diseases of civilization; literary references
Curschmann, Heinrich (1846–1910) 66
Curtis, H. Holbrook 74
cytolytic reactions 123

Dale, Henry (1875–1968) 19, 48–50, 98
Dalrymple, Theodore 198, 213
death, of von Pirquet 54–5
see also mortality and morbidity rates
Dekker, Hermann 168, 169
delayed sensitivity 123
Dermatophagoides pteronyssinus 168–71
desensitization 22, 56–7, 69–76, 83–5, 93–5, 194–8
detergent industry 141–2, 166
developing countries 111, 148, 151
diagnosis and treatment 92–7, 201–2
    of asthma 66–7, 74, 87–8, 94–5, 107–8, 115, 135–6
    drug-free 138, 199–200
    disagreements on 91–2, 194–200, 206–8
    of hay fever 130
    pharmacological 127–39
    see also desensitization
Dickens, Charles (1812–1870) 67, 69
diets 174–5, 201, 202
diphtheria antitoxin 30
diseases, allergy-related 43–4, 82–3, 110–16, 117, 120–22, 186–7, 209
    see also infectious diseases; respiratory diseases
'diseases of civilization' 13–16, 23, 141–7, 178–84
    asthma as 66–9
    hay fever as 59–60, 61–5, 216
    trends in 185–6, 216–20
    see also class; cultural factors; environmental factors; lifestyles; literary references; socio-economic factors
disodium cromoglycate 136
The Divine Comedy (pop group) 155
domestic allergens 139–41
drug allergies 120, 147
drug-free treatments 138, 199–200
drug therapies 127–39
    see also names of drugs
Dubos, René (1901–1982) 15, 142, 150, 152, 184, 188–9, 219
Dunbar, Helen Flanders (1902–1959) 86
Dunbar, William P. (1863–1922) 30, 60–61, 63, 72, 75
Durham, Oren C. (1889–1967) 79, 80
dust 120, 139–41, 167, 168–73

Eastern Society (US) 77
ecological factors 16–17, 23–4, 186–90
ecology, clinical 200–08

economic factors *see* cultural factors; socio-economic factors
eczema 44, 110, 120, 121, 133
egg intolerance 74
Ehrlich, Paul (1854–1915) 18, 30, 50
Elias, Norbert (1897–1990) 15
Elliotson, Sir John (1791–1868) 57–8
Emanuel, Michael 20
Emerson, Alfred Edwards (1896–1976) 202
emotions, and allergy 87–90
emphysema 106–7
environmental endocrine hypothesis 186–7
environmental factors 16–17, 149–52, 154–66, 181, 204–8, 218
    see also climate therapy; indoor environment; nature; pollen
Environmental Protection Agency 163–4
enzymes, in detergents 141–2
ephedrine 127–8
Escherich, Theodor 34
Europe, studies of allergy in 59, 80, 114
European Academy of Allergology and Clinical Immunology 99
Ewan, Pamela 132, 194

family size 176–7
Feingold, Benjamin F. (1900–1982) 145
Felsol 129
fenoterol 108
film (cinematic) 182–3
Fisons 136
Fleck, Ludwik (1896–1961) 16, 20, 36
Flindt, Michael 141–2
Floyd, H. Hugh 207
Floyer, Sir John (1649–1734) 28–9, 65
food allergy 28, 47, 74, 144–7, 200, 202–3, 205–6, 207–8
food industries 12, 145–7, 174
Forster, E. M., *Howards End* (novel) 64–5, 212
Forward, Charles W., *The Golden Calf* 95, 137
fragrances 142
Francis, Alexander 46
Frankland, A. W. 82, 84–5, 94, 97, 98, 172, 194
Franol/Franol-Plus 128, 131
Frazier, Claude 114, 180
Freeman, John (1876–1962) 50, 70–74, 74–5, 76–7, 81–2, 89–90, 90–94, 97, 176–7
    see also St Mary's Hospital, London
Frew, A. J. 196
fungal spores 159–60

Gabbay, John 20, 66
Gandy, Matthew 183
Gell, P.G.H. (b. 1914) 122–4

286

Use of Bech, with writing — a bit weak?